AF538475

Manual of Otolaryngology—Head and Neck Therapeutics

Manual of Otolaryngology—Head and Neck Therapeutics

Arnold E. Katz, Editor

Department of Otolaryngology
Tufts University School of Medicine
New England Medical Center
Boston, Massachusetts

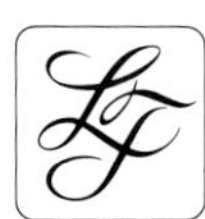

Lea & Febiger 1986 *PHILADELPHIA*

Lea & Febiger
600 Washington Square
Philadelphia, PA 19106-4198
U.S.A.
(215) 922-1330

Library of Congress Cataloging in Publication Data

Manual of otolaryngology—head and neck therapeutics.

Includes bibliographies and index.
1. Otolaryngology—Handbooks, manuals, etc.
I. Katz, Arnold E. [DNLM: 1. Otorhinolaryngologic
Diseases—therapy—handbooks. WV 39 M294]
RF56.M36 1985 617′.51 85-238
ISBN 0-8121-0957-0

Copyright © 1986 by Lea & Febiger. Copyright under the International Copyright Union. All rights reserved. This book is protected by copyright. No part of it may be reproduced in any manner or by any means without written permission from the publishers.

PRINTED IN THE UNITED STATES OF AMERICA

Print No. 4 3 2 1

In Memory of
Julius Katz

Preface

The specialty of Otolaryngology—Head and Neck Surgery is both a medical and a surgical discipline. Many of the patients referred to the otolaryngologist require a diagnostic evaluation; and in most practices, less than 20% eventually require surgery. It is this blend of medicine and surgery in patients of all ages that makes the practice of Otolaryngology—Head and Neck Surgery so rewarding. It is unfortunate that medical schools and even some residencies devote so little of their curriculum to the medical aspects of otolaryngology.

This manual presents in outline form a meticulous approach to therapeutic problems of the head and neck. It presents a thorough, logical diagnostic and therapeutic evaluation of various diseases of the head and neck, stopping short of a discussion of surgical technique. Many of the chapters deal with local signs of systemic disease and their therapeutic implications.

The 34 eminent contributors were carefully selected from 20 medical centers throughout the country to describe areas of their expertise. They were asked to present their clinical "pearls" and describe how they would evaluate and treat their patients. Several of the authors are presently chairmen of their own departments and many of the contributors have achieved national and/or international recognition for their work.

The manual has been designed for the first year resident in Otolaryngology—Head and Neck Surgery, although it should also be useful for medical students and primary care physicians. Many of the 38 chapters deal with problems commonly seen by the internist, the pediatrician, the physician's assistant, and the nurse practitioner.

The form of the manual was designed so that it could be carried easily in the house officer's coat pocket and be readily available for use in the emergency room, the ward, or the clinic. The material is concisely presented; taking care to discuss basic science subjects, such as anatomy, physiology, and biochemistry, *only* if they have *therapeutic* implications. The material is presented in outline form so that it is easily retrievable in the clinical situation, and hopefully will allow for improved care of patients with these disorders.

Boston, Massachusetts Arnold E. Katz, M.D.

Acknowledgments

"We are like dwarfs seated on the shoulders of giants. If we see more and further than they, it is not due to our own clear eyes or tall bodies, but because we were raised on high and upborne by their gigantic bigness."

Bernard of Chartres, 1119 A.D.[1]

Throughout my medical career, I have been taught by many gifted and inspired teachers. Dr. Carl V. Moore, Dr. Dean M. Lierle, Dr. Barry J. Anson, and Dr. Scott N. Reger are now deeply missed, but their works still benefit us and our patients. Dr. Brian F. McCabe continues the traditions of those great teachers, instilling his residents with an unquentiable thirst for excellence, whether in the clinic, the operating room, or the laboratory. While I was studying with Dr. McCabe, his staff included Dr. Janusz Bardach, Dr. Leslie Bernstein, Dr. Lee A. Harker, Dr. Charles J. Krause, Dr. Ward B. Litton, Dr. Jacob Sadé, and Dr. Maxwell Abramson. "If we see more than they. . . it is. . . because. . . we (are). . . upbourne by their gigantic bigness."

It would be impossible to complete a work such as this without family support. My wife, Lillian, and my children, John David, Rachell Anne, Jennifer Ruth, and Jason Aaron, have sacrificed and in their own ways contributed to the production of this manual. My mother, Rose, and my brothers, Robert and Raymond, have been an unending source of encouragement when I was convinced that I had undertaken more than I could possibly accomplish.

The many contributors to this manual were carefully selected and gave unselfishly of their expertise, so that we could pass on to those who follow us that which we have received from our teachers.

Finally, this work could not have been completed without the assistance of my friend and colleague, Ms. Bess Arick.

Arnold E. Katz, M.D.
Boston, Massachusetts

---

[1] McCabe, B.F.: Barry J. Anson. Ann. Otol. Rhinol. Laryngol., *84*:131, 1975.

Contributors

Howard B. Ashby, M.D.
Staff Psychiatrist, Sacred Heart Medical Center, Spokane, Washington

Shan Ray Baker, M.D., F.A.C.S.
Associate Professor, Department of Otolaryngology—Head and Neck Surgery, University of Michigan, Ann Arbor, Michigan

Don B. Blakeslee, LTC, MC, USA
Otolaryngology—Head and Neck Service, Fitzsimons Army Medical Center, Aurora, Colorado; Clinical Assistant Professor of Surgery, Uniformed Services University of the Health Sciences, Bethesda, Maryland; Clinical Assistant Professor, Department of Otolaryngology, University of Colorado Health Science Center, Denver, Colorado

Robert M. Bumsted, M.D., F.A.C.S.
Professor, Department of Otolaryngology—Head and Neck Surgery, University of Iowa Hospitals and Clinics, Iowa City, Iowa

Victor E. Calcaterra, M.D.
Assistant Professor of Otolaryngology, Tufts University School of Medicine; Senior Surgeon, New England Medical Center, Boston, Massachusetts

Barbara Carter, M.D.
Professor of Radiology and Otolaryngology, Tufts University School of Medicine; Chief of CT Scanning and ENT Radiology, New England Medical Center, Boston, Massachusetts

Werner D. Chasin, M.D., F.A.C.S.
Chairman and Professor of Otolaryngology, Tufts University School of Medicine; Otolaryngologist-in-Chief, New England Medical Center, Boston, Massachusetts

Roger L. Crumley, M.D., F.A.C.S.
Clinical Professor, Department of Otolaryngology—Head and Neck Surgery, University of California, San Francisco, California

Julius Damion, M.D.
Chief Resident in Otolaryngology, Departments of Otolaryngology, Boston University and Tufts University Schools of Medicine, Boston, Massachusetts; Associate Attending Staff, Maine Medical Center, Portland, Maine

R. Kim Davis, M.D.
Assistant Professor of Surgery, University of Utah College of Medicine, Division of Otolaryngology—Head and Neck Surgery, University of Utah Medical Center, Salt Lake City, Utah

J. Kevin Fortson, M.D.
Clinical Instructor, Department of Otolaryngology, University of California at San Diego College of Medicine, San Diego, California; Chief of Otolaryngology, Kern Medical Center, Bakersfield, California

Marie G. Gauthier, M.D.
Active Fulltime Staff, Bay Medical Center; Consulting Staff, Midland Hospital, Bay City, Michigan

Hubert L. Gerstman, D. Ed.
Associate Professor of Rehabilitation Medicine and Otolaryngology Tufts University School of Medicine; Instructor of Oral Biology, Tufts University School of Dental Medicine; Chief, Speech, Hearing and Language Center, New England Medical Center, Boston, Massachusetts

Robert H. Gilman, M.D., D.M.D.
Clinical Instructor, Departments of Otolaryngology and Plastic Surgery, Boston University School of Medicine, Boston, Massachusetts

Charles J. Hodge, Jr., M.D.
Professor of Neurosurgery, State University of New York; Upstate Medical Center, The Veterans Administration Medical Center, Crouse-Irving Medical Center, Syracuse, New York

Waun Ki Hong, M.D.
Professor of Medicine, Chief, Head and Neck Medical Oncology, The University of Texas System Cancer Center, M.D. Anderson Hospital and Tumor Institute, Houston, Texas

Ellen M. Howard, R.N.
Staff Nurse, Department of Otolaryngology, New England Medical Center, Boston, Massachusetts

Roger L. Hybels, M.D., F.A.C.S.
Clinical Assistant Professor of Otolaryngology, Boston University School of Medicine, Boston, Massachusetts; Staff, Lahey Clinic Medical Center, Burlington, Massachusetts

Matthew J. Jackson, D.M.D., M.S.D.
Assistant Clinical Professor, Tufts University School of Dental Medicine; Consultant in Maxillofacial Prosthetics, University Hospital, Boston University Medical Center; Clinical Instructor, Boston University School of Graduate Dentistry; Chief, Prosthodontics and Maxillofacial Prosthetics, Boston Veterans Administration Medical Center, Boston, Massachusetts

Collin S. Karmody, M.D., F.A.C.S.
Professor of Otolaryngology, Tufts University School of Medicine; Senior Surgeon, New England Medical Center, Boston, Massachusetts

Arnold E. Katz, M.D., F.A.C.S.
Associate Professor Otolaryngology, Tufts University School of Medicine; Instructor of Otolaryngology, Boston University School of Medicine; Senior Surgeon, New England Medical Center; Senior Staff, Boston Veterans Administration Medical Center, Boston, Massachusetts

Charles F. Koopmann, Jr., M.D., F.A.C.S.
Associate Professor of Surgery, University of Arizona College of Medicine; Staff, University Medical Center, Tucson Medical Center, St. Joseph's Hospital, Northwest Hospital, El Dorado Hospital, Tucson Veterans Administration Medical Center, Tucson, Arizona

Charles J. Krause, M.D., F.A.C.S.
Professor and Chairman, Department of Otolaryngology—Head and Neck Surgery, University of Michigan, Ann Arbor, Michigan

Donald A. Leopold, M.D.
Assistant Professor, Department of Otolaryngology, State University of New York; Staff, Upstate Medical Center, The Veterans Administration Medical Center, Crouse-Irving Medical Center, Syracuse, New York

Barbara A. MacLean, R.N., B.S.
Staff Nurse, Department of Otolaryngology, New England Medical Center, Boston, Massachusetts

W. Frederick McGuirt, M.D., F.A.C.S.
Associate Professor of Surgery, Section on Otolaryngology, Bowman Gray School of Medicine, Wake Forest University Medical Center, Winston-Salem, North Carolina

Russell Noyes, Jr., M.D.
Professor of Psychiatry, University of Iowa College of Medicine, Iowa City, Iowa

Max E. Reddick, M.D.
Assistant Clinical Professor of Dermatology, Baylor College of Medicine; Staff, Methodist Hospital, The Bentaub Hospital, Memorial City Medical Center, Houston, Texas

David E. Schuller, M.D., F.A.C.S.
Professor and Chairman, Department of Otolaryngology, College of Medicine, The Ohio State University, Columbus, Ohio

Stanley M. Shapshay, M.D., F.A.C.S.
Assistant Professor, Department of Otolaryngology, Boston University School of Medicine, Boston, Massachusetts; Chairman, Department of Otolaryngology—Head and Neck Surgery; Director, Eleanor Naylor Dana Laser Research Laboratory, Lahey Clinic Medical Center, Burlington, Massachusetts

M. Stuart Strong, M.D., F.A.C.S.
Professor and Chairman, Department of Otolaryngology, Boston University School of Medicine; Chief of Otolaryngology, University Hospital, Boston, Massachusetts

April E. Tuck, M.S., C.C.C.
Instructor, Team Teacher, Emerson College; Teaching Affiliate, Tufts University School of Medicine; Speech and Language Pathologist, Speech, Hearing and Language Center, New England Medical Center, Boston, Massachusetts

Glenn H. Weissman, M.D., F.A.C.S.
Chief, Department of Otolaryngology, San Gabriel Community Hospital, San Gabriel, California

Moshe Ziv, M.D.
Active Medical Staff, Grant Medical Center; Associate Staff, Mt. Carmel Medical Center, Columbus, Ohio

Contents

PART I: TRAUMA

PART II: EAR

PART III: NOSE AND SINUS

PART IV: ORAL CAVITY AND LARYNGOPHARYNX

I.

TRAUMA

1

SOFT TISSUE TRAUMA

ROGER L. HYBELS

The evaluation and treatment of injuries to the soft tissues of the face and neck should be approached with respect. The examination should be unhurried and thorough. Most often, the head and neck surgeon is called to the emergency suite to treat specific neck and facial injuries after other physicians have assessed the general condition of the patient and have assumed overall care. If the head and neck surgeon is asked to accept primary care of the patient because soft tissue damage is judged to be the "only" injury, however, he should evaluate the patient personally and not accept the diagnostic conclusions of others without verification. This principle is not only medically and legally sound, but also it is in the best interest of the patient.

One should obtain a thorough history of the circumstances of the injury if possible, including the place and time of the accident, the mechanism of trauma or the offending object, and its direction. This information is carefully documented by direct quotations from the patient and witnesses both for medicolegal reasons and for insight into the injury itself. Photographs should be taken of all injuries before repair; in time, patients and their families may forget the magnitude of an injury.

Facial injuries present a wide range of problems. Some principles, such as wound healing and suturing technique, have general applicability, but the unique anatomy of the face and its importance in one's body image add a special dimension to these injuries. The surgeon should avoid optimism with respect to final outcome in discussions with the patient and the family. In fact, it is good policy to inform them that a revision will most likely be necessary in 6 to 12 months.

I. INITIAL CARE AND EVALUATION

A. Emergency Considerations

1. Airway

a. *Obstruction* The airway is the first consideration in most emergency situations. Otolaryngologists are uniquely qualified to evaluate and to deal with this problem. Normally, immediate distress is obvious and will have been treated in some manner, usually by intubation, before the otolaryngologist arrives. Some patients, however, have an apparently patent airway that later becomes stridulous. The otolaryngologist should foresee this problem and should treat such patients before an emergency develops. Anticipation of these problems is aided by a complete examination of the head and neck and a thorough medical history. Airway obstruction is most common in association with fractures of the mandibular and maxillary skeleton or neck trauma. Traumatically created deformities are not the only cause of airway obstruction; blood, teeth, and foreign bodies may fill the mouth or pharynx.

b. *Nonobstructive respiratory distress* The otolaryngologist should not approach respiratory distress with "tunnel vision" because the upper airway is not the only source of difficulty. Other possible causes are pneumothorax including the tension type, flail chest, sucking injuries, and hemothorax. Brain injury can lead to central apnea. Not all pulmonary distress is immediate; in some patients, it develops over several hours, as in shock lung.

2. Hemorrhages should be stopped appropriately. Most active bleeding will have been controlled by the body's own hemostatic mechanisms by the time the patient is transported to the emergency facility. If such is the case, the surgeon should be gloved and should have hemostats ready before exploring and cleansing the wound. It is common for the inexperienced physician to clean the clots from a wound only to find severe hemorrhage. In general, simple pressure should be used for the initial control of hemorrhage. Uncontrolled clamping into a poorly visualized wound is to be condemned. Occasionally, large amounts of blood are lost from a transected named vessel, and rapid exploration with precise control of the vessel is required. Shock is uncommon with facial injuries, but when present, injuries of the chest, the abdomen, the vessels of the neck or lower extremities must be suspected.

3. Central nervous system A nervous system injury should be suspected in anyone receiving trauma to the head and neck. Knowing the mechanism of the injury is helpful in determining the probability of nervous system involvement. Many of these injuries cause appreciable flexion and extension of the cervical spine, at times enough to induce fracture. It is reasonable to assume that every patient has a fracture of the cervical spine until proved otherwise by physical examination and radiography. Neurologic consultation should be obtained without hesitation.

B. Initial Inspection

The initial assessment of the wound after emergency or lifesaving procedures accomplishes several objectives. Diagnostic studies are chosen and a treatment plan is formulated at this time. The presence of fractures should be determined before undertaking any repair of soft tissue because fixation should be performed through the open wound if possible. One may explore the wound gently in a sterile manner while irrigating it; the full extent of soft tissue damage is difficult to determine in a wound obscured by clotted blood. Instruments to control larger blood vessels should be at hand. At this time, visible contamination and foreign bodies may be removed. If injuries to other regions of the body are so serious that repair of soft tissue is impossible or is of secondary importance, the wounds can be cleansed and dressed. Tissue flaps are assessed for vascularity and are placed in untwisted positions. This evaluation may be more comfortable for the patient if local anesthesia is administered; however, the state of the patient's motor and sensory nerves should be determined before one injects an anesthetic agent.

C. Timing of Repair

As a general rule, the earlier a wound can be repaired, the better the result. Closure within 6 hours is a reasonable goal, but primary closure is possible up to 24 hours. Cosmetic considerations must play a secondary role in the patient with multiple trauma, and repair may have to be delayed in such persons.

1. **Patients with no other injuries** When the patient has no other injuries or only minor ones, the repair can normally be performed in the emergency suite, with the patient under local anesthesia, as soon as diagnostic studies have been completed. When a wound is seen late and when the degree of contusion and devitalization is considerable, closure may be delayed. This procedure involves necessary debridement, application of wet dressings, and administration of antibiotics until the wound appears clean, with little edema and inflammation.
2. **Patients with associated injuries requiring general anesthesia** When major associated injuries require surgical intervention, the facial and neck injuries can be repaired concurrently without adding significant anesthesia time. When anesthesia time is short, expeditious closure may consist primarily of wound toilet and debridement, elimination of dead space, and rapid skin closure with a continuous running suture or with staples if necessary.
3. **Patients with associated injuries not requiring general anesthesia** In patients who have major associated injuries but who do not require general anesthesia, wounds should be

cleansed thoroughly, packed, and dressed under pressure for later closure. Occasionally, a few strategically placed sutures align the wound edges in adequate, temporary approximation. Delayed repair can often be performed at the bedside, when the patient's condition has stabilized, 24 to 48 hours later.

D. Tetanus Immunization

These guidelines have been adapted from the recommendations of the Committee on Trauma of the American College of Surgeons, as revised in 1979.

1. **General** Basic immunization is accomplished in adults and older children by 3 injections of tetanus toxoid, with booster injections given every 10 years thereafter. For children under 7 years of age, 4 immunizing doses are given.
2. **Previously immunized patients**
   a. ***Booster within 10 years***
      i. No booster dose is given when the chance of tetanus is small.
      ii. A booster dose is given if more than 5 years have elapsed since the last booster and if the wound is prone to the development of tetanus. If the patient has had excessive previous toxoid injections, the booster may be omitted.

   b. ***Booster more than 10 years previously*** These patients should be given 0.5 ml tetanus toxoid.
3. **Inadequate previous immunization,** that is, either none or one previous injection or when the patient's history of immunization is unknown.
   a. ***For non-tetanus-prone wounds,*** one should give 0.5 ml toxoid and follow-up with additional injections to complete immunization.
   b. ***For tetanus-prone wounds,*** one should give 0.5 ml toxoid and 250 U *human* tetanus antitoxin. Equine antitoxin is indicated only when human antitoxin is unavailable and when the possibility of tetanus is greater than the risk of reaction to horse serum. Prophylactic antibiotics may be considered.

II. ANESTHESIA

A. Local

Whenever possible, local anesthesia should be used for patients, including children, with soft tissue injuries. Parenteral narcotic-barbiturate combinations provide supplementary sedation for children. Adults may benefit as well from an intramuscular or intravenously administered narcotic or tranquilizer, as long as an injury to the central nervous system is not suspected. Lidocaine (Xylocaine), 1 or 0.5%, with 1:100,000 or 1:200,000 epinephrine, is used; the latter combination is preferred if large amounts are required.

Bupivacaine hydrochloride (Marcaine) is also useful, and its effects last longer than those of lidocaine. The anesthetic solution should be injected slowly into the wound edges or through previously anesthetized skin using a small, 27- to 30-gauge needle. Massaging the tissues gently spreads the solution. Regional block is helpful even when a local anesthetic is injected. Many nerves of the head and neck are amenable to this type of block. A period of 10 to 15 minutes should be allowed between injection and repair, to attain maximal anesthesia and vasoconstriction.

B. General

General anesthesia is required for extensive or specialized repairs, when flaps or grafts are necessary, and in children. Good judgment dictates when this form of anesthesia is indicated. Unlike patients undergoing elective surgical procedures, trauma patients are not "prepared" for operation. When the patient's medical history reveals significant food or alcohol ingestion or both, a delay before induction of anesthesia may be justified. When a patient suspected of retaining food in the stomach is taken to the operating room, a prudent anesthesiologist will elect to perform the intubation with the patient awake. A large-bore stomach tube is useful for decompression, to minimize the risk of aspiration of gastric contents.

III. WOUND PREPARATION

A. Toilet

Before definitive repair, the wound is irrigated copiously with sterile saline solution; too much irrigation is impossible. During irrigation, the wound is inspected carefully, and foreign bodies are removed. In especially dirty wounds, additional irrigation with povidone-iodine (Betadine) solution may be helpful. Infection can destroy the result of even the most outstanding soft tissue closure.

B. Debridement

Although obviously devitalized tissues should be removed, debridement in the head and neck can be more conservative than in other areas because of the superior blood supply. When the site of injury is away from specialized facial structures, the wound edges can be trimmed without fear of altering the patient's appearance. In irregular or beveled lacerations, this technique is useful in achieving linear, sharp wound edges, which always give a better cosmetic result. In effect, debridement turns a wound into a clean incision. Removal of 2 mm of the wound edge is more critical in delayed closure because it eliminates tissue at risk for bacterial colonization. When an anatomic structure is included in the tissue disruption, debridement should be minimized, and surgical revision should be performed after full healing if the cosmetic result is unsatisfactory. Revisions are made easier when the maximal amount of local tissue remains available. In cosmetically critical areas, pieces of tissue with minimal remaining attachment are sutured in place and essentially become a free graft. These pieces often survive in some form.

IV. TYPES OF INJURY

A. Abrasions

Cleansing with removal of foreign bodies is the main treatment for abrasions as long as extensive tissue loss is not present. Often, foreign bodies are not obvious, but must be sought if a pigmented scar is to be avoided. Brushing is sufficient in most instances. Occasionally, in patients with deeply embedded foreign particles, a stiff brush or a dermabrader can be useful. The use of solvents, such as acetone or ether, may be necessary to remove embedded materials that are not water soluble. Dressings are important and should be of the water-soluble type, not ointments. In patients who have lost full-thickness skin, procedures to move tissue into the area may be necessary. When the patient's condition does not allow this procedure to be accomplished expeditiously, time can be bought by using split-thickness skin grafts or simply by applying wet dressings.

B. Contusions

Contusions of soft tissue require little therapy if the underlying structures are not injured. What appears to be a minimal injury can obscure serious bone damage. Diffuse bleeding can result when the tissues are loose, as in the periorbital region. Occasionally, a more localized hematoma can develop, such as in the subgaleal plane of the forehead; such a wound should be aspirated and covered with a pressure dressing. Otherwise, elevation of the involved area and application of ice packs constitute adequate treatment.

C. Lacerations

1. Soft tissue technique

a. ***General principles*** Careful application of the basic techniques of soft tissue repair provides major benefits when dealing with facial trauma. The necessity for later revision may be eliminated or may be simplified as a result. Because wound healing characteristics vary among individuals, the goal of repair is to obtain the best possible result in a given patient.

b. ***Incision*** The surgeon performing an elective procedure can place the incision in a favorable cosmetic position. The surgeon repairing a soft tissue injury must accept the "incision" as it is and should resist the temptation to alter the direction of the wound during primary repair. These techniques are saved for surgical revision.

c. ***Undermining of wound edges*** The goal of all soft tissue techniques is to place the corresponding layers of tissue on each side of the wound exactly opposite and in contact with one another. Undermining of the wound edges, which contributes to layer closure and relieves wound tension, must be done carefully to avoid injury to important structures or landmarks. The use of tooth forceps on subcutaneous tissues and of skin hooks on the epidermis is advocated to minimize further damage to already traumatized tissues. All bleeding points must be controlled to prevent hematoma, a major antagonist of any wound. Undermined areas should be sutured, and muscle layers should be closed with absorbable suture to eliminate dead space.

d. ***Dermal and subcutaneous closure*** Although a layer of sutures in the subcutaneous tissues is necessary, the most important layer for closure catches the lower aspect of the dermis as well as the subcutaneous tissues. These knots should be buried; that is, the knot should be tied at the lowest point of the suture in the subcutaneous tissues. This layer of closure relieves the epidermis of tension and contributes to eversion of the edges. Although the epidermis is cosmetically important, it need not hold the wound together.

e. ***Suturing*** The interrupted suture is standard for cosmetic closures. The experienced surgeon can attempt variations. The continuous intradermal suture is valuable, with or without reinforcement with skin tapes. Skin tapes alone without suture can be used in selected patients. Any stitch chosen should evert the wound. Everted scars flatten during contracture of the wound, but they do not spread. When using interrupted sutures, one enters the skin at a 90° angle or less with respect to the wound edge and thereby includes more deeper tissues in the bite than superficial tissues. The vertical mattress suture is excellent for eversion and can be used when interrupted sutures fail. The half-buried horizontal mattress suture is useful in approximating a pointed area. Sutures are placed 2 to 3 mm apart and 1 to 2 mm from the wound's edge. A small diameter suture is chosen (5-0 or 6-0) of nylon or polypropylene (Prolene). When suture removal is undesirable, 6-0 mild chromic catgut can be used in the skin. Monofilament materials are preferred, to minimize epithelial ingrowth. The surgeon's technique is more important than the size or material of suture chosen.

f. ***Final closure*** The knot should be closed gently, preferably with a small needle holder intended for plastic surgical procedures. The tissues contained within the suture should not blanch and should accommodate posttraumatic edema.

g. ***Cleansing*** After closure, the wound should be cleaned of dried blood, which provides a nidus for bacterial growth.

2. **Simple lacerations** In general, the repair of simple lacerations is straightforward. When it has been cleansed adequately, the wound is closed carefully in layers: muscle and fascia, subcutaneous tissues, dermis, and epidermis. The principles of closure as previously discussed are followed. When the laceration crosses an anatomic landmark, the sutures of all layers must be placed with the proper orientation of this structure in mind. These areas include the eyebrows, the vermilion border of the lip, the alar rim of the nose, hairlines, prominent skin creases, and the pinna. The first skin suture should be placed at the edges of these structures, to ensure proper approximation. An excellent wound closure is ruined when these landmarks are not aligned. Parents of injured children should be warned that the scar will remain red and will maintain a hypertrophic character for a long time.

3. **Stellate (irregular) lacerations** These injuries are often the result of blunt trauma and are characterized by an irregular shape. It is difficult to achieve an ideal result because of the multiple flaps and the associated contused soft tissues. When the injury is in an area of mobile skin, it may be possible to excise the flaps and to convert the wound into a linear laceration, with a better cosmetic result. If such is not possible, the many corners of the wound should be joined with a buried subcuticular suture. The wound can be revised after healing.

4. **Avulsions**

    a. ***Flaps*** Traumatically created flaps of skin, typically "U" shaped, are problems because the flap may become necrotic or the cosmetic result may be poor. During healing, contracture of the scar occurs, and the skin flap assumes an elevated, visible position. A thin flap is similar to a split-thickness skin graft and can be held in place by selected sutures and splinted. If the skin flap is thick, the method of closure will depend on beveling of the margin. If the angle approaches 90°, the wound can be closed by trimming any small, irregular edges. In suturing, the bites taken on the flaps should be shallower than those on the wound's edge, to compensate for the bevel. When the angle is acute and thus creates a thin margin to the flap, the edges are trimmed back, and a right angle is created on both the flap and the wound margin. Undermining the tissue surrounding the flap may be useful in creating countertraction to balance the forces generated by healing. Later revision of avulsion flaps is often necessary.

    b. ***Tissue loss*** Lost tissue must be replaced in some manner. Small areas, if properly preserved in iced saline solution, may be sutured back into place if the tissue occupies a portion of a facial structure that would be difficult to reconstruct, such as a pinna, an alar margin, or an eyebrow. If a specific landmark is not involved, but the tissue loss covers a large area, it is most prudent to cover the area with a split-thickness skin graft. This technique provides immediate, physiologic protection for the wound and gives one time to plan and to perform reconstruction. If the area is small, undermining and primary closure are easily accomplished. Local skin flaps can be used judiciously during initial repair by the experienced surgeon, but major movement or transfer of tissues is best avoided during the initial treatment of an acute injury.

D. Burns

1. Thermal

a. *Fire* The treatment of burns is a major subspecialty within surgery, and no attempt is made to be inclusive here. Basically, treatment is the same as for burns on any area of the body, although opinions do vary. These cosmetic injuries should be treated vigorously and with great respect. A major problem is stenosis of the various orifices of the head during healing of a burn. Contracture of the eyelid may lead to exposure keratitis, and early grafting may be necessary. Perichondritis is possible wherever cartilage underlies the skin and is particularly a problem in burns of the pinna. When this complication occurs, treatment should be instituted rapidly because significant deformities result. Patients with major facial burns should be referred to surgeons experienced in their treatment. Patients with burns of the head and neck may also have significant thermal injury of the lower respiratory tract with resulting respiratory distress.

b. *Frostbite* Extremities, including the nose and ears, are susceptible to frostbite. These injuries can be insidious, and the patient may be unaware of the process. The involved areas are often covered with a whitish film and are colder to the touch than the surrounding normal face. These areas should be warmed as rapidly as possible at just above body temperature, 40 to 42° C. They should be cleansed and protected against trauma. When the pinna is involved or when the injury is extensive, antibiotics may be indicated. Debridement is avoided until the irreversibly injured areas are well defined.

2. Electrical The commonest electrical injury occurs when a child bites into a live wire. Deep burns of the lips, often involving the commissures, result. The wound should be kept as clean as possible. Most surgeons treat these injuries conservatively, debriding and reconstructing the commissures when the full extent of necrosis has been determined and when healing has taken place. Feeding can be a problem, and a nasogastric tube may be necessary.

E. Bites

Animal and human bites are common and differ in their treatment. Animal bites can be extensive injuries resulting from mauling. Human bites are typically not extensive, but the organisms introduced may be more pathogenic. Vigorous cleansing and irrigation are in order for either type of bite. Ordinarily human bites are not primarily repaired unless tissue is amputated. Antibiotics and moist dressings are indicated. Wounds created by animals can be approached more directly and can be repaired in the acute stage. Tetanus immunization guidelines should be followed closely. The possibility of rabies should be entertained in patients with animal bites, and the local animal control authority should be properly notified.

V. SPECIAL ANATOMIC CONSIDERATIONS

A. Eye Region

When trauma occurs in the region of the orbit, the status of the globe and the patient's vision should be documented carefully before any procedure is performed. Corneal abrasion is common. Ophthalmologic consultation should be sought if any question exists. A protective lens should be placed over the cornea during repair.

1. Eyelids

a. ***When full-thickness skin is lost*** from the lower lids, immediate grafting should be performed if primary closure would produce an ectropion. This tissue can be obtained from the upper lid, if the graft is small, or postauricularly, if large. The upper lid is not often a problem because excess tissue is common in this area, but the same principles apply.

b. ***Through-and-through losses*** of the lower lid of less than a quarter of its length can be closed primarily. The edges can be trimmed carefully, to leave a "V"-shaped wound. A suture is placed through the gray line at the margin of the lid and is useful for traction. A 6-0 nylon suture placed in a subcuticular manner approximates the conjunctiva and the tarsal place and can be pulled out later. A fine absorbable suture tied in an interrupted manner with buried knots accomplishes the same end. Fine catgut joins the orbicularis oculi muscle. The skin is closed with carefully placed interrupted sutures. When larger areas are lost, the sophisticated techniques required should not be attempted by a beginner.

c. ***For losses of less than a quarter of its length,*** the upper lid can be closed similarly to the lower lid. The procedure changes for greater losses because of the functional requirements of the upper lid. The general principle is to use portions of the lower lid to replace the upper, and then to reconstruct the resulting lower lid deficit with other tissues. If possible, disruptions of the levator palpebrae superioris muscle should be repaired, to prevent ptosis.

2. **Eyebrows** A frequent result of closure of an eyebrow laceration is loss of a strip of hair follicles along the wound, leaving an unhidden scar. The edges of the wound can be trimmed on each side parallel to the shafts of the hairs, to avoid this problem. This adjustment of the wound edges should be kept to an absolute minimum or should be saved for a later revision. When portions of the eyebrow are lost, it is best to obtain coverage with a split-thickness skin graft and to perform a reconstruction later.
3. **Lacrimal system** Injuries of the eyelids medial to the lacrimal puncta may disrupt the lacrimal duct system. The continuity of these ducts can be determined with fine probes. When transections are found, the duct is splinted over a nylon suture, which is brought through the skin over the lacrimal sac and is tied. Fine polyethylene tubing can also be used.
4. **Canthus**
   a. ***Disruptions of the medial canthus*** without bone injury can be repaired by simple suturing; however, fractures are usually accompanying features. If the ligament remains attached to a bone fragment, reduction of the fracture will place the ligament in its proper position. This procedure may require through-and-through wires over a button on the opposite side of the nose. These injuries may be complicated by lacrimal injuries. Unrecognized canthal trauma leads to the significant cosmetic deformity of traumatic telecanthus.
   b. ***Lateral canthal injuries*** are more easily handled because the ligament can be sutured to the periosteum of the frontal process of the zygoma.

B. Nose

Lacerations of the nose, including through-and-through injuries that involve the vestibule or mucosa without tissue loss, are repaired primarily in layers as in any other area. Special care should be taken when the alar margin is involved to minimize notching, which always occurs to some extent. Lost tissue is immediately replaced if primary approximation would cause distortion. Small full-thickness skin grafts can be obtained from loose postauricular or supraclavicular tissues. Small local flaps may be useful as an alternative to skin grafts. When the lost tissue is greater than 2 cm in diameter and contains both external and internal lining, the skin is closed to the mucosa, and secondary repair is planned. If the original tissue is available, one may attempt to suture it into position after thorough cleaning. Major reconstructions are not performed during primary repair.

C. Oral Region

1. Lips

a. An important point in closure of lip injuries is *careful approximation of the muscle layer,* to minimize notching. The mucosa is closed with silk or catgut suture; catgut is preferable when suture removal may be difficult, as in children. The catgut chosen should be larger than might seem necessary, such as 3-0. Mattress sutures are helpful to evert both the mucosa and the vermilion border, which have a natural tendency to inversion.

b. ***When lip substance is lost,*** the wound can be converted to a wedge shape and may be closed primarily. This procedure can be performed for up to 30% of the lip's length. If the loss is up to 50%, the uninvolved lip can supply the necessary tissue. Greater losses require sophisticated repair techniques. In the lips, unlike in other areas, local flaps have a place in primary closure. Losses of vermilion tissue can be replaced with flaps or free grafts of mucosa. In severe injuries to the lips or cheeks, for example, gunshot wounds, debridement and mucosa-to-skin closure should be the primary treatment.

2. Oral cavity

a. ***Mucosal lacerations*** can be repaired if they are extensive or associated with overlapping skin injuries. Silk is the best suture material unless removal would prove difficult. Small injuries may be left open to heal secondarily and may be kept clean by irrigations or gargles of saline solution or hydrogen peroxide, or both.

b. ***Tongue lacerations*** should be repaired using 2-0 chromic catgut sutures; one should take large suture bites and bury the knots.

c. ***Soft palate injuries*** should be repaired in three layers with emphasis on the muscle layer, similar to repair of the lip.

d. ***Floor of mouth*** Unlike the parotid duct, the duct of the submaxillary gland does not need repair. Disruption of this duct normally leads to harmless fistulization into the floor of the mouth.

D. Parotid Region

1. **Parenchyma of gland** In patients with lacerations in the region of the parotid gland, one should suspect interruption of the duct or branches of the facial nerve. These injuries should be ruled out by careful, deliberate evaluation. Injury to the gland tissue itself is not a major problem, except for the possibility of postoperative salivary collections or leakage. If the injury is small, skin and subcutaneous tissues may be closed,

and pressure may be applied. If collections of saliva appear, sterile aspiration or expectant observation will be indicated. If the injury is extensive, it is prudent to anticipate such a problem and to drain the wound into the oral cavity, where a fistula will not present a problem.

2. **The parotid duct** runs parallel to and 1 cm inferior to the zygomatic arch from the anterior edge of the ramus of the mandible to a point inferior to the lateral edge of the eye. If the duct has been transected, the distal portion can be found by probing through the orifice of the duct, and the medial part by applying pressure to the gland parenchyma to force saliva from the cut end. A microscope can be useful. The duct is repaired over a polyethylene catheter, which is sutured to the buccal mucosa for 10 days. The buccal branch of the facial nerve is often injured along with the duct.

3. **Facial nerve** Injuries to the facial nerve are suspected by the location of the injury. Each of the important branches should be checked: that of the forehead, of the eye, the buccal branch, and that of the corner of the mouth. The wound should be explored, and the ends of the nerve should be approximated with 7-0 or 8-0 nylon sutures placed through the epineurium. The distal ends of the nerve can be found with a nerve stimulator, but the proximal ends may be difficult to locate. In 72 hours, the nerve loses its ability to be stimulated. Because the terminal branches of the nerve are small and reinnervation is often spontaneous, it is impractical to attempt repair.

E. Pinna and External Auditory Canal

1. **In patients with laceration of the pinna,** cartilage may need trimming, to allow adequate skin coverage. Suture of the cartilage is usually unnecessary. Skin losses over cartilage may be covered with a flap from the postauricular skin. If the loss is extensive, the area of denuded cartilage can be drawn back and buried in a postauricular subcutaneous pocket. If only the posterior skin is lost, the raw surface can be sutured to a corresponding denuded area postauricularly. Another method is to suture the raw edge of the pinna to an incision in the postauricular skin. Both methods require secondary reconstruction.

2. **Lacerations extending through the external auditory canal** should be closed in any way possible, with stenting of the canal for 2 to 3 weeks. When the injury is circumferential, longer stenting is required.

3. **Patients with exposed cartilage** should be given prophylactic antibiotics, such as oxacillin. The wound should be irrigated copiously. Application of moist cotton to conform to the lateral and medial surfaces of the pinna and held by a mastoid dressing is a useful way to splint and to protect the ear. Hematomas

are a significant problem because they form between the nutrient perichondrium and cartilage, with subsequent necrosis of the cartilage. Hematomas should be drained. and a pressure dressing should be applied.

VI. CARE FOLLOWING REPAIR OF INJURY

A. Dressings

Dressings can provide pressure, protection, and splinting. Pressure can benefit every wound by limiting the collection of fluid and the formation of a hematoma. Elastic bandages with adhesive on one surface are available in various sizes and are a convenient method of providing pressure. The dressing keeps the patient away from the wound and, by covering it, minimizes the distress of the family. One potential problem with dressings is that the wound is unseen and may be forgotten. Contaminated wounds should be inspected within 24 hours. Furthermore, wet dressings or fine mesh gauze may contribute to debridement in these potentially infected wounds. Application of bacitracin ointment twice a day is helpful as protection and minimizes the crusting that contributes to stitch marks and a poor cosmetic result.

B. Antibiotics

Antibiotics are not routinely indicated, but in certain situations they appear to be justified, as in contaminated wounds, cartilage injuries, oral cavity injuries, and bite wounds. Antibiotics cannot replace proper cleaning of the wound.

C. Suture removal

Sutures are removed in the head and neck in 3 to 5 days. In areas such as the eyelids, and where tension is not present, sutures may be removed early. If the dermal layer has been closed properly, early removal of sutures will not present a problem. Skin tapes are useful to provide epidermal support when the sutures have been removed. A continuous intradermal suture may be left in for up to 3 weeks.

2

FACIAL FRACTURES

SHAN R. BAKER

I. GENERAL TREATMENT MEASURES

A. Assessment of the Airway

Such assessment is the first and most important measure in the management of patients with facial fractures. The unconscious patient develops respiratory obstruction because the tongue falls back into the pharynx. Similarly, bilateral anterior mandibular fractures allow the tongue to fall posteriorly, occluding the pharynx. Secretions, blood, vomitus, and foreign bodies such as loose teeth and broken dentures may obstruct the airway. Blunt trauma or penetrating injuries of the neck may cause respiratory difficulties because of edema or fracture of the larynx or trachea. Associated thoracic injuries may impede normal respiration and may lead to alveolar hypoventilation.

1. **Suctioning of secretions and placement of an oropharyngeal airway** usually maintain a patent airway in patients with severe facial fractures. When such a device is not immediately available, upper airway obstruction can be generally relieved by anterior traction on the tongue. Pulling the mandible anteriorly is helpful and is best achieved by placing one's index finger inside the patient's mouth and pulling superiorly on the symphysis or by placing one's hands posterior to the angle of the mandible bilaterally and lifting anteriorly.
2. **Oroendotracheal intubation** may be necessary when facial edema is massive. Similarly, when patients are intoxicated or unconscious, concern exists not only for the airway, but also

for the possibility of aspiration of mucus and blood. In such instances, oroendotracheal intubation is preferred.

3. **Tracheotomy** is indicated in patients with severe midfacial fractures that require intermaxillary fixation and reduction of nasal fractures and nasal packing. Trauma to the larynx or trachea dictates immediate tracheostomy inferior to the site of injury.

B. Determination of Other Injuries

A search for other injuries that require immediate care must be made prior to directing attention to facial fractures. Blunt trauma to the chest and abdomen may result in pneumothorax, hemothorax, or ruptured or herniated abdominal viscera. Correction of shock should be simultaneous with the establishment of an adequate airway.

1. **Hypovolemic shock** can rarely be attributed to facial fractures, except when large scalp lacerations are present. Intrathoracic or intra-abdominal bleeding should be suspected when facial fractures are associated with hemorrhagic shock. Fractures of the extremities may lead to hypovolemic shock. Immobilization and fluid replacement must be attended to promptly.
2. **Neurogenic shock** may be the result of injury to the head or cervical spine. Permanent neurologic deficit may be caused by manipulation of the patient's neck while the airway is secured or facial fractures are assessed. Any facial fracture can be associated with a fracture of the cervical spine. When spinal injury is suspected, the patient's head should be immobilized until confirmatory roentgenograms are obtained. Intracranial bleeding may occur early, or it may be delayed subsequent to head trauma. Neurologic checks should be made frequently during the first 24 hours following injury.

C. Treatment of Facial Lacerations

If more serious injuries are not present and if the treatment of airway obstruction and of shock is satisfactory, one may treat facial lacerations. All facial lacerations can be closed primarily despite the time lag between injury and treatment. The excellent vascularity of the face usually prevents infection. When lacerations are grossly contaminated with foreign debris, limited debridement of the wound and the use of appropriate antibiotics are indicated. One should search for damaged facial nerve branches or salivary gland ducts. Repair of these structures is concurrent with closure of lacerations.

D. Diagnosis of Facial Fractures

The diagnosis of a facial fracture is established by a history of recent trauma and by physical examination.

1. **Inspection** may reveal swelling, ecchymosis, distortion of the

facial contour, displacement of the mandible, and malocclusion of the teeth. Eye mobility may be impaired.

2. **Palpation** may demonstrate tenderness, crepitus, subcutaneous emphysema, step-off of a bony contour, or motion of a normal stationary segment.

3. **Roentgenograms** should supplement, but not replace, the physical examination in the documentation of facial fractures. Radiographic signs of recent facial fractures include paranasal sinus air-fluid levels, soft tissue swelling, subcutaneous air, and intraorbital air. Disruption of suture lines and bony cortices may be noted. An increased density from overlap or rotation of bony fragments is another sign of recent or old facial fracture.
   a. ***The Caldwell view*** provides an excellent evaluation of the orbit. The anterior, medial, and posterior portions of the orbital floor are seen on end. With this view, the neck of the mandibular condyle is clearly visible.
   b. ***The Waters view*** allows radiographic assessment of the nasal cavity and arch and is best for the maxillary sinuses and zygomatic bones. The articular surface of the mandibular condyle is clearly seen.
   c. ***The lateral view*** demonstrates the anterior and posterior walls of the frontal sinus. The sphenoid sinus and the pterygomaxillary fossa are well visualized. In addition, the nasal spine is clearly visible.
   d. ***The submental vertex view*** enables the evaluation of the anterior and posterior ethmoid air cells. The sphenoid sinus is well outlined, as are the zygomatic arches.
   e. ***The orthopantomogram*** offers a composite view of the entire mandible and provides the best overall visibility. The angle and body of the mandible and subcondylar areas are particularly detailed.
   f. ***Nasal bone roentgenograms*** are obtained, primarily for medicolegal reasons. Such films are not necessary for the diagnosis or treatment of nasal fractures.

E. Treatment of Facial Fractures

The treatment of facial fractures is not an emergency. Nasal fractures evaluated early may be reduced immediately. Reduction of other types of fractures may be delayed up to 10 days after injury, to allow facial edema to subside. Edema complicates palpation and identification of fracture sites, and ascertaining normal facial and nasal contours may be difficult. The isolation of bony fragments may also be a problem when facial swelling is present.

The treatment principles for facial fractures are similar to those for long bone fractures. Realignment of the bone fragments and immobilization during healing are indicated to restore contour and function. The key to reduction of mandibular and maxillary fractures is re-establishment of the patient's pretraumatic dental occlusion.

1. **Closed reduction** is usually adequate for most nasal and mandibular fractures. Occasionally, minimally displaced zygomatic fractures are treated with closed reduction. Immobilization is achieved by intranasal packing and an external splint for fractures of the nasal bones. Arch bars, dental splints, and interosseous wiring provide suitable immobilization for fractures of the mandible.
2. **Open reduction and fixation of bone fragments** with internal wiring are required for the majority of maxillary and zygomatic fractures. Unfavorable mandibular fractures (discussed later in this chapter) and compound nasal fractures may require open reduction as well.

II. NASAL FRACTURES

A. Cause and Diagnosis

Nasal fractures occur from direct blows to the nose. The external appearance of the nose may be minimally altered or grossly deformed. Small chip fractures frequently occur along the edges of the pyriform aperture and along the lower border of the nasal bone. These injuries rarely cause external deformity. Moderate blows can displace one of the nasal bones into the nasal cavity. More severe blows may move the entire nasal pyramid off the midline or may cause the nasal bones to telescope posteriorly into the ethmoid sinuses.

1. **Medical history and examination** Inquiry should be made into the cause of injury, the direction of the blow, and the extent of nasal hemorrhage. Patients may report the inability to breathe through one or both sides of the nose. They may complain of significant deviation or a change in configuration of the nose following trauma. External deviation or flattening of the nasal bones may be observed. Deformity and asymmetry of the upper and lower lateral cartilages, nasal tip, and columella must be noted.
2. **Palpation** demonstrates tenderness and crepitus along fracture lines; however, edema and ecchymosis may obscure some of the physical findings. The nasal interior may reveal mucosal lacerations and septal injuries. Fracture dislocation of the septal cartilage can occur without fracture of the nasal bones. Septal cartilage may fracture and may telescope posteriorly, causing duplication. When this phenomenon occurs, thickening of the septum, shortening of the nose, and retraction of the columella are noted on examination.
3. **Roentgenograms** of the nasal bones are seldom necessary and should not unduly influence the diagnosis of a nasal fracture. Normal suture lines may be interpreted as fracture lines, or

gross nasal displacement may be present without radiographic evidence of a fracture.

B. Emergency Treatment

Initial treatment of nasal fractures requires control of hemorrhage. The nasal passages must be cleared of blood clots, to allow visualization of the septum. Hematomas should be drained by an incision through the mucosa and compressed with nasal packing. Septal cartilage dislocation must be reduced and supported with intranasal splints. Large mucosal lacerations are closed with absorbable sutures. Appropriate antibiotics are indicated if nasal packing is required for longer than 48 hours.

Swelling and hemorrhage dictate delay of the fracture reduction. If edema is minimal, closed reduction may be attempted after topical application of cocaine to the nose. One should insert a blunt instrument under the depressed nasal bone and elevate it while simultaneously applying external pressure on the laterally displaced opposite nasal bone. The reduction is stabilized with an external splint and intranasal packing as needed.

C. Untreated Nasal Fractures

Nasal fractures that remain untreated can cause external nasal deformity and nasal obstruction. Adhesions between the septum and the nasal turbinates may obstruct the nasal passage. In patients who have had considerable damage to the mucous membranes of the internal nose, webbing and stenosis may result. This deformity can be difficult to correct later. Septal hematomas that are not recognized and treated early may cause absorption of the septal cartilage, with a resultant loss of nasal support and saddling of the nasal dorsum.

III. NASOETHMOID FRACTURES

A. Diagnosis

The diagnosis of nasoethmoid complex fractures involves assessment of the nasal, ethmoid, maxillary, and frontal bones. The cribriform plate, the nasolacrimal system, and the orbital contents must also be evaluated.

1. **Cause** Nasoethmoid fractures are usually associated with a history of a direct blow to the nose in a posterior or posteroinferior direction. Nasal bleeding is present, and the patient usually has associated lacerations over the nasal bridge.
2. **Appearance** Examination demonstrates comminution and displacement of the nasal bones and septum posteriorly into the ethmoid sinus. The central third of the face is flattened. Spreading of the medial canthus and lateral displacement of the palpebral fissures result from the tearing of the attachments of the medial palpebral ligaments.
   a. ***Patency and continuity of the nasolacrimal ducts*** may

be determined by placing fluorescein dye in the eye and by observing the dye as it exits through the inferior meatus of the nose.

b. ***Cerebrospinal fluid (CSF) leaks into the nose*** are caused by tears of the dura along the cribriform plate or the fossa ethmoidalis. The leak may be copious or sparse. A technique for CSF identification is the "halo" test. Blood and fluid are allowed to drip onto a paper tissue. The fluid separates as it diffuses into the tissue. Blood remains in a central ring; mucus is displaced slightly farther, and spinal fluid diffuses the farthest, to produce a halo around the central pink area.

c. ***Examination of extraocular muscle function*** is necessary. Pupillary distances from the midline should be measured. Cranial nerve assessment is important, to determine supratrochlear and supraorbital nerve impairment.

3. **Confirmation of the diagnosis** Plain roentgenograms are not usually helpful in the diagnosis of nasoethmoid fractures. Frequently, polytomographic examination is required to document fractures of the cribriform plate and the medial orbital walls.

B. Initial Treatment

Early treatment includes care of the nasal and septal injuries. Nasal hemorrhage may be severe, requiring anterior and, occasionally, posterior nasal packing. Packing should be avoided if possible when a CSF leak is present. Lacerations are closed, and antibiotics are administered. To lessen facial edema, the patient should remain in a high semi-Fowler position if other injuries permit. Ophthalmologic consultation is imperative. Reduction of fractures requires a surgical procedure. Recognition and early repair of disrupted medial canthal ligaments are essential, to avoid hypertelorism.

C. Complications

Complications following nasoethmoid fractures include injury to the eye resulting in blindness, diplopia, epiphora, and dacryocystitis. Meningitis may result if the dura mater is disrupted. Hypertelorism and broadening of the nasal bridge are common. Chronic sinusitis or mucoceles of the frontal sinus may develop when the nasofrontal duct has been injured.

IV. Zygoma Fractures

A. Zygomatic or Malar Bone Fractures

Sometimes referred to as tripod fractures, these fractures usually involve a break through articulation sites between the zygoma and the other facial bones with which it articulates. Fracture usually occurs at the infraorbital foramen, along the floor of the orbit, into the frontozygomatic suture, and through the zygomatic arch. By necessity, such a fracture occurs across the anterior, lateral, and posterior walls of the maxillary antrum. Herniation of orbital contents in the direction of the antrum may occur.

1. **Medical history and symptoms** A history of significant trauma to the prominence of the cheek is obtained. The patient may complain of diplopia and hypoesthesia in the distribution of the infraorbital nerve because of disruption of the orbital floor and injury of the infraorbital nerve, extraocular muscles, or portions of the third cranial nerve. Numbness of the maxillary teeth is caused by avulsion of the dental nerves in the antral walls. Unilateral epistaxis results from bleeding into the maxillary antrum at the time of fracture.
2. **Signs** Observation of the patient demonstrates flattening of the involved malar eminence with asymmetry of the face and periorbital ecchymosis. The lateral canthus of the eye may appear to be more inferiorly placed than normal because the lateral canthal ligament is attached to the zygoma and is displaced with the bone. In conjunction with this finding, one may see inferior displacement of the pupil and apparent ptosis of the upper eyelid from herniation of orbital contents.
   a. ***Examination often documents tenderness*** and disruption of the inferior and lateral orbital rims. The zygomatic arch usually appears flattened. Similarly, upward pressure on the undersurface of the malar eminence from intraoral palpation causes pain. A fracture line across the face of the maxilla can usually thus be palpated.
   b. ***Occlusion is not disturbed*** because the alveolar ridge of the maxilla is uninvolved; however, limitation of mandibular motion can occur from impingement of the coronoid process by a depressed zygomatic arch.
3. **Radiologic features** Roentgenograms in the Waters projection provide the best overall view of the zygoma. Displacement of the inferior and lateral orbital rims may be seen, as well as cloudiness of the maxillary antrum due to extravasation of blood into the sinus. Submental-vertex and tangential views are useful in evaluating the zygomatic arch.

B. Goals of Treatment

The goals of zygomatic fracture repair are to restore normal facial contour and to prevent limitation of mandibular excursion. The pupils must be level, and eye muscle function should be restored. Repair should be delayed to minimize local edema and to allow time for adequate medical evaluation, including ophthalmologic consultation. The application of ice packs and maintenance of a semi-Fowler position hasten regression of edema.

C. Unrecognized or Unrepaired Zygomatic Fractures

Such fractures may produce marked flattening of the malar eminence. Permanent trismus may result from impingement by the zygoma on the coronoid process. In addition, all the complications that ensue from an unrecognized orbital floor fracture may occur.

V. BLOWOUT FRACTURES

A. Location

Blowout fractures occur in the orbital floor or, less commonly, on the medial wall of the orbit. By definition, the orbital rim is left intact.

1. **Medical history and symptoms** A history is obtained of blunt trauma to the eye. The object striking the eye is usually larger than the globe. Smaller objects generally lacerate or injure the globe directly. The patient frequently complains of diplopia on upward gaze and may have hypoesthesia in the distribution of the infraorbital nerve on the involved side. Unilateral epistaxis may be seen.
2. **Evaluation of the patient** reveals periorbital ecchymosis. Narrowing of the palpebral fissure may occur, and orbital emphysema may be present. Diplopia, a finding in approximately 70% of cases, may be due to entrapment of the inferior rectus or inferior oblique muscles, to injury to the oculomotor nerve, or to hematoma and edema, which interfere with movement of the globe. Orbital herniation may cause ptosis and enophthalmos. Fracture often occurs in the area of the infraorbital foramen and injures the nerve.
   a. ***The traction test*** may help to differentiate muscle entrapment from paresis due to nerve or muscle injury. A few drops of 0.5% tetracaine are placed in the involved eye. Conjunctival forceps are used to grasp the insertion of the inferior rectus muscle. The globe is lifted superiorly with the forceps. Muscle entrapment is unlikely if the globe moves freely.
   b. ***Enophthalmos*** occurs in approximately 15% of blowout fractures and is frequently masked by edema and hematoma immediately following injury. The mechanism of enophthalmos is herniation of periorbital tissue into the maxillary sinus and subsequent fibrosis and periorbital fat absorption.
   c. ***Severe associated injuries*** of the globe are common in patients with blowout fractures. Hyphema, posterior chamber hemorrhage, retinal detachment, and perforation of the globe may occur. Early ophthalmologic consultation is indicated in all blowout fractures.
3. **Radiographic studies,** using the Waters and Caldwell views, are helpful in assessing fractures of the orbital floor, but these studies confirm the diagnosis in only 50% of cases. Polytomographic studies may be indicated when the diagnosis is in question. The typical radiographic finding is a bulging inferiorly

of the orbital floor into the maxillary antrum, indicating a blowout fracture with herniation of periorbital tissue. This sign may be obscured by a cloudy maxillary sinus. Cloudy ethmoid sinuses and orbital emphysema are additional radiographic signs of a blowout fracture.

B. Treatment

The goals of blowout fracture repair are to restore normal eye mobility and to prevent or relieve enophthalmos. Surgical correction is indicated when diplopia does not disappear within 2 weeks following injury and when enophthalmos is present. Immediate therapy should include assessment of the patient's vision and ophthalmologic evaluation. Lacerations of the eyelids should be closed.

C. Complications

Orbital injury, blindness, permanent diplopia, and enophthalmos are complications of blowout fractures. Enophthalmos may be a delayed sequela, occurring weeks after the injury. Rarely is surgery totally successful in the correction of enophthalmos, even when the operation is performed soon after the eye injury.

VI. MAXILLARY FRACTURES

A. Cause and Classification

The paired maxillae and the palatine bones considered together make up the maxilla. Most fractures of the maxilla are from automobile accidents causing a head-on injury that drives the maxillae posteriorly. The force of the blow and the pull of the pterygoid muscles drag the maxillae posteriorly and inferiorly, producing an open bite anteriorly.

1. **Observation and the patient's medical history** reveal bilateral periorbital ecchymosis and edema. Bilateral epistaxis is common. The patient's face is long and flat. One may note apparent ptosis in one or both eyes, and the patient may complain of diplopia on upward gaze. An open-bite deformity or complaint of malocclusion is common. Bilateral hypoesthesia in the distribution of the infraorbital nerves may be present. CSF rhinorrhea should be sought carefully.
2. **The LeFort classification** of maxillary fractures is helpful in assessing the extent of injury to the maxilla. Frequently, however, patients with major facial injuries have various combinations of midfacial, zygomatic, and orbital fractures. For example, the patient may have a LeFort I fracture of one maxilla and a LeFort II fracture of the other.
   a. ***A LeFort I fracture*** is essentially a separation of the hard palate and the lower portions of the pterygoid processes from the rest of the cranial skeleton. If one grasps the anterior portion of the patient's maxilla between one's

thumb and forefinger, the palate will be freely movable in an anteroposterior direction. If dentition is present, the patient will have malocclusion. The posterior teeth meet, but the anterior teeth do not.

b. ***LeFort II (pyramidal) fractures*** of the maxilla are a result of separation of the palate and midportion of the facial skeleton from the cranial skeleton. The fracture line extends through the pterygoid plates across the junction of the maxillae with the zygomatic bones and across the nasal bridge. The midface, nasal bones, and palate are mobile as a unit. Inferior orbital rim irregularities are palpable bilaterally. All the findings associated with blowout fractures of the orbit may be present. The patient has ecchymosis, tenderness, and a palpable fracture line in the superior buccal sulcus bilaterally.

c. ***LeFort III fractures*** are defined as a separation of the entire facial skeleton from the cranium. The fracture line extends across the pterygoid plates adjacent to the base of the skull and across the lateral and medial orbital walls and nasal bridge, separating the maxilla and both zygomatic bones from the skull. Manipulation of the palate causes both malar eminences and the nasal bones to move. Lateral orbital rim irregularities are palpable bilaterally. An infraorbital rim step-off is noted in the presence of a concomitant zygomatic fracture, which separates the zygomatic bone from the maxilla. Massive facial edema is frequently present from laceration of the internal maxillary artery. The patient's face is elongated and flattened.

3. **Plain roentgenograms** usually underestimate the extensiveness of the fractures. The Waters view shows displacement of one or both orbital rims, opacity of one or both maxillary sinuses, and disruption of the nasal arch. Massive soft tissue edema is visible on all facial bone roentgenograms. Polytomographic study is frequently necessary to assess the integrity of the cribriform plate.

B. Treatment

Severe maxillary fractures are commonly associated with impairment of the airway. As in any injured patient, the airway must be maintained. Tracheotomy is generally required, either initially or at the time of operation for LeFort II and III fractures. Associated head, chest, and abdominal injuries must be treated immediately. Internal, ophthalmologic, orthopedic, and neurosurgical injuries take precedence over facial injuries.

1. **Initial measures** When possible, the patient should be placed in a semi-Fowler position. Intravenous antibiotics should be administered, especially if nasal packing is required to control epistaxis or if a CSF leak is present.

2. **Fracture repair** LeFort I fractures can usually be repaired

by closed reduction using interdental fixation. More severe maxillary fractures require open reduction. Fixation is achieved superiorly by suspension wires to the cranium. Interdental wiring and fixation to the mandible inferiorly stabilize the entire facial skeleton.

C. Unrecognized or Unrepaired Maxillary Fractures

Such fractures may lead to malunion of the bony structures of the face. Marked disturbance in occlusion, trismus, permanent diplopia, and deforming facial contours may result. All the sequelae of nasal injury may occur in patients with LeFort II and III fractures.

VII. MANDIBULAR FRACTURES

A. Cause and Diagnosis

The mandible is more commonly fractured than any bone of the face except the nasal bone. The condylar process, composed of the thin neck and the condyle, is the most common location of a mandibular fracture. Trauma to the point of the chin may result in bilateral fractures of the condylar processes. Blows to the side of the mandible typically fracture the ipsilateral body and the contralateral neck of the mandible.

1. **Signs and symptoms** Patients with mandibular fractures complain of pain and malocclusion. An open-bite deformity is observed in bilateral condylar fractures because the external pterygoid muscles pull the mandible anteriorly and cause premature contact of the molars. The degree of swelling, ecchymosis, and drooling may be considerable. Trismus is always present. The patient may have hypoesthesia of the lower lip from injury of the inferior alveolar nerve.
2. **Examination** discloses asymmetry of the jaw. Tenderness and bony crepitus are noted along the fracture line. Pushing on the symphysis causes pain near the ear in patients with fractures of the condylar process. Intraoral lacerations with exposure of the bone are common in fractures of the body and the angle of the mandible, as well as in fractures of parasymphyseal areas.
   a. ***Displacement of bony fragments*** depends on the pull of the muscles that attach to the mandible. The anterior group of muscles displaces the anterior fragment inferiorly, whereas the posterior group displaces the posterior fragment superiorly and medially.
   b. ***Direction of fracture line*** Favorable mandibular fractures occur when the fracture line runs in a direction that allows the muscles to pull the bony fragments toward each other. When the fracture line is in a direction that enables the muscles to distract the bony fragments, the fracture is considered unfavorable.
3. **Radiographic features** Oblique x-ray views of the mandible

offer excellent visualization of the temporomandibular joint and the body of the mandible. The Caldwell view allows assessment of the ramus and the neck of the mandible. Occlusal roentgenograms demonstrate alveolar and parasymphyseal fractures. The orthopantomogram projects the entire mandible on a flat surface and gives the best overall view.

B. Treatment

Bilateral parasymphyseal fractures allow the tongue to fall posteriorly into the pharynx. Airway obstruction must be avoided. Missing or avulsed teeth should be accounted for because they may have been aspirated.

As soon as the patient's condition permits, one should reduce the fractured mandible, to make the patient more comfortable and to lessen the chances of infection. Favorable fractures can frequently be managed conservatively with arch bars and intermaxillary fixation. Unfavorable fractures may, in addition, require open reduction and internal wiring.

C. Complications

Trismus, malocclusion, and loss of teeth are the possible sequelae of mandibular fractures. Malunion and fibrous union may cause pain on eating and deformity of the jaw. Although uncommon, osteomyelitis of the mandible may occur.

VIII. FRONTAL SINUS FRACTURES

A. Cause and Diagnosis

Frontal sinus fractures usually occur from blunt trauma to the forehead. Automobile accidents account for the majority of these injuries. Fractures may be confined to the anterior or the posterior frontal sinus wall. Similarly, the fracture may be limited to the nasofrontal duct area.

1. **Consciousness** Attention must be directed to the patient's level of consciousness. If conscious, he may complain of headache and visual problems. The patient's forehead contour may be depressed. Whether the injury is open or closed, a CSF leak must be suspected. Lacerations about the forehead are common in such injuries.

2. **A complete neurologic examination** is imperative, with careful notation of the level of consciousness and cranial nerve function. If one suspects injury to the dura mater or to the brain, a neurosurgical consultation should be obtained.

   Displaced fractures of the anterior wall cause a depressed area of the forehead. Exploration of compound fractures may allow visualization of the interior of the sinus. This procedure allows one to assess the posterior wall of the sinus for fractures and CSF leaks. Periorbital ecchymosis and edema are common.

Ocular mobility may be limited. Nasal examination can reveal the presence of CSF or of blood.

3. **Roentgenographic studies** should include the Caldwell, Waters, and lateral views. Frontal sinus fractures are not always visible on plain films and may require polytomographic study for confirmation. Posterior wall fractures may be associated with air in the anterior cranial fossa.

B. Treatment

All patients with frontal sinus fractures should be treated with broad-spectrum antibiotics, especially patients with compound fractures or fractures of the posterior wall. If a CSF leak is present, antibiotics should be continued until the leak stops, and nasal packing should be avoided.

1. **Simple nondisplaced fractures** of the anterior wall may be followed by serial roentgenograms. Lacerations should be closed immediately.
2. **Depressed or compound fractures** and fractures involving the posterior wall or the nasofrontal duct require surgical exploration. Such an approach allows assessment and repair of any lacerations in the dura mater of the anterior cranial fossa. Depressed fragments are elevated and are wired in place if unstable. Fractures in the nasofrontal duct often require obliteration of the frontal sinus with fat.

C. Complications

Early complications of frontal sinus fracture include meningitis, brain abscess, acute sinusitis, and osteomyelitis. Repeated episodes of meningitis may represent delayed sequelae. It often takes years before mucoceles and pyoceles manifest themselves as complications of frontal sinus fractures.

3

TRAUMA TO THE EAR AND TEMPORAL BONE

MOSHE ZIV

Trauma to the ear and the temporal bone is common following head injuries, especially those resulting from automobile accidents. The injury may be external through the auricle or the external auditory canal, but it may also involve the middle ear, inner ear, and the facial nerve. The damage to the inner ear secondary to the concussion of the labyrinth in the absence of external ear or middle ear injuries is often underestimated.

I. AURICULAR LACERATIONS

Lacerations of the auricle and hematomas are consequences of direct trauma to the auricle. The rich blood supply to the auricle promotes healing. One should therefore attempt to reconstruct the auricle primarily even in patients with severe lacerations. Debridement should be minimal, to avoid undue loss of tissue.

A. Anesthesia

Local anesthesia is sufficient for reconstructive procedures of the auricle in adults and in youngsters over 15 years old. In children under 15 years of age or in nervous patients, general anesthesia is indicated. One may use 1% lidocaine (Xylocaine) with 1:100,000 epinephrine, to be injected at the following points: (1) anterior to the tragus superiorly, to anesthetize the auriculotemporal nerve; and (2) posterior to the auricle, along the mastoid process in three points, to block the great auricular nerve and the lesser occipital nerve. In addition, one should inject the lateral surface of the external auditory canal to anesthetize the branches of the vagus and auriculotemporal nerves.

B. Technique

Cleansing of the ear should be thorough, with minimal debridement only when obvious necrotic tissue is present. The wound must be closely approximated, to preserve the normal anatomic appearance of the auricle. Suturing should be performed with 5-0 or 6-0 nylon on both surfaces of the skin of the auricle. Once the suturing is completed, an otoplasty dressing should be applied, with cotton impregnated with antibiotic ointment to fill in the shape of the auricle both laterally and medially. This procedure is followed by the application of sponges to absorb bloody discharge. The dressing should be kept on for 2 to 3 days and then changed, to allow one to check wound healing. The same type of dressing should be reapplied. Sutures may be removed in 5 to 6 days.

II. AURICULAR HEMATOMA

An auricular hematoma should be incised and drained. A Penrose drain should be left in position. An otoplasty dressing should be applied and changed daily. Systemic antibiotics should be administered in the presence of infection; a specimen should be taken for culture and sensitivity testing. In the absence of infection, systemic antibiotics are not indicated.

III. EXTERNAL AUDITORY CANAL

Injury to the ear may also involve the external auditory canal, sometimes in conjunction with auricular injury. Injury to the external auditory canal may include soft tissue as well as the bony canal. Fracture of the anterior wall of the external auditory canal may occur secondary to injury to the mandible or fracture of the temporal bone. X-ray studies of the temporal bones are necessary before treating an injury of the external auditory canal if fracture is suspected. Lateral tomograms of the ear canal and the temporal bone provide useful information. Anteroposterior tomograms are optional. Clinical evaluation of the patient's hearing is necessary, and hearing testing is recommended prior to treatment.

A. Anesthesia

In adults and in older children, one can administer local anesthesia following appropriate premedication. The points of injection are the same as for auricular anesthesia, with additional injections of: (1) the external auditory canal at its four quadrants; (2) the ear canal superiorly, close to the junction of the bony and cartilaginous canal; and (3) the external auditory canal inferiorly. In patients with substantial lacerations of the external auditory canal, local anesthesia may not be effective, and general anesthesia may be required.

B. Technique

Sterile preparation and draping are followed by exploration using the surgical microscope. If the ear canal is too narrow, one may expose it with an endaural incision. If the anterior wall of the external auditory canal is fractured, one may use a Lempert or nasal speculum to widen the external auditory canal and to reposition the fractured fragments. This maneuver should be avoided when the mastoid bone is fractured because of the risk to the facial nerve. The ear canal should be suctioned, to remove debris and accumulated blood. Soft tissue flaps should be approximated and placed in their original position. Irrigation with saline solution warmed to body temperature should be performed and the ear canal should be packed. The packing should remain in place for about 2 weeks. Many patients have a combination of auricular lacerations and ear canal injury, and both must be treated.

IV. TYMPANIC MEMBRANE PERFORATIONS

Perforation of the tympanic membrane may occur secondary to explosions, either in civilian life or in wars, blunt trauma to the ear, or incidental injury to the tympanic membrane, such as with a cotton swab or while water skiing. Perforation of the tympanic membrane is usually an isolated injury, but it may involve damage to the ossicular chain as well. Clinical examination of the ear with an otologic microscope is necessary. Cleansing of the ear should be performed by suctioning. Hearing tests should include determinations of pure tones, speech reception thresholds, and discrimination of sounds prior to any treatment procedure. In many instances of traumatic rupture of the tympanic membrane, cochlear damage is also present. Each type of tympanic membrane perforation requires a different approach.

A. Traumatic Perforation with a Cotton Swab

This type of perforation of the tympanic membrane is usually small, without inversion of tympanic membrane flaps, and the wound is generally clean. Any debris in the ear canal should be suctioned. One should avoid ear drops; most antibiotic drops are ototoxic. In patients with a healthy mucous membrane of the middle ear, absorption may occur, and inner ear damage may result. Systemic antibiotics are not usually necessary. Most of these traumatic perforations heal spontaneously; one should follow them clinically and audiologically on a weekly basis. If infection develops, systemic antibiotics may be necessary, in conjunction with cleansing by suctioning.

B. Blast Perforation

The degree of damage to the tympanic membrane, middle ear, and inner ear following blast injury depends on the type of explosive, the proximity to the source of explosion, and the direction of the ear canal in relation to the source of the blast. The size of this perforation may range from small, less than 20%, to large, more than 50% of the tympanic membrane. Clinical and audiologic studies are necessary prior to management. The ear should be evaluated with a microscope and then suctioned, to remove debris from the ear canal. The management of blast perforations of the tympanic membrane depends on the size of the perforation and on the presence of inverted flaps.

1. **Perforations without inverted flaps** Perforations of less than 20% of the tympanic membrane may require no specific management beyond suctioning. Ear drops should be avoided. The ear needs to be kept clean and dry. One may place an external patch in the form of a small disc of sterile rubber taken from a surgical glove or a small disc of sterile gel film. Antibiotic ointment may help to adhere the disc to the tympanic membrane. The advantage of external patching is to lessen the patient's slight conductive hearing loss and occasional tinnitus. If the perforation is larger than 20% of the tympanic membrane, both suctioning and external patching are indicated.

2. **Perforations with inverted flaps** Patients with inverted flaps of the ruptured tympanic membrane require suctioning of debris from the middle ear, elevation of the flaps, and placement of absorbable gelatin sponge (Gelfoam) in the middle ear to support these flaps. Careful alignment of the flaps is important. One should apply an external patch using a disc of sterile gel film or of some other sterile material. Additional pieces of Gelfoam should be placed lateral to the patch. This procedure must be done under local anesthesia in adults and general anesthesia in children. In 2 weeks, the patient should be given ear drops to soften or to dissolve the Gelfoam, and 10 days later, the Gelfoam may be suctioned from the ear canal. One may be able to follow the healing of the perforated tympanic membrane through the transparent gel film. The gel film may be removed a month after placement.

   The prognosis for blast perforations of the tympanic membrane, as well as for most other traumatic perforations, is good. About 85 to 90% of tympanic membrane perforations in blast injuries heal when treated in the foregoing manner. The few perforations that fail to close following this treatment may require tympanoplasty at a later date.

V. OSSICULAR DISRUPTION FOLLOWING TRAUMA

The most common sites of injury of the ossicular chain are the incudostapedial joint and the long process of the incus. In some instances, the stapedial crura may be fractured. One may also see a fracture of the footplate of the stapes with an oval window fistula. The malleus is the most resistant ossicle to traumatic damage. In case of severe temporal bone injury, the ossicles may be dislocated or fractured. In such injuries, the foregoing principles of treatment may be applied. Appropriate clinical and audiologic evaluations, as well as x-ray studies, are required. If a temporal bone fracture is suspected, tomographic evaluation of the temporal bones is indicated as part of the workup in addition to conventional roentgenograms. When ossicular trauma occurs, one must suspect an injury to the temporal bone that may also affect the inner ear. One should not correct an ossicular disruption in the acute phase. Rather, one should assess the general status of the patient, and then one should treat the other injuries related to the ear and the temporal bone. The patient with an ossicular discontinuity may have a ruptured tympanic membrane that requires treatment, as described previously. Many patients with an ossicular disruption also have sensorineural hearing loss secondary to cochlear concussion. One should wait approximately 6 months to a year before attempting to correct this ossicular dysfunction.

VI. INNER EAR DAMAGE FOLLOWING TRAUMA

Sensorineural hearing loss and vertigo are common following trauma to the temporal bone, with or without fracture. In the absence of temporal bone fracture, the damage to the inner ear may be due to concussion of the inner ear, with microruptures and tears of membranes as well as increased pressure in the inner ear secondary to the piston effect of the stapes. The skull and the ossicular chain may not move in the same direction at the same time of the blow, and pressure in the inner ear may be increased. Otolithic dislocation is another possibility at the time of head injury. Sensorineural hearing loss is a frequent sequela of head trauma. Most commonly affected are the high frequencies, including 4000 and 6000 Hz, but the patient's ability to hear the low frequencies may also be impaired. The vestibular system is often affected in the acute phase following head trauma. Compensation generally occurs in about 2 weeks to a month. Some degree of unsteadiness may persist for a longer time. Some patients develop benign paroxysmal positional vertigo resulting from head trauma. Patients with head injuries require an audiologic workup, especially patients who complain of hearing loss, tinnitus, or dizziness. Vestibular evaluation with an electronystagmographic recording is indicated if the patient complains of vertigo or unsteadiness. In the acute phase, the management of vertigo includes rest and symptomatic medication. If the patient has sensorineural hearing loss or a fluctuation in hearing accompanied by dizziness that persists unchanged for more than 10 days despite rest, one should suspect a fistula of the oval or round window. In such patients, exploration of the middle ear is indicated. The obliteration of the site of fistula is primarily helpful in overcoming the vestibular symptoms and in improving lower-frequency hearing loss. High-frequency hearing losses seem to be irreversible.

VII. FACIAL NERVE PARALYSIS DUE TO TEMPORAL BONE FRACTURE

Facial nerve paralysis may occur secondary to fracture, either horizontal or longitudinal, of the temporal bone. The longitudinal fracture is the most common, but only about 25% are associated with facial nerve paralysis. On the other hand, approximately 50% of horizontal fractures of the temporal bone are accompanied by facial nerve paralysis. Temporal bone fractures also cause cochlear and vestibular damage and, possibly, middle ear injury. Many patients with temporal bone fractures are in critical condition because of intracranial injury or injury to other parts of the body. As soon as the patient's general status allows, one should proceed with a neuro-otologic workup. Clinical evaluation of the ear with the otologic microscope is indicated, as well as tomographic evaluation of the temporal bones; facial nerve evaluation including topographic diagnosis should also be performed. Immediate facial nerve paralysis following head injury is usually an indication for complete transection of this nerve. Facial nerve paralysis of late onset may be due to secondary edema or to hematoma. Early diagnosis of temporal bone fractures is important. The diagnostic evaluation includes clinical, audiologic, and radiographic workups. Electrodiagnostic tests of the facial nerve are indicated following the injury. Facial nerve paralysis of delayed onset usually has a good prognosis. If electrical tests demonstrate evidence of degeneration, facial nerve exploration should be planned as soon as the general condition of the patient permits. In most instances, the lesion of the facial nerve is situated in the horizontal section in the middle ear or in the descending portion of the vertical part in the mastoid bone. See Chapter 26.

A. Immediate Onset of Facial Nerve Paralysis

After complete otologic, audiologic, and radiographic evaluation and topographic diagnosis of the facial nerve lesion, facial nerve exploration, decompression, and grafting, if indicated, should be planned. This procedure often cannot be performed at an early stage because of the patient's general status. If the patient's condition allows a tympanomastoid procedure, the facial nerve should be explored by means of a tympanomastoidectomy. Decompression includes opening the nerve sheath. If the facial nerve is dissected or crushed, cable grafting may be necessary. The optimal time for intervention is 2 to 3 weeks after the initial injury. Temporal bone fracture and facial nerve injury may occur in the internal auditory canal. If the greater superficial petrosal nerve is involved and if the patient has substantial loss of lacrimination on that side, a middle fossa approach combined with mastoidectomy may be required.

B. Delayed Onset of Facial Nerve Paralysis

This disorder usually has a good prognosis for spontaneous recovery. The function of the facial nerve should be followed on a daily basis. At the earliest sign of degeneration, decompression of the facial nerve should be considered.

VIII. FISTULA OF THE OVAL AND ROUND WINDOWS

Fistula of the oval or round window may result from major head trauma, as well as from minor trauma such as physical strain or barotrauma in divers or aviators. Symptoms include sensorineural hearing loss or fluctuation in hearing, tinnitus, and vertigo. The most common finding with this type of fistula is hearing loss. Approximately 75% of these patients also have tinnitus, and about 50% have vertigo.

Following clinical, audiologic, and radiographic studies, bedrest with head elevation is recommended for 7 to 10 days. Every few days, the patient should be re-evaluated clinically and audiologically. If no improvement is noted in hearing, vertigo, or tinnitus, one should surgically explore the middle ear. Autograft tissue should be used to close a fistula. One may use tragal perichondrium or temporalis muscle fascia. The patient should receive prophylactic broad-spectrum antibiotics for 10 days. Physical activity is restricted for several months, as well as air travel and trips to high altitudes. Diving is also contraindicated. The foregoing treatment regimen successfully controls vertigo, and about 50% of these patients report an improvement in hearing, although high-frequency losses are usually irreversible.

4

HEAD TRAUMA

DONALD A. LEOPOLD AND CHARLES J. HODGE, JR.

The otolaryngologist frequently sees patients with head injuries. Early identification of neurologic trauma with appropriate documentation of signs, selection of diagnostic studies, and treatment minimize the possibility of permanent damage. The otolaryngologist must be particularly alert for the injuries of the brain and skull commonly associated with facial trauma.

I. INITIAL MANAGEMENT

A. Maintenance of Vital Functions

1. **Airway** Maintenance of an adequate airway is of primary importance. Although oral suction and placement of an oral airway are usually sufficient, endotracheal intubation or even emergency tracheotomy may be needed. The status of the patient's cervical spine must be considered. Patients with frontal basilar fractures should not receive positive-pressure respiration with a mask lest contaminated material be forced into the cranium.
2. **Blood pressure** Hypotension, rarely a result of cranial injury, is an indication to search for other areas of post-traumatic hemorrhage such as the chest, abdomen, or pelvis. Increased intracranial pressure is often accompanied by hypertension and bradycardia.
3. **Spinal integrity** All patients with significant head trauma should be treated as though they had a cervical spinal fracture until radiographic evidence confirms the integrity of the cervical spine through C7.

B. Placement of Intravenous Lines

Intravenous lines should be placed, and appropriate blood studies, such as a complete blood count and determinations of electrolytes, alcohol level, type, and crossmatch, should be obtained.

1. **Medications or blood transfusions** may be administered by this route.
2. **Isotonic fluids** are given initially at about 75% of maintenance levels if loss of blood or other fluids is not significant.

C. Prohibition of Oral Feeding

1. **A surgical procedure** may be indicated.
2. **Prevention of aspiration** is essential.
3. **A nasogastric tube** should be placed if patient is vomiting; particular care must be taken in patients with frontal basilar fractures.

D. Catheterization of the Bladder

1. **Renal perfusion** must be assessed.
2. **Possible genitourinary system trauma** should be investigated.
3. **Diuretics** Catheterization is necessary prior to administering diuretics such as mannitol or furosemide to an unconscious patient.
4. **Neurologic damage to the spine** may preclude normal bladder function.
5. **Bladder distension** may cause the patient discomfort and unnecessary agitation.

E. Determination of Level of Consciousness

One must rapidly evaluate the injured patient's level of consciousness; one should write down whether the patient is awake and alert, obeys commands, or responds only to pain.

F. Monitoring of the Patient

One must make sure that the patient is always accompanied by someone who can maintain an airway and can monitor vital signs and level of consciousness.

II. EVALUATION OF THE PATIENT'S CONDITION

A. Injuries Other than Head Trauma

Prior to making detailed neurologic and otolaryngologic evaluations, one must examine other potentially injured areas, such as the thorax, abdomen, spine, and extremities.

B. Neurologic Evaluation

The importance of the initial neurologic examination cannot be overemphasized because it is the standard against which future changes will be measured. One must usually repeat major aspects of the examination several times during the initial evaluation, to determine whether the patient is deteriorating or improving neurologically. The cause of neurologic deterioration must be rapidly identified and treated. Common causes of progressive neurologic worsening in patients with head injuries include intracranial hemorrhage (subdural, epidural, or intracerebral), cerebral swelling, and metabolic factors such as hypoxia, hyponatremia or hypotension.

1. **Level of consciousness** This determination is the most important part of the neurologic examination and should be repeated frequently. When describing the patient's level of consciousness, one should note exactly both the type of stimulus necessary to obtain a response from the patient, such as commands or pain, and the best response obtained, such as coherent speech or agitation. Ambiguous terms such as "semicomatose" should be avoided. Deterioration of the level of consciousness is the first and most sensitive indication of a worsening neurologic status, regardless of whether the cause is a mass lesion or a metabolic disorder. A depressed level of consciousness indicates either bilateral hemisphere dysfunction, which is common in patients with cerebral contusion, or brain-stem dysfunction. Brain-stem dysfunction occurs frequently as a result of transtentorial temporal lobe herniation secondary to a mass lesion such as a subdural or epidural hemorrhage.
2. **Speech** In a conscious patient, the ability to speak coherently and to understand spoken commands should be tested.
   a. ***The inability to speak*** indicates a dominant, usually left-sided, frontal lobe lesion.
   b. ***The inability to understand complex sentences,*** often accompanied by meaningless "word salad" type of speech, indicates damage to the posterior dominant temporal lobe.
3. **Cranial nerves**
   a. ***Olfactory nerve (I)*** This most commonly injured cranial nerve can be easily evaluated using the patient's ability to smell vanilla, soap, tobacco, or any other mild odorant.
   b. ***Optic nerve (II)*** If the patient is awake, visual acuity should be tested. Visual field testing of each eye individually should be done using a confrontation technique. Ophthalmoscopic examination of the optic disc and retina is also indicated. The presence of retinal hemorrhages or of papilledema usually indicates increased intracranial pressure. The absence of these findings does not mean that intracranial pressure is normal, however.
   c. ***Oculomotor, trochlear, and abducens nerves (III, IV, and VI)*** Testing of extraocular movements is a crucial part of the neurologic examination. If the patient is awake, deficiency in eye movements can be tested by using voluntary gaze. In the unconscious patient, eye movements are evaluated by moving the patient's head. If the brain stem and the third, fourth, and sixth cranial nerves are intact, the eyes will remain fixed in direction when the head is moved.

Thus, the movement of the eyes in the head may be assessed. Globe malposition from external forces such as proptosis, enophthalmos, and hematomas may limit eye movement. A third-nerve lesion is indicated by lack of medial, superior and inferior deviation of the affected eye. A sixth-nerve lesion causes lack of lateral deviation of the affected eye. Pupillary response to light must be carefully evaluated; shining a bright light in either eye should cause both pupils to constrict briskly. In lesions of the third nerve, the affected pupil is larger than the unaffected pupil, and neither pupil constricts in response to light shined in the eyes. Complete third-nerve paralysis causes a fully dilated, unresponsive pupil. A third-nerve lesion, which is characterized by a lack of medial eye deviation and a large, unresponsive pupil, associated with a decreasing level of consciousness indicates an expanding mass lesion in the head on the same side as the larger pupil. The reason is that a mass lesion causes herniation of the medial temporal lobe with consequent distortion of the ipsilateral third nerve. Other causes of abnormalities of eye movement and pupils include direct trauma to the globe, orbital fractures, eye drops, or systemic medications such as opiates.

d. ***Trigeminal nerve (V)*** Evaluation of the fifth cranial nerve should include, when possible, testing of the corneal reflex, of masseter function, and of facial sensation. An absent corneal reflex may represent damage to the fifth cranial nerve (first division), to the brain stem, or to the contralateral hemisphere. The most common source of decreased facial sensation after head and facial trauma is damage to peripheral branches of the nerve (infraorbital, mental, or supraorbital) secondary to fractures through the appropriate foramina.

e. ***Facial nerve (VII)*** Facial paralysis or weakness involving the lower part of the face only indicates damage to supranuclear motor pathways and is a common sequela of contralateral cerebral contusions or of compressive mass lesions such as epidural or subdural clots. Paralysis of the upper and lower portions of the face indicates a peripheral facial-nerve lesion, most commonly following petrous bone fracture. Delayed peripheral facial-nerve paralysis may result from basilar skull injuries; the time between injury and paralysis may be minutes, hours, or even days. **The status of this nerve must be documented immediately** because therapy for delayed paralysis is different than that for immediate paralysis. See Chapter 26.

f. ***Vestibulocochlear nerve (VIII)*** The patient's ability to hear a calibrated whisper or a spoken voice is the easiest and quickest way to check this function. Testing with a tuning fork, at 256 or 512 Hz (Weber and Rinne testing), highlights a conductive or a neural loss, either of which can result from head trauma. Recent loss of vestibular function causes nystagmus; if the patient's tympanic membrane is intact, cold caloric testing unilaterally evaluates this function.

g. ***Glossopharyngeal and vagus nerves (IX and X)*** Both are important for cough reflex and adequate swallowing. The vagus nerve controls the movement of the vocal cords and may be evaluated by either direct or indirect laryngoscopy, as during endotracheal intubation. Vocal-cord paralysis after trauma is usually the result of soft tissue injuries of the neck.

h. ***Accessory nerve (XI)*** This nerve, which supplies the sternocleidomastoid and trapezius muscles, is damaged most commonly by penetrating posterior neck injuries.

i. ***Hypoglossal nerve (XII)*** This nerve controls tongue movement and may be damaged by basilar skull fractures or in its peripheral course through the neck. Tongue deviation is common after contralateral cerebral contusions causing damage to supranuclear pathways.

4. **Motor patterns** Adequate neurologic examination should include an evaluation of motor patterns. Contralateral hemiparesis, involving the arm and hand more often than the leg, is common after cerebral contusion or as a result of compressive mass lesions. As motor function is lost during neurologic deterioration from mass lesions or metabolic disorders, motor responses change from purposeful to decorticate posturing, which is characterized by flexion and internal rotation of the upper extremity and extension of the lower extremity and indicates a lack of cortical function, and then to decerebrate posturing, which is characterized by extension of both upper and lower extremities and indicates a loss of basal ganglia and cortex. Severe brain-stem (pons and medulla) dysfunction is characterized by flaccidity of the patient's extremities. Abnormal motor patterns are usually accompanied by increased tone, hyperactive reflexes, and a positive Babinski response.

5. **Respiratory patterns** Bilateral hemisphere dysfunction causes Cheyne-Stokes respiration. Neurologic worsening with upper brain-stem compression is often accompanied by neurogenic hyperventilation, whereas dysfunction of the lower brain stem is manifested by agonal hypoventilation or apnea.

6. **Examination of the head** All scalp lacerations should be explored with a gloved finger, to identify retained foreign bodies or underlying fractures. The presence of bilateral periorbital ecchymoses (panda bear eyes) often indicates a frontal basilar skull fracture and should alert the examiner to the possibility of cerebrospinal fluid (CSF) rhinorrhea or carotid cavernous fistula. Hemotympanum, CSF otorrhea, or Battle's sign usually

indicates basilar skull fracture with its associated risk of meningitis. An orbital bruit is a common sign of carotid cavernous fistula.

III. TYPES OF HEAD INJURIES

A. Concussion

Concussion is characterized by a transient loss of consciousness with subsequent antegrade and retrograde amnesia of variable duration. No focal neurologic findings exist, although patients frequently complain of headaches and an inability to concentrate for several weeks after the injury.

B. Contusion

Cerebral contusion, the most common severe head injury, is usually characterized by alterations in level of consciousness and by focal hemispheric findings; brain-stem (eye movement, pupillary, and corneal) reflexes are normal, however. Severe contusion can result in progressive swelling of the brain with brain-stem compression and eventual death. Treatment is directed at the maintenance of adequate pulmonary function and the control of intracranial pressure. In patients with progressive neurologic dysfunction, surgical decompression may be required.

C. Subdural Hematoma

Acute subdural hematoma is usually associated with underlying brain contusion. It is characterized by progressive neurologic deterioration made manifest by a decreased level of consciousness, by worsening movement patterns, and commonly by ipsilateral third-nerve dysfunction. The treatment is surgical decompression.

D. Epidural Hematoma

This type of injury is most common in children with an associated skull fracture crossing venous or arterial channels. Clinically, the patient usually has a mild concussion followed by a lucid interval of minutes to hours; then one sees rapid neurologic worsening, with depression of the level of consciousness, ipsilateral third-nerve dysfunction, and abnormal motor and respiratory patterns. Treatment is surgical evacuation of the blood clot.

E. Intracerebral Hematoma

This disorder is usually associated with cerebral contusion. These clots, which may not appear until several days after the injury, often cause a marked focal deficit, such as hemiplegia or aphasia and may lead to brain-stem compression with obtundation and third-nerve dysfunction.

F. Skull Fractures

1. **Closed fractures** may be linear, stellate, or diastatic. No specific treatment is indicated.

2. **Open fractures** may be associated with overlying lacerations or communications with sinus, nose, or middle ear. These fractures are usually treated by observation. If a CSF leak is present, high doses of antibiotics should be given. Nose blowing should be avoided. The patient's ear should be examined and should be cleaned under sterile conditions. If a CSF fistula fails to close, or if late-onset meningitis occurs, the skull defect and the dural laceration will require operative repair.

3. **Depressed fractures** may be closed or compound. Closed depressed fractures are generally elevated; all compound depressed fractures must be explored and debrided.

G. Temporal Bone Fracture

The facial nerve is the motor nerve most commonly injured by trauma to the head. Fracture of the temporal bone may impair the function of cranial nerve VII or VIII. This loss of function may be either immediate or delayed. Fractures can be transverse (10%) or longitudinal (90%) or both. Polytomographic studies may be needed to diagnose the exact course of the fracture. Immediate loss of facial function with progressive degeneration usually indicates loss of nerve continuity; one should surgically explore the nerve when the patient's condition is stable and allows general anesthesia. An immediate loss of function without degeneration usually resolves spontaneously. Patients with a delayed loss of facial function and progressive degeneration comprise a small group. In such patients, measurement of submandibular gland flow can help the decision whether to explore the nerve surgically. A decrease of 30 to 40% on the affected side, as compared to the normal side, is an indication for surgical intervention. The majority of patients have a neurologic impairment of delayed onset without degeneration; this condition usually resolves spontaneously. See Chapter 3.

IV. DIAGNOSTIC STUDIES

A. Skull and Cervical Spine Roentgenograms

These studies are indicated in any patient who has been or is unconscious as a result of a head injury, as well as when a depressed fracture or a CSF leak is suspected.

B. Computed Tomographic (CT) Scanning

CT scanning is the diagnostic procedure of choice for any patient with neurologic deficit as a result of head injury. Intracranial clots or contusion can be rapidly and reliably detected. The use of CT scanning obviates the need for most emergency angiographic studies.

C. Lumbar Puncture

This study has no place in the diagnostic evaluation of head injuries, and it may be dangerous in the presence of intracranial mass lesions.

V. DRUG THERAPY

A. Cerebral Edema

1. **Dexamethasone,** 10 mg IV and then 4 mg q6h, is normally given to patients with focal or diffuse neurologic deficit as a result of head injury. The efficacy of this drug in diminishing post-traumatic cerebral edema is controversial.
2. **Mannitol,** 1.0 to 1.5 g/kg, is given in the presence of neurologic deterioration. A much more profound diuresis may be induced if furosemide, 40 mg, or ethacrynic acid, 25 mg, is given at the same time. After the use of mannitol, definitive diagnostic studies or surgical procedures are necessary because diuresis can transiently mask the effects of an intracranial mass.
3. **Hyperventilation** is an effective method to lower intracranial pressure transiently, although the associated decrease in cerebral blood flow may further compromise cerebral function.

B. Prevention of Meningitis

Patients with compound or basilar skull fractures with CSF leakage are usually treated with antibiotics, but the efficacy of this treatment in preventing meningitis is unclear. We recommend cefazolin sodium, 1 g q6h, or oxacillin sodium, 1 g q6h, with tobramycin sulfate, 80 mg IM q8h.

C. Post-traumatic Seizures

Diazepam, 10 to 20 mg IV, and phenytoin sodium, 300 to 500 mg IV (slowly), are used to treat acute seizures. Because the antiepileptic effect of diazepam has a shorter duration than its sedative effect, this drug must frequently be combined with phenytoin sulfate or barbiturates to control seizures.

D. Agitation

The patient with head injuries is frequently agitated or combative, and diagnostic studies are therefore impossible to complete. Diazepam, 10 to 20 mg IV, usually quiets these patients long enough to obtain satisfactory roentgenograms or scans. Respiratory support systems and facilities for endotracheal intubation of the patient must be available if such sedative drugs are to be used. **Agitation may be the result of hypoxia, and this disorder must be ruled out with studies of blood gases before sedation is administered.**

5

NECK TRAUMA

GLENN WEISSMAN

Acute trauma to the neck can be difficult to manage and to evaluate. A systemic and thorough approach must be used to determine the nature of injuries because the decisions and treatment during the initial period affect the patient's outcome. Some principles of management remain controversial. This chapter attempts to offer a succinct method of evaluation and some preliminary steps in management of neck trauma. Of paramount importance is the understanding of the general anatomic features and the different fascial planes that are often traversed in penetrating injuries.

I. ANATOMY

Various fibrous connective tissue layers invest the muscles, vessels, and major organs of the neck and bind the neck into functional units. The potential spaces and planes are both clinically important and remarkably constant. See Chapter 28.

A. Superficial Cervical Fascia

This fatty fibrous layer encloses the platysma muscle. Superiorly, this fascial layer inserts into the muscles of the face, and inferiorly, it extends to the shoulder, clavicle, and axilla.

B. Deep Cervical Fascia

1. **The superficial layer** of the deep fascia surrounds the neck and encloses the parotid and submandibular glands, the trapezius and sternocleidomastoid muscles, and the posterior triangle of the neck and suprasternal space of Burns. This su-

perficial layer of deep fascia also contributes to the carotid sheath.

2. **The middle layer** of the deep fascia, also known as the visceral layer, encloses the larynx, trachea, esophagus, thyroid gland, and strap muscles and contributes to the carotid sheath.
3. **The deep layer** of the deep fascia consists of two divisions, the alar and the prevertebral fascia. It also contributes to the carotid sheath.

C. Miscellaneous Spaces

1. **The carotid sheath** contains the carotid artery, the internal jugular vein, and the vagus nerve.
2. **The pharyngomaxillary space** is a funnel-shaped area with its base at the base of the skull. Its apex is at the greater horn of the hyoid bone. The styloid process divides this space into two compartments, the anterior prestyloid area, which contains connective muscle and lymph nodes, and the retrostyloid compartment, which contains the great vessels and the cranial and sympathetic nerves.
3. **The pretracheal space** is the area anterior to the trachea and extending from the thyroid cartilage and the hyoid bone inferiorly to the superior mediastinum.
4. **The retrovesical space** is the area posterior to the pharynx and extending from the base of the skull to the mediastinum. The superior portion of this space is commonly known as the retropharyngeal space.
5. **The submandibular space** is where the glandular substance and lymph nodes are located. This area is bounded by the superficial layer of fascia and the mylohyoid muscle.

II. TYPES OF INJURIES

A. Penetrating Injuries

It is important to know the type of instrument that caused the injury.

1. **Gunshot wounds** One must differentiate between handgun and shotgun wounds. One of the most important factors in shotgun injuries is the distance between the muzzle of the gun and the victim. At a distance of over 6 to 7 meters, injuries are usually superficial; a distance of less than 3 meters is associated with more severe trauma. Other considerations of shotgun injuries are the length of the barrel, the bore, the choke, and the range of the gun. Bullets, which are usually comprised of small, irregular fragments, do not traverse the neck in a straight plane. Bullets are easily deflected by the bony structures of the neck, such as the cervical spine, and may leave small, metallic foreign bodies along the path of injury. The lead particles deposited in the neck are readily seen radiographically. Radiographs are helpful in ascertaining the path

of the missile; one may thus determine which structures may have been injured.

2. **Knife wounds** differ from gunshot wounds in that the site of penetration and the path of injury are usually in a straight line. The length of the instrument used and the depth of penetration are important.

B. Crushing Injuries

Crushing injuries present a significant problem. Careful inspection, palpation, and general physical examination are important. One should distinguish between open and closed crush injuries. In most cases, open crush injuries require surgical exploration. A systematic approach is used to evaluate the patient's airway, circulation, swallowing function, and central nervous system. Possible associated injuries such as cervical spinal trauma should be kept in mind.

III. GENERAL EMERGENCY MANAGEMENT

A. Maintenance of the Airway

On arrival of the patient in the hospital emergency room, the first priority is the establishment and security of the airway. If the patient's airway is unstable, endotracheal intubation, cricothyrotomy, or tracheostomy may be necessary. If respiratory distress persists once the airway has been established, a pneumothorax or other chest disorder should be suspected. At this point, one should examine the patient for other possible injuries, such as an unrecognized cervical vertebral fracture. Careful inspection and palpation of the neck are important. Significant deviation of the normal neck architecture or any marked discoloration of the skin of the anterior neck denotes severe trauma. Hoarseness, stridor, or dysphagia should also be noted.

B. Control of Hemorrhage

The next important consideration is uncontrolled hemorrhage. Blind clamping of vessels in a hospital emergency room should be discouraged unless absolutely necessary. Hemorrhaging should be controlled by pressure packing until more definitive, operative management is possible. One important note is the inspection and evaluation of the level of bleeding. Typically, the neck is divided into three regions: the base of the skull, the midneck region, and the supraclavicular area. Vascular injuries at each level of the neck require different techniques of management.

C. Restoration of Blood Volume

The third consideration is the restoration of circulating blood volume. Initially, one should place large-bore intravenous lines and possibly a central venous pressure line. It is advisable to place a peripheral intravenous line in the antecubital fossa opposite the site of the neck injury. Circulating blood volume should be maintained with normal saline solution and with plasma expanders such as normal serum albumin (Albumisol) until banked blood becomes available. Blood should be obtained for hematocrit, type and cross-match, and blood-gas analysis. Radiographs of the lateral neck, chest, and cervical spine should be obtained.

IV. RADIOGRAPHIC EVALUATION

Once general emergency measures have been taken and the patient's condition is considered stable, more definitive contrast-radiographic studies can be performed. Lateral radiographs of the neck are important in evaluation of the airway. The physician should also look for deviation of the air column and any unexplained shadows that might represent foreign bodies or hematomas. The cervical spine should be inspected and evaluated for possible subluxation or fractures. Inadvertent manipulation of an unstable or unrecognized spinal cord injury may cause complete quadriplegia. When a cervical fracture or subluxation is present in a patient with respiratory distress, transoral intubation and hyperextension of the neck are contraindicated.

A. Contrast Barium Study

A contrast barium swallow is useful to document violation of the hypopharyngeal or esophageal mucosa. Water-soluble contrast material is preferred if disruption of the hypopharynx and esophagus is suspected because it allows temporary staining of the soft tissues of the neck, as opposed to permanent staining with oil-soluble contrast material. Extravasation of dye usually confirms such a violation, but the lack of extravasation does not rule out the possibility of a tear. If clinical suspicion is high, contrast studies may be bypassed, and endoscopic examination may be performed.

B. Computed Tomographic (CT) Scanning

CT scanning of the neck is useful for the delineation of normal and abnormal anatomic structures. In the emergency setting, this procedure is academic if the patient's condition is unstable.

C. Arteriography

Arteriography, a useful diagnostic aid, is helpful in localizing lacerations and transections of major vessels. When obvious arterial injuries are found during physical examination, direct surgical exploration is the primary form of management. When the site of the vascular injury is obscure and the patient's condition is stable, arteriographic study may be helpful. Arteriographic techniques may also define some of the early and later complications of vascular injuries.

V. MANAGEMENT OF THE AIRWAY

A. Initial Considerations

Patency of the airway is the first consideration in patients with penetrating or blunt trauma to the neck. A succinct medical history should be obtained whenever possible. Physical examination should be performed, with special attention to various clinical signs. One must check the external landmarks of the neck and note any deviation of the normal anatomic structures. Significant signs such as crepitus, dyspnea, stridor, dysphagia, aspiration, and hemoptysis may be indications for surgical exploration. When the hyoid, thyroid, or cricoid cartilage is painful to palpation, a fracture is likely. Flattening or deviation of the thyroid gland represents significant laryngeal or tracheal trauma.

B. Assessment of the Cervical Spine

Most laryngeal injuries occur secondary to automobile accidents. Because of the rapid deceleration on impact in these accidents, the head and neck are thrown forward in an extended position, fixing the laryngeal structures on the cervical vertebrae. It is therefore important to examine the cervical vertebrae in such patients. Once the examination has been completed, the patient's airway must be established, preferably by endotracheal intubation, provided the cervical spine is stable. If the cervical spine is unstable, the patient's head should be immobilized; in many cases, a cricothyrotomy or a tracheostomy must be performed. Direct laryngoscopic examination is indicated at some point during the initial management of these injuries.

C. Conservative Treatment

Most laryngeal injuries require operative intervention. An indirect laryngoscopic examination should be undertaken first, if the patient's condition is stable. The usual measures of conservative management include voice rest, humidification, and bedrest. Antibiotics are of little value during the initial period. The short-term use of steroids is effective, and these drugs are recommended for initial treatment.

D. Surgical Treatment

More aggressive treatment is required when the patient has evidence of airway obstruction, subcutaneous emphysema, or exposed or fractured cartilage. Primary closure of the mucosal tears and repositioning of the displaced fractured cartilage with internal splinting help to prevent or to reduce the risk of laryngeal stenosis.

VI. MANAGEMENT OF VASCULAR INJURIES

A. Hemorrhage

The most devastating complication of these injuries is uncontrolled hemorrhage. On arrival in the hospital emergency room, all patients should undergo placement of large-bore intravenous lines, as well as central venous pressure lines in the antecubital fossa opposite the site of the neck trauma. Blood for hematocrit determinations and for type and crossmatch for multiple units of whole blood should be obtained. Blind clamping of briskly bleeding vessels is contraindicated because vital structures such as the vagus or phrenic nerve may be damaged.

B. Bruits

A bruit or a rapidly expanding pulsatile mass in the neck is usually an absolute indication for surgical exploration. When a change in consciousness is noted or when the patient has associated hemiplegia, aphasia, or diminished vision, reanastomosis of the transected blood vessels may transform an anemic brain infarct into a hemorrhagic brain infarct.

C. Location of Injury

1. **Base of the skull** Vascular injuries at the base of the skull require different treatment from those in the midneck or the base of the neck. On physical examination, it is important to note the source of bleeding. A clear, milky discharge from the wound usually represents a leakage of chyle. Vascular injuries at the base of the skull are difficult to treat, and it is wise to consult a neurosurgeon to assist with such a patient. It may be necessary to obtain proximal and distal control of hemorrhage through the transtympanic route. Venous injuries in this area can be dealt with by ligation at the level of the foramen.
2. **Midneck region** In the midneck region, major arterial lacerations or injuries should undergo primary repair. If this method is not feasible, a variety of vascular-surgical techniques may be employed. Lateral repair, end-to-end repair, or vein grafting have all been successful. The use of a synthetic graft in the contaminated neck wound is contraindicated because of the high risk of infection.
3. **Base of the neck** Wounds at the base of the neck are by far the most challenging of neck injuries. One must be prepared to perform a sternotomy to obtain distal and proximal control of bleeding. One should consult a thoracic surgeon.

D. Late Complications

Some late complications of neck trauma are important, such as embolization, thrombosis, or arteriovenous fistula following repair. Pseudoaneurysm or true aneurysm can also occur 7 to 21 days after a neck injury. Anticoagulation therapy, intravascular embolectomy, and arteriotomy should be considered if these complications arise.

VII. UPPER DIGESTIVE TRACT TRAUMA

A. Diagnosis and Mortality Rates

Recognition of upper digestive tract laceration and trauma is usually not difficult. Early signs are crepitation of the neck, severe dysphagia, drooling, and hemoptysis. A contrast barium swallow is helpful, but not always diagnostic. An endoscopic examination should be performed when suspicion of such an injury is strong. The mortality rate in patients with untreated perforations in the upper esophagus or hypopharynx formerly was 70%. With the advent of antibiotics, the mortality rate dropped to 40 to 50%. Today, with the use of broad-spectrum antibiotics and surgical drainage, the mortality rate has dropped to 10 to 20%.

B. Management

Mucosal injuries of the nasopharynx and oropharynx do not usually require aggressive treatment. Penetration of these anatomic regions is not associated with extravasation of saliva or deep infections. In contrast, mucosal injuries to the hypopharynx and the upper esophagus require immediate surgical exploration, repair, and drainage. Treatment consists of a complete physical examination and a contrast esophagram if the patient's condition is stable, followed by a full endoscopic examination. A perforation or a tear found during the endoscopic study should be repaired. The necrotic edges of the tear should be cleaned and drained externally. Lacerations or perforations more than 24 hours old should be drained. In either case, broad-spectrum antibiotics are indicated.

VIII. MANAGEMENT OF NERVOUS SYSTEM INJURIES

Any neurologic structure that traverses the neck may be injured by blunt or sharp trauma. Extreme care should be taken in transporting these patients. Routine roentgenograms should be taken if one suspects a cervical spinal injury. Inspection of the entire nervous system is important, including all the cranial nerves, the long tracts, and the sympathetic and parasympathetic systems. Lesions of the central nervous system can usually be distinguished from those of the peripheral nervous system by changes in the patient's level of consciousness, by aphasia, or by visual disorders. Frequently missed are brachial plexus injuries. One should seek neurologic consultation during the initial evaluation of such a patient. See Chapter 4.

IX. INDICATIONS FOR SURGICAL EXPLORATION

This subject is controversial. Some institutions practice routine surgical exploration of all neck wounds, whereas other institutions follow strict criteria for such exploration. The mortality rates in patients who undergo selective neck exploration do not differ from those in patients who undergo routine neck exploration. In an excellent review by May, criteria have been set forth for selective surgical exploration (Laryn-

TABLE 5–1

Indications for Neck Exploration
1. Airway compression
2. Uncontrolled hemorrhage from neck
3. Previous hemorrhage from neck with hypotension
4. Acute oral bleeding without visible oral injury
5. Expanding hematoma
6. Bruit
7. Vertebral artery or subclavian artery injury confirmed by arteriography
8. Progressive central nervous system deficit due to impaired cerebral circulation or thrombosis of major vessels
9. Chyle leak
10. Widening of mediastinum
11. Progressive neck infection or development of an abscess
12. Mediastinitis

goscope, *85*:55, 1975). Of significant importance is the initial examination. The physician must be thorough in making an initial assessment. Table 5–1 gives indications for selective surgical exploration of neck wounds.

II.

EAR

6

EAR PAIN

WERNER D. CHASIN

The cause of pain in the ear can be determined in the majority of patients. Not all ear pain is caused by otitis media or external otitis, and routine treatment should not include the use of antibiotics and ear drops. Rational treatment of otalgia depends on an accurate diagnosis of the cause of the pain. The otalgia produced by disorders of structures within the temporal bone is termed intrinsic otalgia. Pain that is perceived in and around the ear but due to disorders of structures outside the temporal bone is termed extrinsic neuralgia. This latter term includes referred otalgia.

I. INTRINSIC OTALGIA

The disorders that produce intrinsic otalgia are summarized in Tables 6–1 through 6–4.

A. Intrinsic Inflammatory and Infectious Conditions of the External Ear (Table 6–1)

1. **Acute external otitis—diffuse** This condition usually represents a bacterial infection due to one or a variety of microorganisms. Treatment begins with a thorough cleaning of the ear canal of all exudate and epithelial debris. If the ear canal is patent, treatment consists of the instillation of ear drops containing a combination of neomycin, polymyxin B, and hydrocortisone. In patients with a history of contact allergy to neomycin, one should administer a solution that does not contain neomycin. If the ear canal is so swollen that ear drops cannot enter, a wick impregnated with Ergophene or Ichthammol ointment should be inserted by the physician. The

patient should remove this wick 24 hours later and should then begin to instill the ear drops. In diabetics or in other immunosuppressed individuals, a culture of the ear canal should be obtained, and both topical ear drops and a parenteral antibiotic should be prescribed accordingly.

2. **Acute external otitis—circumscribed** A furuncle of the external auditory canal can be strikingly painful. In most instances, this inflammatory condition responds to the insertion of a cotton or gauze wick impregnated with Ergophene ointment. During the 24 hours that the wick is left in the ear canal, the patient is instructed to apply hot soaks to the ear as often as is practical. When this treatment fails, incision and drainage of the furuncle are usually effective. One should not confuse an exostosis of the inner half of the external auditory canal with a furuncle. Furuncles are located in the outer or cartilaginous portion of the ear canal.
3. **Chronic external otitis in exacerbation** This disorder is treated in the same manner as diffuse or circumscribed acute external otitis. If the condition is recurrent in the same ear, the physician should make a special effort to search for an occult tympanic membrane perforation. A recurrent unilateral external otitis may be due to irritation of the skin of the external auditory canal by exudate issuing from the middle ear through a perforation.
4. **Malignant external otitis** This condition is not neoplastic. It is a particularly severe bacterial infectious disorder of the auricle and external canal in diabetics and in other immunosuppressed individuals. The offending micro-organism is usually Pseudomonas aeruginosa. These patients require intensive hospital care with intravenous antibiotics directed against the Pseudomonas organism. If unchecked, this infection can lead to extensive necrosis of skin, cartilage, and bone and may be lethal.
5. **External otitis—fungal** Symptoms are similar to those of bac-

TABLE 6–1

Intrinsic Otalgia—Infectious and Inflammatory Conditions of External Ear
1. Acute external otitis—diffuse
2. Acute external otitis—circumscribed
3. Chronic external otitis—acute exacerbation
4. Malignant external otitis
5. External otitis—fungal
6. External otitis—parasitic
7. Perichondritis of auricle
8. Ramsay Hunt syndrome
9. Relapsing polychondritis
10. Infected ear lobe

terial external otitis. The fungus appears clinically as a black, blue-green, or white-yellow "fuzz" in the ear canal. Treatment consists of a thorough cleaning of the ear. Ideally, the outer epithelial layer of the ear canal skin should be removed with the debris. Treatment continues with the twice-daily instillation of ear drops containing acetic acid or aluminum subacetate. The patient should be re-examined within 4 days of the initial examination, for possible further cleaning of the ear canal.

6. **External otitis—parasitic** Maggots and helminths can cause a painful external otitis with severe swelling of the skin and spontaneous bleeding of the ear. Patients with this type of infection usually feel something moving around in the ear. Topical antibiotic drops are ineffective until the parasites are killed or removed from the external auditory canal.

7. **Perichondritis of the auricle** This disorder may result from a spreading infection of the skin or the ear canal, infected bites, infected hematoma, and lacerations, and it may also be a complication of mastoid and tympanoplastic surgical procedures. The skin and subcutaneous tissues of the auricle are red, swollen, and tender, and the normal ridges of the auricle are camouflaged. Treatment must be aggressive, to prevent a permanent deformity of the auricle. The condition requires treatment with oral or parenteral antibiotics, according to culture obtained from the external auditory canal. Subperichondrial accumulations of fluid must be aspirated, and a pressure dressing may be required to prevent reaccumulation of fluid. On occasion, continuous suction is required for this purpose.

8. **Ramsay Hunt syndrome** This painful, vesicular eruption in the ear canal and on the auricle is caused by the Herpes zoster virus. Patients afflicted with this infection may also suffer a sudden cochlear and vestibular catastrophe if the virus affects these structures. The skin eruption does not require special treatment, but the physician should remain in communication with the patient in the event that cochlear or vestibular complications occur.

9. **Relapsing polychondritis** This condition, probably an autoimmune disorder, is characterized by recurrent, painful, red swelling of the auricle. Although auricular involvement may occur alone, more often other cartilaginous structures, such as the nose, larynx, and ribs, are also involved. The patient may have evidence of rheumatoid arthritis or systemic lupus erythematosus. Treatment is with corticosteroids.

10. **Infected ear lobe** This condition is almost invariably associated with an infection following an ear-piercing procedure for earrings. The infection may occur either shortly after the procedure or in well-established stud holes. It may represent a bacterial infection or a contact reaction to the metal in the earring. Treatment consists first in omitting the wearing of the

earring. Application of warm compresses and frequent cleaning of the ear lobe with isopropyl alcohol usually clear the infection. When the infection is severe and associated with surrounding cellulitis, an antibiotic chosen according to culture results may be required.

B. Intrinsic Otalgia due to Noninflammatory Disorders of the External Ear (Table 6–2)

1. **Carcinoma** Basal cell carcinomas usually are limited to the auricle. Squamous cell carcinomas may involve either the auricle alone or the external auditory canal and even the middle ear and the mastoid process. Although these tumors are painless at first, they may become continuously painful once they invade the perichondrium or the periosteum. The physician should consider the possibility of squamous cell carcinoma of the external auditory canal in an individual with stubborn, unilateral external otitis, especially with localized or diffuse skin swelling. The diagnosis is made by biopsy. Treatment consists of either surgical excision, radiation therapy, or both. Small lesions of the auricle are managed by excisional biopsy, without the need for a prior biopsy.
2. **Other tumors** In children, a painful polyp or tumor in the ear canal may be a rhabdomyosarcoma. Other tumors that may produce ear pain include meningioma, chemodectoma, and choristoma. These tumors may be diagnosed by appropriate x-ray study and biopsy. The physician should bear in mind that chemodectoma is a vascular tumor, and biopsy may be followed by hemorrhage. Biopsies, therefore, should be performed only under appropriate conditions. The treatment of these tumors depends on the cell type. Rhabdomyosarcomas are treated primarily with radiation therapy and chemotherapy; meningiomas and choristomas, by surgical excision. Chemodectomas are often treated by preliminary arterial embolization, to reduce their vascularity prior to surgical excision.
3. **Histiocytosis X** Both the Letterer-Siwe variant and the eosinophilic granuloma may manifest themselves as painful tumors in the ear canal or the middle ear. Diagnosis is made by x-ray study and biopsy, and treatment consists of radiation therapy

TABLE 6–2

Intrinsic Otalgia—Noninflammatory Disorders of External Ear
1. Carcinoma
2. Other tumors
3. Histiocytosis X
4. Traumatic and post-traumatic pain
5. Frostbite of the auricle
6. Keloid of the ear lobe

and, sometimes, immunosupportive therapy with calf-thymus extract.

4. **Traumatic and post-traumatic pain** Patients with fractures of the temporal bone may experience pain in the ear for many weeks or months thereafter. This pain may become worse with atmospheric and climatic changes. No special treatment exists for this type of pain except mild analgesics and reassurance. Sometimes, detailed radiographs of the ear, such as tomograms or computed tomographic (CT) scans, disclose a previously undiagnosed fracture in patients with post-traumatic ear pain.

5. **Frostbite of the auricle** The treatment of frostbite of the auricle consists of rapid rewarming of the ear by means of wet saline compresses at 38 to 42° C. Because the rewarming process produces pain, the patient may require an analgesic medication. Any skin injury including insertion of needles and incision should be avoided, lest a secondary infection be produced. Any tissue that becomes devitalized once the effects of the injury have subsided will require surgical excision and reconstruction.

6. **Keloid of the ear lobe** almost always represents a complication of piercing for earrings. Although not limited to black people, keloids occur most often in that group. A keloid is a firm, painful, and often tender swelling, usually on the posterior aspect of the ear lobe. The condition may be treated either by intralesional injection of triamcinolone or by excision followed by steroid injection to prevent a recurrence. Patients with this condition should be advised to avoid further ear piercing.

C. Intrinsic Otalgia due to Infectious and Inflammatory Disorders of the Middle Ear and Mastoid (Table 6–3)

The treatment of the disorders listed but not discussed in this section is detailed in Chapter 9 of this book.

1. **Acute otitis media** See Chapter 9.

2. **Eustachian tube obstruction—negative middle ear**

TABLE 6–3

Intrinsic Otalgia—Infectious and Inflammatory Disorders of Middle Ear and Mastoid

1. Acute otitis media
2. Eustachian tube obstruction—negative middle ear pressure
3. Eustachian tube obstruction—middle ear effusion
4. Chronic otitis media—acute exacerbation
5. Acute otitis media—dural irritation
6. Chronic otitis media—dural irritation
7. Acute mastoiditis
8. Gradenigo's syndrome
9. Wegener's granulomatosis

pressure In both children and adults, middle ear pain may be produced by the following sequence of events. An inflammatory obstruction of the eustachian tube results in inadequate ventilation of the middle ear, and the gases in the middle ear are absorbed by the mucous membranes. This process causes a partial vacuum, which may produce pain. The condition is best diagnosed by impedance audiometry. Such ears may look perfectly normal to otoscopic examination. Treatment consists of attempts to inflate the middle ear either by Valsalva maneuver, politzerization, or eustachian tube catheterization followed by inflation. The condition is self-limiting. It is not clear whether nose drops and sprays or oral decongestants are helpful in patients with eustachian tube obstruction.

3. **Eustachian tube obstruction—middle ear effusion** This condition results from a protracted obstruction of the eustachian tube. In both children and adults, the condition is sometimes associated with intermittent ear pain in addition to blockage, autophony, and hearing loss. If the effusion fails to clear spontaneously within 1 to 2 weeks, it may be relieved by myringotomy, either alone or with the insertion of a ventilating tube. The physician must carefully evaluate the nasopharynx for the possible presence of a tumor that may obstruct the eustachian tube. In such instances, the pain may be due directly to the tumor, which causes referred otalgia, rather than to the presence of the fluid in the middle ear.

4. **Chronic otitis media—acute exacerbation** See Chapter 9.

5. **Acute otitis media—dural irritation** See Chapter 9.

6. **Chronic otitis media—dural irritation** See Chapter 9.

7. **Acute mastoiditis** See Chapter 9.

8. **Gradenigo's syndrome** See Chapter 9.

9. **Wegener's granulomatosis** This autoimmune disorder commonly involves the middle ear and mastoid process, either as an initial manifestation or subsequent to prior involvement of other portions of the respiratory tract. Ear involvement is characterized by intense and persistent pain that does not respond to treatment that is usually effective in cases of ordinary acute or subacute otitis media. Nothing is characteristic about the otoscopic appearance of the ear. The physician diagnoses the condition only by suspecting it and by performing a biopsy of either the middle ear or mastoid mucosa or some other affected portion of the upper respiratory tract. Treatment consists of administration not only of appropriate antibiotics for the secondary infection, but also of cyclophosphamide and prednisone. The prognosis for this disorder has improved since the introduction of this therapeutic regimen.

D. Intrinsic Otalgia due to Noninflammatory Disorders of the Middle Ear and Mastoid (Table 6–4)

Ear pain in these conditions results from irritation of the nerve endings in the periosteum or mucoperiosteum.

1. **Primary carcinoma** Although not a common tumor in the ear, a primary epidermoid carcinoma may arise in the middle ear and mastoid mucosa, sometimes after pre-existing chronic otitis media. Superficially, the condition mimics chronic otitis media with otorrhea, otorrhagia, hearing loss, increased pressure, and deep-seated pain. On otoscopic examination, a tumor mass resembling an aural polyp is usually seen. The presence of periauricular and cervical lymphadenopathy should make the physician especially suspicious of the presence of a tumor. Such patients require a careful evaluation with radiographs and biopsy, as well as prompt and aggressive management with a combination of surgical techniques and radiation therapy.
2. **Metastatic carcinoma and sarcoma** Neoplasms from other parts of the body, especially breast, prostate, and parotid gland, may metastasize to the temporal bone and may cause otalgia. The metastatic tumor may not be visible otoscopically and may be detectable only on appropriate radiographs of the temporal bone. Treatment depends on the type and involvement of the metastasizing tumor.
3. **Other tumors** that arise within the temporal bone or spread from adjacent sites include chemodectoma, meningioma, rhabdomyosarcoma, and choristoma. Any of these tumors may produce ear pain from irritation of nerve endings in the periosteum or mucoperiosteum of the temporal bone. They may not be detectable otoscopically and may require radiographs for their detection. At the present time, computed tomographic (CT) scanning of the temporal bone is probably the best method for detecting such lesions. Treatment depends on the type, extent, and location of the tumor.
4. **Histiocytosis X** This bone-destroying lesion, which may occur in children as well as in adults, is characterized by per-

TABLE 6–4

Intrinsic Otalgia—Noninflammatory Disorders of Middle Ear and Mastoid
1. Primary carcinoma
2. Metastatic carcinoma and sarcoma
3. Other tumors (chemodectoma, meningioma, rhabdomyosarcoma, choristoma)
4. Histiocytoma X
5. Bell's palsy
6. Acoustic neuroma
7. Aural neuralgia

sistent otalgia. Although it is most often diagnosed by the detection of a polypoid mass in the ear canal, radiographs may be required if the lesion remains hidden within the osseous parts of the temporal bone. The disorder is diagnosed by biopsy, and after staging is treated with localized radiation therapy.

5. **Bell's palsy** Also known as idiopathic facial paralysis, this disorder is frequently associated with pain and tenderness in and around the tip of the mastoid process. Occasionally, the pain precedes the paralysis by a day or two; in such cases the cause of the ear pain is virtually impossible to diagnose. The otalgia of Bell's palsy is self-limiting and usually requires only analgesics. If pain is particularly severe, a short course of an oral corticosteroid may reduce its intensity.

6. **Acoustic neuroma** In some patients with an acoustic neuroma, deep-seated ear pain is a significant symptom. The cause of this pain may be irritation of the nervus intermedius within the internal auditory canal. Although pain is not the most characteristic symptom of acoustic neuroma, the author has seen patients with otalgia as the first symptom of this lesion. Therefore, any patient with ear pain of an obscure nature should undergo appropriate testing for an acoustic neuroma, including audiometry, vestibular examination, and radiography.

7. **Aural neuralgia** This rare disorder produces pain in the middle ear and is presumed to be due to a neuralgia of the fibers of the tympanic plexus. The otoscopic examination is negative. The condition can be diagnosed only: (1) by first ruling out the many more likely causes of intrinsic and extrinsic otalgia; and (2) by being able to abolish the pain by instilling lidocaine (Xylocaine) into the middle ear through a small-gauge needle pierced through the drumhead without preliminary injection of the skin of the ear canal wall. If the condition is diagnosed with confidence, the pain may be permanently abolished by performing tympanic neurectomy by means of a formal tympanotomy.

II. EXTRINSIC OTALGIA

In patients with obscure otalgia and in whom no evidence indicates that the pain is due to intrinsic disease of the temporal bone, the physician must explore the possibility of pain referred to the ear. The nerves that innervate the ear include the trigeminal, facial, glossopharyngeal, and vagus nerves, as well as the upper roots of the cervical nerves. The territory of each of these nerves must be examined in a logical sequence.

A. Referred Otalgia Mediated by the Trigeminal Nerve (Table 6–5)

The trigeminal nerve mediates the most common and frequent causes of referred otalgia.

1. **Dental disorders** Pain may be referred to the ear from dental caries, pulp infection, gingival disorders, and periapical infections of the posterior teeth, from unerupted wisdom teeth, and from a subperiosteal infection of the upper or lower jaw. When the teeth or gums are suspected of being the probable cause of otalgia, the patient should be referred to a dentist.
2. **Temporomandibular joint disorders** Disorders of the muscles and ligaments of the temporomandibular joint and, to a lesser extent, intrinsic disorders of the joint are a common cause of referred otalgia. The condition often results from bruxism, dental malocclusion, excessive chewing of gum, or contraction of the jaw muscles due to psychic tension. Intrinsic joint disorders are due to systemic arthritis affecting the temporomandibular joint, extrinsic trauma, congenital anomalies, and degenerative changes in the articular cartilage and ligaments. When a temporomandibular joint disorder is diagnosed as the probable source of otalgia, the patient should be referred to a physician, dentist, or temporomandibular joint clinic; such persons have the experience and interest in working with these patients and their problems. Such disorders, which are often difficult to treat and protracted, require much time and extensive physical and psychosocial management.
3. **Paranasal sinus irritation** Inflammatory and neoplastic irritation of branches of the trigeminal nerve in the paranasal sinuses, especially the maxillary sinuses, may produce referred otalgia. In the absence of obvious clinical findings of sinus disease, patients with obscure otalgia require radiographs of the sinuses. Treatment depends on the nature of the sinus disorder. See Chapter 15.

TABLE 6–5

Extrinsic Otalgia—Trigeminal Nerve
1. Dental disorders
2. Temporomandibular joint disorders
3. Paranasal sinus irritation
4. Oral cavity lesions
5. Salivary gland disorders
6. Disorders of the jaws (tumors, cysts, histiocytosis X)
7. Nasopharyngeal tumors
8. Temporal arteritis
9. Irritation of dura mater
10. Tumors in infratemporal fossa
11. Schwannoma of trigeminal nerve

4. **Oral cavity lesions** Inflammatory and especially neoplastic lesions of any portion of the oral cavity are commonly associated with otalgia mediated by either the maxillary or mandibular divisions of the fifth cranial nerve. Usually, the patient has more obvious symptoms of these lesions. Some patients are unaware of the presence of such a lesion and complain mainly of the referred otalgia. The diagnosis is made by a thorough examination of the oral cavity, using inspection and palpation. Special attention must be focused on the retromolar trigone, the posterior portion of the floor of the mouth, the tongue, and the mucosal surfaces covering the most posterior portions of the mandible. Treatment consists of management of the oral cavity lesion. See Chapter 16.

5. **Salivary gland disorders** Inflammatory, obstructive, and neoplastic disorders of the submandibular, sublingual, and especially the parotid salivary glands may produce otalgia. In cases of obscure otalgia, one should pay special attention to the sublingual gland and the deep lobe of the parotid gland, both of which may harbor malignant tumors that are not outwardly apparent. CT scanning, coupled with sialography, has provided an unprecedented rate of detection of occult neoplasms of these glands. Treatment depends on the nature of the disorder. See Chapter 20.

6. **Disorders of the jaws** Benign and malignant tumors of the jaws, expanding cysts, and histiocytosis X of the jaws may produce otalgia referred by either the maxillary or the mandibular nerves. Diagnosis is made by radiographs and biopsy, and treatment depends on the nature of the growth.

7. **Nasopharyngeal tumors** The anterior portion of the nasopharynx derives its sensory innervation from the maxillary nerve. Carcinoma of the nasopharynx may produce referred otalgia with few, if any, symptoms and signs to call attention to a disorder in this part of the throat. Therefore, whenever the physician is faced with a patient with obscure otalgia, a careful examination of the nasopharynx must be made. Occasionally, persistent, unilateral otalgia in the absence of any other findings may justify the biopsy of an otherwise normal-appearing nasopharynx. Biopsy is mandatory if the patient also demonstrates a persistent middle ear effusion. A malignant tumor is treated with irradiation.

8. **Temporal arteritis** In older individuals, the temporal arteries may become painful as they are involved by a granulomatous inflammation. The pain is located just anterior to the ear and in the temple. The diagnosis is made by finding a tender, firm temporal artery and an elevated erythrocyte sedimentation rate; it is confirmed by a biopsy of the affected vessel. The disorder usually responds favorably to treatment with oral corticosteroids.

9. **Irritation of the dura mater** The dura mater of the brain is innervated by the trigeminal nerve. Irritation by infection or tumor of the dura mater of the middle or posterior cranial fossa, including the dura that encloses the lateral and sigmoid venous sinuses, may produce ear pain. In most instances, other symptoms and signs predominate over otalgia and lead the physician to an accurate diagnosis. Ear pain, however, is sometimes the dominant symptom, especially when a tympanomastoiditis has been partly suppressed by antibiotic therapy, and the patient is developing either a perisinal abscess of the sigmoid sinus or a localized pachymeningitis in the dura mater over the tegmen of the middle ear or mastoid. The diagnosis is made by a careful medical history, otologic examination, neurologic examination, and CT scanning. Treatment depends on the cause of the dural irritation.

10. **Tumors in the infratemporal fossa** The main neural occupants of this space, which is located beneath the base of the middle cranial fossa and medial to the zygomatic arch, are the mandibular and lingual nerves. The fossa is located in such a position that adjacent tumors from the nasopharynx, deep lobe of the parotid gland, parapharyngeal space, orbit, pterygomaxillary fossa, and retromolar trigone can invade it. Patients with such tumor extension have deep pain in the side of the face and ear and may have trismus if the pterygoid muscles are involved. The diagnosis is suspected on finding hypesthesia in the territory of the lingual nerve (floor of mouth and side of the tongue) and mandibular nerve (skin overlying the mandible) and weakness or wasting of the masseter muscle. The diagnosis is confirmed by CT scanning of the infratemporal fossa. Management depends on finding the site and nature of the primary neoplasm and ordinarily includes radiation therapy.

11. **Schwannoma of the trigeminal nerve** A benign or malignant schwannoma may arise from the sheath of the intra- or extracranial portions of the trigeminal nerve. Although the dominant findings are facial pain and hypesthesia, with muscle wasting if the mandibular nerve is involved, these patients may also experience referred otalgia. Treatment consists of surgical excision and, if the tumor is malignant, radiation therapy.

B. Referred Otalgia Mediated by the Facial Nerve (Table 6–6)

The facial nerve, primarily a motor nerve, is closely associated with the nervus intermedius or nerve of Wrisberg, also referred to as the sensory root of the facial nerve. This sensory root is thought to include somatic sensory fibers that innervate the cavum and eminence of the concha, as well as the skin of the posterior bony canal wall and posterior portion of the drumhead.

1. **Acoustic neuroma** Ear pain from acoustic neuroma has al-

TABLE 6–6

Extrinsic Otalgia—Facial Nerve
1. Acoustic neuroma
2. Bell's palsy
3. Ramsay Hunt syndrome
4. Aberrant vascular loop syndrome

ready been discussed in the section of this chapter on noninflammatory intrinsic disorders of the ear.

2. **Bell's palsy** has previously been discussed in the section of this chapter describing intrinsic noninflammatory pain.
3. **Ramsay Hunt syndrome** This disorder, also known as herpes zoster oticus, has been discussed in the section of this chapter on intrinsic inflammatory disorders of the external ear.
4. **Aberrant vascular loop syndrome,** which involves the pressure of an aberrant vascular loop on the intracranial neurovascular bundle destined to enter the internal auditory meatus, has not yet been clearly described. On the basis of a few cases in which such a loop has been found, the author feels obliged to add this entity to the list of disorders that might cause referred otalgia by the nervus intermedius. Currently, this diagnosis should be considered only when the patient exhibits an atypical audiovestibular syndrome in addition to the symptom of deep pain in the ear. A clear method of diagnosis of this disorder is not yet available. The treatment, which is justified only when a more pressing indication exists for an exploratory suboccipital craniotomy, consists of separating the vascular loop from the nerve bundle. A tumor found in the cerebellopontine angle must, of course, be treated.

C. Referred Otalgia Mediated by the Glossopharyngeal Nerve (Table 6–7)

1. **Tonsillitis** Infections of the tonsil and tonsillectomy commonly produce otalgia. The ear pain disappears after adequate

TABLE 6–7

Extrinsic Otalgia—Glossopharyngeal Nerve
1. Tonsillitis
2. Peritonsillar abscess
3. Malignant tonsillar neoplasm
4. Stylalgia (Eagle's syndrome)
5. Lingual tonsillitis or abscess
6. Foreign body in tonsil or base of tongue
7. Carcinoma of base of tongue
8. Carcinoma of nasopharynx
9. Glossopharyngeal neuralgia

treatment of the tonsillitis, and post-tonsillectomy pain usually subsides within 9 days of the operation.

2. **Peritonsillar abscess** Ipsilateral otalgia is experienced by virtually every patient with this infection. The pain disappears after the successful treatment of the pharyngeal infection.

3. **Malignant tonsillar neoplasm** When a patient has persistent otalgia of obscure origin, the physician must scrutinize and palpate the tonsil thoroughly. Sometimes, a neoplasm is located beneath the mucosal surface or even in the lateral aspect of a tonsil. If such a tumor is suspected, only a complete tonsillectomy and examination of the specimen by a pathologist will disclose the diagnosis. The subsequent treatment may consist of either radiation therapy, further surgical excision, or a combination of the two, depending on the type and stage of the tumor.

4. **Stylalgia** This disorder, also called Eagle's syndrome, occurs in patients who have had a previous tonsillectomy and who now have pain in the lateral oropharyngeal wall with radiation to the ipsilateral ear. The treatment is transpharyngeal amputation of the styloid process.

5. **Lingual tonsillitis or abscess** may occur in isolation or as part of an infection of all components of Waldeyer's ring. The condition, which produces throat pain and otalgia, can be diagnosed only by performing a mirror examination of the base of the tongue. Treatment consists of antibiotics chosen according to the results of culture.

6. **Foreign body in the tonsil or base of the tongue** A foreign body such as a fishbone or pencil point may become lodged in the depths of the lymphoid tissue of the faucial or lingual tonsil and may produce pharyngeal and ear pain. The diagnosis is made by obtaining a careful medical history, by a thorough mirror examination, and, if necessary, by x-ray study. Extraction of the foreign body relieves the symptoms.

7. **Carcinoma of the base of the tongue** Patients with carcinoma of the base of the tongue may have ear pain as the dominant symptom. When a patient has ear pain of obscure origin, one must make a most thorough evaluation, both visually and by palpation, of the base of the tongue. If the lesion cannot be detected, but if the physician remains suspicious, a CT scan with intravenous contrast enhancement may disclose the neoplasm. The diagnosis is confirmed by multiple and deep biopsies performed with the patient under general anesthesia. Treatment involves radiation therapy; surgical excision is employed only in the less-common, smaller tumors in this area.

8. **Carcinoma of the nasopharynx** This condition has already been discussed under otalgia mediated by the trigeminal nerve.

It is listed again here because the more posterior areas of the nasopharynx are innervated by the ninth nerve.

9. **Glossopharyngeal neuralgia** is a tic-like pain in the sensory distribution of the ninth nerve. Patients with this disorder experience brief but recurrent episodes of excruciating pain in the lateral oropharyngeal wall with radiation to the ipsilateral ear. The neurologic, pharyngeal, and otologic examinations disclose no abnormalities. The mounting evidence now suggests that, as in trigeminal tic, this condition may be caused by an aberrant vascular loop that irritates the intracranial segment of the glossopharyngeal nerve. If the pain is not relieved by carbamazepine (Tegretol), these patients may require suboccipital craniotomy to explore the glossopharyngeal nerve root. Surgical treatment consists of separation of the vascular loop from the nerve or, if such a vessel is not found, intracranial section of the glossopharyngeal nerve root.

D. Referred Otalgia Mediated by the Vagus Nerve (Table 6–8)

The territory of the sensory innervation by the vagus nerve is large, and in determining the cause of referred otalgia, the physician has to evaluate the structures innervated by this nerve.

1. **Pharyngeal infection** Retropharyngeal abscess, epiglottitis, and epiglottic abscess all produce referred otalgia. The diagnosis is usually made by the patient's medical history, by the clinical manifestations, and by radiographs. The otalgia disappears when the infection is treated appropriately.

2. **Hypopharyngeal and laryngeal carcinoma** Carcinoma of the laryngopharynx most commonly occurs in individuals with a long-term history of excessive alcohol consumption and smoking. These persons are accustomed to chronic irritation of the throat. Sometimes, the symptom that occasions their visit to a physician is the new onset of otalgia, and they may

TABLE 6–8

Extrinsic Otalgia—Vagus Nerve

1. Pharyngeal infection
2. Hypopharyngeal and laryngeal carcinoma
3. Laryngeal inflammatory disorders
    a. Contact granulomas
    b. Tuberculosis
    c. Cricoarytenoid arthritis
    d. Laryngopyocele
    e. Laryngitis due to gastroesophageal reflux
4. Esophageal foreign body
5. Carcinoma of esophagus
6. Angina pectoris
7. Tumor in jugular fossa

minimize any throat discomfort that is present. The diagnosis is usually apparent by a careful mirror examination of the laryngopharynx and the pyriform sinus. Management consists of a preliminary biopsy of the lesion followed by surgical excision, radiation therapy, or both, depending on the stage of the tumor. If treatment is successful in controlling the tumor, then the ear pain will subside. Recurring otalgia may be the first indication of a tumor recurrence.

3. **Laryngeal inflammatory disorders**
   a. ***Contact granulomas*** occur in the mucosa of the vocal cords covering the vocal processes of the arytenoid cartilages. They are the result of laryngeal misuse or psychic tension and can be easily overlooked unless the physician focuses on this area of the larynx. These lesions produce dysphonia and referred otalgia. Treatment, which may be difficult, consists of voice rest and possibly voice therapy. The otalgia disappears as these ulcerations heal.
   b. ***Tuberculosis*** Laryngeal tuberculosis occurs secondary to pulmonary infection and characteristically involves the posterior portion of the larynx. The patient has hoarseness, laryngeal pain, and possibly otalgia. The otalgia disappears following appropriate antimicrobial treatment of the infection.
   c. ***Cricoarytenoid arthritis*** Patients with arthritis of the cricoarytenoid and cricothyroid joints have significant otalgia, in addition to dysphonia, laryngeal pain, and odynophagia. The condition is diagnosed from a history of systemic, usually rheumatoid, arthritis and recurrent episodes of laryngeal arthritis. During an acute attack, the mucosa of the arytenoid eminence is red and swollen. The treatment of the acute episode includes voice rest, a soft diet, and antiarthritis medication.
   d. ***Laryngopyocele*** causes painful laryngitis with referred otalgia; it involves an infection of a pre-existing laryngocele. Treatment consists of antibiotics for the infection and subsequent surgical excision of the laryngocele.
   e. ***Laryngitis due to gastroesophageal reflux*** Patients may develop posterior laryngitis due to the reflux of acid gastric juice into the laryngopharynx. In addition to throat discomfort, these patients may experience otalgia. Treatment is directed toward the reflux problem.

4. **Esophageal foreign body** Patients with a foreign body in the cervical esophagus may have otalgia in addition to symptoms of esophageal obstruction. Small, sharp objects such as pins and fish bones may not obstruct the esophagus, but may cause pain. Treatment consists of extraction of the foreign object.

5. **Carcinoma of the esophagus** Otalgia is a prominent symptom in patients with carcinoma of the pyriform sinus and of

the cervical esophagus. Treatment is directed at the esophageal neoplasm.

6. **Angina pectoris** In some individuals with coronary insufficiency, the pain of angina pectoris may radiate to the sides of the neck and toward the ear or ears. Treatment is directed toward the cardiac condition.

7. **Tumor in the jugular fossa** Primary and metastatic tumors in the jugular foramen may irritate the glossopharyngeal and vagus nerves and may produce, among other symptoms, referred otalgia. Treatment is directed against the tumor.

E. Referred Otalgia Mediated by the Cervical Nerves (Table 6–9)

The posterior and part of the lateral aspects of the auricle receive sensory innervation from the second and third cervical nerves (C2-C3). They therefore mediate referred otalgia when these nerves are irritated in the other cervical portions of their territory.

1. **Occipital neuralgia** Patients with this condition complain of pain in the occipital region, with radiation to the postauricular area. Treatment consists of analgesics and, sometimes, cervical section of the occipital nerve.
2. **Cervical lymphadenitis** Referred otalgia may be caused by infection of the upper cervical lymph nodes. Treatment is directed at the infection.
3. **Infected branchial cysts** Once such an infection has been treated, the cyst requires surgical excision.
4. **Thyroiditis** Referred otalgia is a frequent symptom of inflammation of the thyroid gland. Treatment is directed against the thyroiditis.
5. **Infection of cervical fascial compartments** These infections, which are usually secondary to primary foci in the oral cavity or pharynx, produce pain and swelling in the neck and are often accompanied by ear pain. Treatment is directed toward the infection.
6. **Grisel's syndrome** This uncommon disorder of the upper

TABLE 6–9

Extrinsic Otalgia—Cervical Nerves
1. Occipital neuralgia
2. Cervical lymphadenitis
3. Infected branchial cysts
4. Thyroiditis
5. Infection of cervical fascial compartments
6. Grisel's syndrome
7. Cervical arthritis
8. Postoperative pain

cervical spine involves subluxation of the atlantoaxial joint and produces symptoms of upper neck pain, torticollis, and otalgia. It may result from pharyngeal infections and may complicate adenoidectomy. Treatment is directed at the cervical spinal problem.

7. **Cervical arthritis** Patients with arthritic conditions of the upper cervical spine may complain of otalgia among other symptoms. The treatment is directed toward the cervical spinal disorder.

8. **Postoperative referred otalgia** Patients who have undergone neck, parotid, or postauricular operations may experience prolonged otalgia. A frequent cause of this pain is inadvertent injury to the greater auricular nerve in the neck during biopsy of a lymph node or during parotidectomy for removal of a tumor of the gland. An occasional patient experiences prolonged ear pain after a postauricular incision for an ear operation. No specific treatment exists for this type of pain, other than diagnosing it, explaining it to the patient, and reassuring the patient that it will probably subside spontaneously.

7

HEARING LOSS

COLLIN S. KARMODY

The treatment of hearing loss depends on its origin, which may be in the external auditory canal, middle ear, inner ear, internal auditory canal, or cerebral pontine angle. Because each ear is connected to both cerebral cortices, central hearing loss beyond the cerebral pontine angle is difficult to document. Most of the anatomic defects that cause hearing losses are well documented, but little is known about the biochemical and other possible mechanisms. Consequently, therapeutic techniques directed toward mechanical solutions for mechanical problems have been well studied and are now often successful. The therapy of "nonmechanical hearing loss," however, remains mostly empiric. Hearing loss may be divided into two categories, conductive and sensorineural. Acute, subacute, and chronic infections are frequent causes of hearing losses, most commonly of the conductive type. Because the treatment of ear infections is detailed in Chapter 9, this chapter deals primarily with hearing losses caused by noninfectious processes.

I. DIAGNOSIS

A. Medical History

A history of hearing loss is usually given voluntarily by the patient. Parents frequently provide such details for their children. In addition, a history of hearing problems might be obtained from the patient's relatives, spouse, and others who are close to the patient. Some direct questioning may be necessary, as exemplified in the following paragraph.

One should inquire about the mode of onset of the hearing loss, whether sudden or gradual. Is the hearing loss static or progressive? Is pain, otorrhea, tinnitus, vertigo, or imbalance present? Is the hearing loss unilateral or bilateral? One should then inquire about the patient's family history, which is frequently positive in otosclerosis and certain types of sensorineural hearing loss. One should discuss the patient's medical history, noting in particular renal disease, allergy, or systemic diseases. Has the patient undergone previous treatment for hearing loss, for example, for the removal of cerumen? One should inquire about medications: aspirin may cause a sensorineural hearing loss and so may certain of the aminoglycosides and diuretics. Has the patient had recent trauma to the ear or head, or exposure to loud noises, either explosively or on a long-term basis? Has the patient a previous history of ear infections, even as far back as childhood? In what situations is the hearing loss more pronounced and in what situations is it improved? For example, does the patient have difficulty with background noises, as in sensorineural hearing losses, or does the hearing improve when the patient listens to conversation and background noise? This phenomenon is known as paracusis of Willis and is common in otosclerosis. Does the patient hear noises but have difficulty in understanding speech? In young children, one should always respect the observations of their parents, who are surprisingly accurate in the early diagnosis of their children's hearing loss.

B. Examination

1. **Observation** One should observe the patient's responses to a conversational voice across the room during the initial interview. One should look for signs of lip reading, as indicated by the patient's watching the examiner's mouth carefully during conversation. Does the patient respond accurately when the examiner's mouth is shielded? Does the patient wear a hearing aid? Is the patient's pattern of speech flat and monotonal, as is frequent in congenital deafness? Is it intelligible? Does the patient have obvious facial asymmetry from facial nerve dysfunction, or are asymmetric developments of the skull and facial bones visible?

2. **Physical examination** One should examine the patient's ear systematically and carefully, including observing and palpating the pinna for redness, swelling, and tenderness, all of which can indicate infection. One should also palpate the cartilaginous external canal. Is it tender, as in acute external otitis? Then one should palpate the temporomandibular joints.

3. **Otoscopic study** Otoscopic examination must be performed carefully, while one observes the condition of the skin of the external auditory canal for signs of infection or neoplasia. Is the canal of normal width and length, or is it stenosed? This observation is particularly important in young children. Is the canal filled with cerumen? Is the tympanic membrane present? Can it be clearly recognized as such? The absence of the usual landmarks may indicate stenosis of the external auditory canal or a pathologic condition of the tympanic membrane or of the middle ear. One should note carefully the condition of the

tympanic membrane for color, consistency, and mobility. A red and edematous tympanic membrane indicates an acute suppurative otitis media. On the other hand, a yellow and transparent tympanic membrane suggests a serous effusion in the middle ear. A dull, slate-colored membrane is found in patients with a mucoid effusion of the middle ear, a "glue ear." Is a perforation of the tympanic membrane visible? Is it dry or moist? One should note the position of the perforation. An anterior perforation represents a benign chronic otitis media, whereas a posterior or superior perforation or one in the pars flaccida is usually associated with cholesteatoma.

4. **Tuning fork tests** Although results of tuning fork tests are qualitative, not quantitative, they are still important and should be understood by anyone who treats patients with hearing loss. The standard tuning fork tests are Rinne and Weber tests. The Rinne test identifies the difference between conductive and sensorineural hearing losses, and the Weber test indicates the side of a conductive hearing loss (Karmody, C.S.: Textbook of Otolaryngology. Philadelphia, Lea & Febiger, 1983, p. 43). Other tests described by Gellé and Schwabach, although usually found in textbooks, are no longer in routine use. Tuning fork tests should always be repeated with masking. At the present time, using a speaking tube in the affected ear while the normal ear is masked is helpful in evaluating a profound hearing loss. Whenever possible, audiologic assessment is recommended for patients who complain of hearing losses. It is no longer advisable to rely on one's clinical interpretation of such a loss. In addition to the examination of the ears outlined previously, a thorough examination of the nose, mouth, nasopharynx, and all craniofacial nerves should be performed. If one sees an indication of vestibular upset or if a question of neoplasm in the cerebropontine angle exists, then tests of vestibular function must be performed.

II. TREATMENT

A. Congenital Hearing Loss

One should obtain a detailed history of the patient's problem, particularly the cause for parental concern about deafness, and determine the presence or absence of other anomalies. Then one should obtain the details of the family's medical history. Does the family have a history of hearing loss in early life, or a history of renal diseases or pigmentary abnormalities as seen in Waardenburg's syndrome? Was the patient's mother in contact with any infectious diseases during the first trimester of pregnancy? One must perform a thorough physical examination and document all anomalies. Responses to loud noises in the office environment should be noted and should be tested before one attempts to examine the ears. One should note carefully the responses of the child to the voices of the parents. The ears, the rest of the head, and the neck must be examined in the finest possible detail, and all pertinent findings must be carefully documented. One should evaluate the auditory thresholds by behavioral and evoked-response audiometry. One should also use radiographs, particularly computed tomographic (CT) scanning, to assess anatomic disorders. It is important to assess the child's chances for long-term survival. Parents who think that their child has a hearing problem are usually correct. It is therefore the physician's duty to evaluate such a child with great care and as soon as possible. A single test of hearing is not acceptable for diagnosis; two or three or more sessions may be required for confirmation. One must remember that the diagnosis of congenital hearing loss is the beginning of a lifetime of social disability and stigma. The following points apply to all patients with congenital hearing losses.

1. **Counseling** Parents must be counseled, preferably by experts, about their child's problems and must be given emotional support by physicians and auxiliary personnel.
2. **Hearing aids** should be prescribed for all patients initially, regardless of the type of hearing loss. As soon as a congenital hearing loss becomes obvious, such as caused by the absence of the external auditory canal, the patient should be fitted with one or two hearing aids. Hearing aids are successful in patients with congenital hearing losses, and nothing is gained by delaying the fitting of hearing aids to any child suspected of having a congenital hearing loss.
3. **Educational programs** must be planned as soon as the diagnosis is made.
4. **Speech therapy** The child should be enrolled in speech therapy classes as soon as possible.
5. **Determination of possible causes** One must conduct a vigorous search for possible etiologic factors. These must be addressed as soon as they can be identified. For example, syphilis is one of the few treatable causes of hearing loss.
6. **Stimulation** The child must be maximally stimulated constantly and encouraged to develop the other senses, such as sight, touch, and taste. Parents must be encouraged at every stage because they are the foundation for successful therapy.
7. **Surgical treatment** is considered only for patients with conductive congenital hearing losses, usually only when the loss is bilateral. In unilateral cases, surgical treatment may be indicated if the problem can be corrected by simple maneuvers. Surgical intervention should be contemplated only after careful study of the patient's ears, and the child preferably should be 7 years of age or older. Procedures should be performed in the presence of a well-developed middle ear cleft and mastoid cell system. All these features can be determined by careful

CT study. One should also carefully assess the position of the fallopian canal because damage to the facial nerve is a real possibility. The child and the child's parents must be sufficiently cooperative to undertake postoperative care, particularly in the case of an open mastoidectomy cavity. It is not the intent of this text to describe surgical technique, but the principles are as follows. The technique for surgical treatment of congenital conductive hearing loss depends on anatomic variations. In general terms, most of these patients require the creation of an external auditory canal and reconstruction of the ossicular chain. When aplasia of the canal is the problem, a new channel must be created through the mastoid process. If the external canal is narrow, it must be widened. In most cases, a new tympanic membrane is fashioned from temporalis fascia or by use of a homograft. The ossicular chain is reconstructed using the patient's own available tissues or homografts. In a few cases, a stapedectomy is required. In all patients with congenital aplasia, the facial nerve may be damaged, and the surgeon must take care to identify the nerve early in the procedure.

B. Inflammatory Disorders of the Ear

1. **External otitis** Hearing loss caused by external otitis is usually easily treated by a thorough cleansing of the external auditory canal. All pus and debris are cleared with loops, curettes, or suction devices. The external otitis is controlled by anti-infectious and anti-inflammatory agents such as an otic preparation of drops or ointment containing polymyxin, neomycin, and hydrocortisone. Three drops 2 to 3 times per day are usually effective, and the drops are most effective if instilled at bedtime. The patient lies on the opposite ear for at least 10 minutes, to allow the drops to penetrate the deeper part of the canal.

2. **Chronic external otitis** may cause a long-standing conductive hearing loss from occlusive swelling of the skin of the external auditory canal and accumulated debris. The hearing loss improves only with vigorous treatment of the external otitis. Both acute and chronic external otitis may require the use of a wick made of an absorbent strip of material, such as Nu gauze, inserted into the ear canal and moistened periodically, for example every 6 hours, with an otic preparation containing an antibiotic and hydrocortisone.

3. **Indolent external otitis** sometimes requires surgical removal of all canal skin and squamous epithelium from the lateral surface of the tympanic membrane, widening of the canal by drilling away of excess bone and the creation of a wide meatoplasty, and finally, lining of the widened canal with a split-thickness skin graft taken from the inner aspect of the upper arm or another hairless area.

4. **Malignant external otitis** is a colloquial term for a severe pseudomonas infection of the external auditory canal in middle-aged or elderly diabetics or other immunocompromised patients. The condition is characterized by a painful infection of the cartilaginous external auditory canal that resists all forms of topical therapy and slowly involves the rest of the temporal bone. Such an infection may prove fatal. Treatment is with intravenous gentamicin, carbenicillin, or tobramycin, debridement of the external canal as indicated, and rigid control of existing diabetes. One must rule out the presence of a true neoplasm in these patients; such a tumor could have similar clinical manifestations.
5. **Otitis media** is discussed in Chapter 9.
6. **Suppurative labyrinthitis** is discussed in Chapter 9.
7. **Serous labyrinthitis** is discussed in Chapter 9.
8. **Viral labyrinthitis** is a clinical entity that is poorly defined and is even less understood pathologically. This disorder is probably the major cause of sudden hearing loss and vertigo and can also be associated with other illnesses. The patient may have a positive history of an associated systemic viral infection such as mumps, measles, or an upper respiratory infection. Frequently, however, no clear association exists, and diagnosis becomes conjectural. Because vasoconstriction is a possible causative factor, viral labyrinthitis can be treated with vasodilators such as nicotinic acid, 100 mg after meals or in an amount sufficient to cause flushing. High doses of corticosteroids may be helpful; for example, one may prescribe prednisone by mouth, at an initial dose of 15 mg q6h and a daily dose reduced by 10 mg every second day. Other methods of treatment have been described, including the administration of histamines intravenously and plasma-expanding agents such as dextran 40. Antivertigo medications, for example meclizine and marezine, are given if needed.

C. Traumatic Injury

1. **External auditory canal** Trauma to the external auditory canal is usually caused by foreign objects introduced either voluntarily or inadvertently. Lacerations of the skin of the canal are painful and bleed easily, and accumulated blood may cause a conductive hearing loss. The diagnosis is easily made by thorough examination. Most lacerations occur on the posterior wall of the auditory canal. The majority of lacerations of the external canal heal spontaneously, and infection is uncommon. Therefore, topical or systemic antibiotics should be prescribed only if infection supervenes. Stenosis of the canal, a rare but significant complication of trauma, is more frequent after mastoidectomy or tympanoplasty. Stenoses cause a substantial conductive hearing loss. Most stenoses consist of either a mass of

fibrous tissue or a thin web-like diaphragm. Such lesions are treated surgically. The stenosing tissue is removed, and the raw area is grafted with a split-thickness skin graft. Concomitantly, the canal is widened by a meatoplasty. Postoperatively, a splint of nonreactive material such as acrylic can be inserted until the lumen shows no further tendency to constrict.

2. **Tympanic membrane** Acute traumatic perforation of the tympanic membrane as an isolated injury usually causes a mild conductive hearing loss and requires no treatment. Both the perforation and the hearing loss heal spontaneously. The area should be kept clean and dry, and eardrops and antibiotics are not necessary unless infection supervenes. If the perforation is large and the edges are rolled, the edges may be unrolled during the first 24 hours and splinted across the perforation with a piece of Gelfoam. Occasionally, the external canal or the tympanic membrane is damaged by chemicals such as strong acids. Relief of symptoms and healing are promoted by the use of a wick impregnated with an antibiotic-steroid preparation such as polymyxin, neomycin, and hydrocortisone, preferably as a cream or ointment. The wick should be changed at least once a day until the canal is dry and healing.

3. **Ossicles** Hearing loss caused by traumatic ossicular discontinuity is usually diagnosed late, that is, some time after the event. Traumatic ossicular discontinuity can be caused by a transcanal injury with pens or pencils, for example, introduced into the canal, usually for the purpose of scratching. Alternatively, ossicular discontinuity may occur in association with fractures of the temporal bone. Traumatic ossicular discontinuity requires surgical correction. Briefly, an exploratory tympanotomy is performed, and the pathologic features are identified. Because fractures of the human ossicles do not heal, ossicular continuity must be re-established by repositioning of the ossicles and interposing of bone and cartilage or by the use of a replacement prosthesis. See Chapter 3.

4. **Noise injury** The majority of hearing losses from noise are temporary (temporary threshold shift) and recover spontaneously within a few hours. Loud explosions, however, cause greater losses that tend to be permanent. Acoustic trauma characteristically causes a sensorineural hearing loss, maximally at 4 kHz; with continued exposure, hearing of other frequencies is affected. Treatment of the hearing loss consists primarily of the use of an appropriate hearing aid. Simultaneously, the patient should avoid exposure to loud noise. If such exposure must be continued, however, ear protectors should be used. These apparatus come in many patterns, but the headphone type of ear protector is generally most efficient.

D. Neoplasms

1. External auditory canal

a. ***Exostoses*** These smooth, white, bony growths in the bony part of the external auditory canal occur more frequently in people who swim in cold water than in other persons. These neoplasms characteristically occur in the roof of the canal close to the tympanic membrane and cause problems of recurrent external otitis or hearing loss if they become large enough to obstruct. Exostoses are removed surgically, but only if they produce significant symptoms. Other benign neoplasms of the external canal are less common and are treated by surgical excision.

b. ***Malignant neoplasms*** of the external canal are usually extensive when diagnosed. Most are squamous cell carcinomas, and presenting symptoms are persistent pain and a purulent, possibly bloody discharge. In the early stages, however, no pain may be present, and the patient may have the symptoms and physical findings only of chronic external otitis. The canal is at first thickened, firm, and granular; the neoplasm becomes obvious later. One should suspect such a neoplasm or fulminating external otitis when external otitis is recalcitrant to the usual therapeutic regimens. Biopsy is indicated early because these tumors spread rapidly. Treatment is by wide surgical excision followed by radiation therapy. For patients with large tumors, the prognosis is poor.

2. Chemodectoma, the commonest benign tumor of the **middle ear**, originates in a glomus body. In the middle ear, glomus bodies are found in the adventitia of the jugular bulb (glomus jugulare) and on the promontory (glomus tympanicum). Chemodectomas can be multicentric, and roughly 10% of patients with glomus tumors of the temporal bone have concomitant chemodectomas elsewhere, particularly carotid body tumors. Four percent of these tumors are malignant. The presenting symptom is a pulsating tinnitus synchronous with the patient's pulse. Conductive hearing loss, serous middle ear effusion, cranial nerve palsies, and bleeding occur later. Clinical findings depend on the stage of the disease at diagnosis and the point of origin of the tumor. Characteristically, one sees a smooth, red mass behind the tympanic membrane that may blanch under positive pressure applied with a pneumatic otoscope. The mass, however, may be pale or may not be visible on otoscopy. Large tumors may appear as polypoid lesions in the external canal. Further diagnosis is confirmed by CT scanning with simultaneous intravenous contrast techniques and by angiography. Biopsy is performed with great caution. Small lesions are treated by excision, and usually tumors of the glomus tympanicum can be removed by the transcanal approach. Larger lesions are treated by excision or radiation therapy.

Tumors of the glomus jugulare, which usually are of significant size when diagnosed, often require an extensive procedure.

3. **Acoustic neuroma** is the most frequent neoplasm involving the **eighth cranial nerve and cochlea**. Most acoustic neuromas arise from the superior vestibular nerve and cause hearing loss by compression of the cochlear nerve or the internal auditory artery. Most patients have a unilateral sensorineural hearing loss characterized by abnormally poor speech discrimination in relation to the levels of pure tone thresholds. Vertigo is not a frequent complaint, but mild unsteadiness is common. Loss of caloric response is often noted in the affected ear. Diagnosis is confirmed by radiologic studies such as CT scanning and contrast studies of the posterior cranial fossa using air or a radiopaque material. Acoustic neuromas grow slowly, but they may attain large, life-threatening dimensions with displacement of the brain stem. Neuromas are usually removed surgically. Small intracanalicular tumors may be approached by way of the middle cranial fossa, but larger tumors may require a translabyrinthine or suboccipital approach. Hearing is seldom preserved postoperatively, except in a few patients with small tumors.

E. Chemically Induced Hearing Loss

1. **Aminoglycoside-based antibiotics** are all potentially toxic, particularly in patients with renal disease. The aminoglycosides in most common use are gentamicin sulfate, tobramycin, streptomycin, and amikacin sulfate. All these antibiotics can cause severe sensorineural hearing losses, dizziness, and ataxia because of damage to the sensory cells of the cochlea and vestibular systems. Once established, hearing loss is permanent and does not respond to the usual therapy. It is possible, however, to prevent ototoxicity by daily monitoring of the vestibular system with caloric tests because the vestibular system seems to be damaged earlier than the cochlea. At the first indication of depression of vestibular function, the drug dose should be lowered or stopped.
2. **Aspirin** High serum levels of salicylates, 30 to 40 mg/100 ml, cause sensorineural hearing losses. Such losses may be as great as 40 to 50 db, but they usually improve when aspirin is discontinued.
3. **Quinine** has been used for the treatment of malaria and has been a common ingredient in many cold preparations and soft drinks. In high doses, quinine causes a permanent sensorineural hearing loss with an accompanying high-pitched tinnitus. The loss may be reversible if the drug is withdrawn at the first sign of toxicity. Quinine also crosses the placenta and can cause congenital hearing loss.
4. **Diuretics** Furosemide and ethacrynic acid are two diuretics

usually reserved for intravenous use. Both can cause sensorineural hearing losses, particularly in patients with severe renal failure. Ethacrynic acid causes a permanent loss, but the loss from furosemide may be temporary and may improve on withdrawal of the drug. If ethacrynic acid must be used in patients with severe renal failure, then doses must be carefully titrated, and hearing should be assessed audiometrically, daily if possible. Once hearing has been lost, the only form of therapy is a hearing aid.

F. Idiopathic Disorders

1. **Otosclerosis,** a familial progressive disease of bone confined to the otic capsule, is found only in humans. Otosclerosis is more prevalent in Caucasians than in others and is more common in females than in males. Its point of origin is around the fissula ante fenestram, a small area close to the anterior rim of the oval window. The patient's main complaint is of a slowly progressive bilateral hearing loss, frequently first noted as a teenager. At first, the hearing loss is conductive because of fixation of the footplate of the stapes. Further expansion of the otosclerotic process eventually causes an additional sensorineural hearing loss. Consequently, most middle-aged to elderly patients with otosclerosis have mixed hearing losses. A particularly active form of otosclerosis may occur in younger adults and may become manifest primarily as a sensorineural hearing loss with a small conductive element. Clinical otosclerosis is sometimes unilateral.
   a. ***Clinical findings*** Usually, no significant diagnostic findings are present on examination, except definition of a conductive hearing loss. In the younger patient with an active focus (otospongiosis), the mucosa over the focus may be hyperemic and may appear as a pink blush behind the tympanic membrane (the Schwartze sign).
   b. ***Treatment*** The conductive hearing loss of otosclerosis can be treated by stapedectomy or with the use of a hearing aid. In a stapedectomy, part or all of the stapes is removed and is replaced by a prosthesis attached to the long process of the incus and extending to the vestibule. The activity of aggressive foci might be reduced by the ingestion of sodium fluoride in high doses, although this therapy is not universally accepted.

2. **Sudden hearing loss** The causative factors of sudden hearing loss are still not known. Some evidence implicates viral labyrinthitis, but other factors such as vascular phenomena, specifically thrombosis or hemorrhage, are probably causative in some cases. A few cases are caused by a spontaneous fistulization through the round or oval windows. Fortunately, sudden loss of hearing is frequently unilateral. Such a loss may be either partial or total; 60% of sudden hearing losses, par-

ticularly partial losses, are recovered spontaneously. Not all patients recover totally. Treatment is empiric. Vasodilators are used on the premise that vasospasm is the cause. Corticosteroids are used as described for viral labyrinthitis. If one suspects a spontaneous fistula, an exploratory tympanotomy should be performed, and the fistula or fistulas should be sealed with a free graft of fat or fascia. See Chapter 8.

8

SUDDEN SENSORINEURAL HEARING LOSS

MOSHE ZIV

Sudden sensorineural hearing loss is the result of multiple etiologic factors that affect the auditory organ. Viruses commonly associated with sensorineural hearing loss include varicella-herpes zoster, mononucleosis, mumps, adenovirus type 2, rubella, rubeola, influenza, and parainfluenza viruses. Apparently, viral infection is the single most common cause of sudden sensorineural hearing loss, and it accounts for about one-third of these cases. Bacterial labyrinthitis is another cause of sudden sensorineural hearing loss, as are Ménière's disease, syphilis, ototoxic substances, trauma to the head, severe acoustic trauma, barotrauma, and blast injury. Sudden vascular insufficiency to the auditory organ creates a sudden hearing loss, as a result of localized obstruction of the internal auditory artery or one of its branches or from a more proximal vascular obstruction. Acoustic neurinoma manifests itself in 10 to 15% of patients with sudden sensorineural hearing loss. Cerebellopontine angle lesions may also cause sudden hearing loss. Ruptures of membranes in the inner ear or in the oval or round window, secondary to strain and elevation of cerebrospinal fluid (CSF) pressure, are other causes of sudden hearing loss. Some of these patients may have a persistent fistula of the oval or round window that may require surgical correction.

The natural history of a sudden sensorineural hearing loss does not allow one to predict the outcome. Approximately half the patients recover rapidly, usually shortly after the onset of the hearing loss. Patients with a downward-sloping audiogram and severe vertigo do not recover useful hearing. Almost all patients with isolated midfrequency sudden hearing loss recover completely. Approximately 70% of patients who have a hearing loss at 4000 Hertz (Hz) that is equal to or greater than the loss at 8000 Hz recover completely or at least retain usable hearing. Between 30 and 40% of all patients with sudden hearing losses recover completely, and about 65% recover usable hearing. On the other hand, if the patient is unable to hear at 8000 Hz, regardless of the hearing at other frequencies, the prognosis of improvement is approximately 30%. Most patients show evidence of recovery during the first 10 days following the initial event of sudden sensorineural hearing loss.

Different therapeutic techniques are used in the management of this type of hearing loss. Most commonly used are bed rest, and vasodilators such as nylidrin hydrochloride, papaverine hydrochloride, nicotinic acid, histamine, atropine, and inhalation of 5% carbon dioxide and 95% oxygen. Blocking of the stellate ganglion, diuretics, anticoagulants, plasma expanders such as dextran, and diatrizoate meglumine injected intravenously are also used sometimes. No scientific evidence to date has proved the efficacy of medication in the treatment of sudden hearing loss.

This author's approach to the management of sudden sensorineural hearing loss is based on the natural history of the disease, the prognostic guidance of the audiologic appearance, and considerations of safety. The management of sudden sensorineural hearing loss is still controversial. Additional basic information regarding the mechanism of the idiopathic form of this disorder, its most common manifestation, will be helpful in determining appropriate therapy.

I. DIAGNOSTIC WORKUP

Hospitalization is recommended for every patient with sudden sensorineural hearing loss. Bed rest is indicated, with head elevation to decrease CSF pressure. The workup is then initiated and should include the following studies.

A. Initial Examinations

1. **Complete audiologic evaluation.**
2. **Neurologic examination.**
3. **Electronystagmography** (ENG), to identify vestibular associated disturbances.
4. **Brain-stem evoked response audiometry.**

B. Radiographic Studies

1. **X-ray studies of the internal auditory canal and cerebellopontine angle,** to rule out acoustic neurinoma or cerebellopontine angle lesion.
2. **Computed tomographic (CT) scanning of the temporal bones,** and if necessary, posterior fossa myelography.

C. Laboratory Studies

1. **Fluorescent treponemal antibody absorption test** for syphilis.
2. **Thyroid function tests.**

3. **Blood glucose and three-hour glucose tolerance test,** to rule out diabetes mellitus.
4. **Triglyceride and cholesterol** determinations, to rule out hyperlipoproteinemia.
5. **Prothrombin consumption test** for hypercoagulable state.
6. **Viral studies** of blood serum, CSF, and stool for seroepidemiologic purposes.

II. MANAGEMENT

A. Idiopathic Hearing Loss

1. **General considerations and exact history taking** are important. The onset of sudden sensorineural hearing loss, as well as precipitating factors, contribute to an understanding of a possible cause. Is the hearing loss isolated, or are other neurologic abnormalities present, such as vertigo, ataxia, or other deficits? The workup is conducted while the patient is hospitalized.
2. **Bed rest and head elevation** are needed to decrease the CSF pressure, as well as the perilymphatic pressure. Tranquilizers may be helpful in decreasing the patient's anxiety.
3. **Daily audiograms** are necessary, to follow the progress of the patient's hearing loss.
4. **Duration of therapy** Bed rest is indicated for about 10 days. At that time, the workup should be completed. When a specific cause is found, the patient should be treated accordingly.

B. Hearing Loss of Defined Origin

1. **Acoustic neurinoma or a cerebellopontine angle lesion** needs neuro-otologic surgical intervention.
2. **Syphilis** requires appropriate antibiotic treatment and corticosteroids. The steroids may be indicated for a long-term therapeutic regimen.
3. **Ototoxic medication** should be discontinued and replaced by a nonototoxic agent if possible. Hearing may spontaneously be restored without any therapeutic intervention, but most sudden sensorineural hearing losses caused by these drugs are not recovered. If the cause of ototoxicity is aspirin or quinine, however, the prognosis is good.
4. **Trauma** For fracture of the temporal bone, blast injury, severe acoustic trauma, and labyrinthine concussion, no specific treatment is required, except bed rest. The most common sequelae of traumatic injury are high-frequency hearing losses and subjective tinnitus.

C. Perilymph Fistula

If the patient's medical history suggests a pre-existing physical strain, labyrinthine membrane rupture and perilymph fistula should be considered. Such a patient cites a specific event, such as a physical strain, barotrauma, diving, lifting, or air travel, followed by symptoms of sudden hearing loss.

1. **Mild-to-moderate hearing loss (25 to 50 decibels)** Bed rest with head elevation and neuro-otologic workup as described are indicated. If the patient has no improvement in hearing or vertigo in 2 weeks, an exploratory tympanotomy should be considered, to look for oval or round window fistula. If the patient's hearing worsens, earlier surgical exploration may be indicated.
2. **Severe hearing loss without vertigo** Bed rest is the only indicated therapy, combined with the diagnostic workup. Surgical intervention is not recommended because the prognosis of this condition is poor.
3. **Severe hearing loss and vertigo** Initially, only bed rest is indicated. If no improvement is noted in 10 days to 2 weeks, one should consider surgical exploration of the middle ear, to rule out fistula, for the purpose of controlling the vertigo. The patient's hearing is not expected to improve. In exploration of the middle ear to look for fistula, one should carefully examine the oval and round windows. Vertigo resolves or improves in about 70% of these patients if one uses fascia or perichondrium to seal the fistula. Results are poor if fat is used, and only about 15% of patients note an improvement. Gelfoam may induce granuloma formation and should not be used.

9

EAR INFECTIONS

WERNER D. CHASIN

I. EXTERNAL EAR

The external ear includes the auricle and the external auditory canal. Table 9–1 lists external ear infections.

A. Furuncle of the Ear Canal

Furuncles occur only in the hair-bearing part of the canal, which is the distal half of the external auditory canal. Diagnosis is based on the finding of tender swelling in the meatus or canal. The ear is sensitive to manipulations on the tragus or to pulling of the auricle inferiorly or posteriorly. Treatment consists of the application of warm compresses around the auricle and measures to reduce the canal swelling, to allow ear drops to enter the ear canal. A wick of cotton or gauze impregnated with Ergophene ointment is gently slipped with forceps into the distal half of the ear canal. Enough of the wick is left protruding from the meatus, so the patient can remove the wick in 24 hours. Thereafter, ear drops containing hydrocortisone and an antibiotic are placed into the ear canal by the patient or someone else 3 times a day. Occasionally, it becomes necessary, in an unresponsive case, to incise and drain the furuncle.

B. Diffuse Infections of the Ear Canal

These infections may represent spreading cellulitis from a furuncle or dermatitis caused by bacteria, fungi, maggots, foreign bodies, or general dermatologic problems. Diffuse canal infections may also be secondary to subacute or chronic otitis media, with the drainage from the middle ear infecting the skin of the canal. Because of this possibility, it is wise to refrain from irrigating the ear

TABLE 9–1

External Infections of the Ear

A. Furuncle of the ear canal
B. Diffuse external canal infection—acute
C. Perichondritis of the auricle
D. Malignant external otitis
E. Eczematous external otitis
F. Ramsay Hunt syndrome
G. Myringitis bullosa
H. Cellulitis of the auricle
I. Insect bites of the auricle
J. Fungal infection of the ear canal

canal. One should remove as much pus and debris as possible from the ear canal by means of a small suction tip or by gentle wiping with small, cotton-tipped applicators. A foreign body should be removed either by suction or with small alligator or ear-dressing forceps. Subsequent treatment depends on whether the infection is localized to the canal or whether it is accompanied by auricular or periauricular cellulitis. If the infection is localized to the ear canal and the debris suggests a fungal organism, as characterized by blue, black, or yellow particulate matter, a solution containing acetic acid should be prescribed. A regimen of 3 drops of VoSol or VoSol HC Otic Solution instilled into the ear 3 times a day is successful in most cases. In bacterial infections, a solution containing hydrocortisone and a broad-spectrum antibiotic is useful. Examples of such drops are Cortisporin and Otobione Otic Suspension. When auricular or periauricular cellulitis is present, or when the ear infection causes a regional lymphadenitis, an oral antibiotic should also be administered. The patient may begin treatment with a penicillin compound, but the ear canal should be cultured and the antibiotic tailored to the micro-organisms identified. Compresses with a cloth repeatedly moistened with warm water or aluminum subacetate solution are helpful when applied frequently to the auricle and the inflamed periauricular tissues. The physician should watch for the presence of perichondritis of the auricle, which requires even more aggressive treatment, as described in the following paragraph.

C. Perichondritis of the Auricle

This disorder can be caused by gram-positive as well as gram-negative bacteria. The auricle is thickened and tender, and the skin is red. The various ridges and fossae of the auricle are obliterated by the swelling of the perichondrium and subcutaneous tissues. The patient should be checked for diabetes. Perichondritis may result in a permanent auricular deformity and hence requires aggressive inpatient hospital treatment. The ear canal infection is treated as described in the foregoing section. The patient is given intravenous antibiotics in accordance with the culture obtained from the ear canal drainage. Unresponding cases may require incision and drainage of the auricle and subsequent debridement of devitalized cartilage.

D. Malignant External Otitis

This diagnosis is made in patients who are diabetic and who have an unresponsive infection of the external auditory canal and auricle, usually caused by gram-negative micro-organisms, especially Pseudomonas aeruginosa. These patients must undergo an intensive attempt to control the diabetes and require prolonged inpatient hospital treatment of the infection with antipseudomonas intravenous antibiotics. Surgical debridement is sometimes required. The term "malignant" refers only to the particularly serious character of the infection and not to any neoplastic process.

E. Eczematous External Otitis

This type of inflammation causes diffuse redness and swelling of the skin of the ear canal, part or all of the auricle, and sometimes even the periauricular skin. The skin is often blistered and seems to weep diffusely. Such infections may be due to an unusual reaction to an ordinary external otitis or to allergy, either to a medication being used by the patient or to another substance such as hair spray, hair dye, or earrings. When the eczematous process merely represents an overreaction of the tissues to an ordinary ear canal infection, it should respond to cleaning of the ear canal, instillation of otic drops, and application of compresses. If these measures fail, then an allergic reaction should be suspected. Although patients may be allergic to almost any topical medication, neomycin, which is a component of most antibiotic-containing ear medications, is the most frequent offender. Neomycin-containing medications should be discontinued, and aluminum subacetate drops and compresses should be given instead. Occasionally, a plain, topical corticosteroid-containing cream hastens the resolution of the eczematoid reaction if the culture is negative. In cases of recalcitrant eczematoid dermatitis of the ears, the patient must discontinue use of all hair sprays and other cosmetics in an attempt to identify the offending allergen. Thereafter, the patient may have to use hypoallergenic cosmetics.

F. Ramsay Hunt Syndrome

This syndrome, which represents a herpes zoster infection of the skin of the ear canal, may be associated with auditory and vestibular signs and symptoms and with facial neuritis. Such a condition must be differentiated from chronic otitis media causing simultaneous inner ear complications and also from secondary external otitis. Tympanic membrane perforation is uncommon in the Ramsay Hunt syndrome, although the tympanum may have vesicles. Treatment of the painful herpetic eruption consists of the application of aluminum subacetate compresses on the herpetic eruption and the prescription of a potent analgesic such as codeine phosphate, 30 or 60 mg q4h. If the condition is complicated by facial paralysis, an ophthalmologic consultation should be obtained both to examine the patient for herpetic involvement of the eye and to assist in protecting the globe while the facial palsy persists. This protection includes the instillation of lubricating eye drops and the closing of the paralyzed superior eyelid, to cover the cornea. In patients with long-lasting palsies, tarsorrhaphy may be required.

G. Myringitis Bullosa

In this viral infection, the tympanic membrane is involved by vesicles that are often hemorrhagic. The condition must be differentiated from acute otitis media, which is sometimes associated with the formation of vesicles on the tympanic membrane. Treatment consists in the correct diagnosis of the condition; no specific therapy is available. The condition is self-limiting, and the crusts that remain on the drumhead when the vesicles have dried normally migrate away from the tympanic membrane as the epithelium is shed.

H. Cellulitis of the Auricle

This disorder is usually secondary to external otitis and is discussed in that section of this chapter. Regardless of the origin of the cellulitis, the auricle becomes painful, red, and swollen. Purulent material should be cultured, and a diagnosis of diabetes should be excluded. Penicillin is the drug of choice until cultures and sensitivities are obtained. An analgesic may be necessary.

I. Insect Bites of the Auricle

Insect bites, a possible cause of cellulitis of the auricle, may even lead to anaphylactic symptoms of varying severity. Antihistamines usually control the itching, although hydrocortisone creams (Hytone 2½%) may offer dramatic relief. Any respiratory or circulatory sequelae must be aggressively treated.

J. Fungal Infection of the Ear Canal

These infections are discussed in Chapter 6.

II. ACUTE INFECTIONS OF THE MIDDLE EAR AND PNEUMATIC CELLS

These infections are listed in Table 9–2.

A. Acute Otitis Media without Complications

Symptoms include pain, a feeling of blockage or pressure, hearing impairment, and sometimes fever. Treatment consists of oral antibiotics, analgesic otic drops, and a nasal spray to aid in decongesting the eustachian tube. When pain is severe, a potent oral analgesic is required, such as codeine phosphate, 30 to 60 mg q3 to 4h, or even meperidine (Demerol), 50 mg q3 to 4h. In adults, acute otitis media is caused mainly by pneumococci, streptococci,

TABLE 9–2

Acute Infections of the Middle Ear
A. Acute otitis media without complications
B. Acute otitis media with complications
1. Facial paralysis
2. Clinical mastoiditis
3. Serous labyrinthitis
4. Suppurative labyrinthitis
5. Sigmoid sinus thrombophlebitis
6. Extradural abscess
7. Meningitis
8. Otitic hydrocephalus
9. Petrositis

and staphylococci, and occasionally by Haemophilus influenzae. The current antibiotics of choice include penicillin G, erythromycin, cephalosporin and amoxicillin. The nasal spray Neo-Synephrine ¼% should be sniffed into the nose 4 times a day; the medication should run into the back of the throat to allow it to contact the inferior end of the eustachian tube and thereby to cause decongestion of the mucous membranes. When the infection fails to respond to this treatment in 48 hours and when pain is severe, a myringotomy should be performed both to drain the infection and to obtain secretions for culture and sensitivity studies. Recurrent infections in the pediatric population should be treated with low-dose prophylactic antibiotics before proceeding with surgical intervention.

B. Acute Otitis Media with Complications

The important complications include facial paralysis (neuritis of the facial nerve), labyrinthitis, clinical mastoiditis, thrombophlebitis of the sigmoid venous sinus, meningitis (extradural abscess and leptomeningitis), encephalitis, and petrositis. Although these complications may occur in otherwise healthy individuals, they are more likely in patients with impaired biologic defenses such as diabetics and persons with chronic illnesses.

1. **Facial paralysis** may complicate acute otitis media and requires aggressive treatment of the otitis media to reverse the paralysis. A myringotomy should be performed as soon as this complication occurs. If the infection fails to respond rapidly after 3 days of oral antibiotics administered according to culture and sensitivity tests, the patient must be admitted to the hospital for intensive treatment with parenteral antibiotics. If the patient requires a mastoid operation for a trapped infection, one should decide whether a facial nerve decompression should be performed at the time of the initial mastoidectomy or whether the patient should undergo a simple mastoidectomy, to be followed by a facial nerve decompression only if

the facial paralysis fails to respond to the antibiotics and the mastoidectomy procedure.

2. **Clinical mastoiditis** refers to an infection of the pneumatic cells severe enough to cause signs and symptoms, such as cellulitis of the skin overlying the mastoid process, a subperiosteal abscess in the same area, intense pain unrelieved by myringotomy, and painful swelling of the skin of the ear canal caused by sagging of the posterosuperior canal wall. When mastoiditis produces such signs and symptoms, the patient should be admitted to the hospital to be treated with intensive parenteral antibiotics, according to the culture and sensitivity test results obtained from the middle ear secretions. If the condition does not respond to such nonsurgical treatment within a few days, then a mastoidectomy will be required. Tissue removed at the time of mastoidectomy should always be submitted for histopathologic examination to check for such unusual conditions as tumor, granulomatous inflammation, and tuberculous infection.

3. **Serous labyrinthitis** complicating acute or subacute tympanomastoiditis is characterized by vertigo, nystagmus, ataxia, and audiologic evidence of cochlear involvement, as demonstrated by elevated bone conduction thresholds. This complication requires an immediate simple mastoidectomy and wide myringotomy, as well as intensive parenteral antibiotics administered according to culture. With such prompt treatment, it may be possible to save the function of the inner ear and perhaps even to reverse the sensorineural hearing loss.

4. **Suppurative labyrinthitis** complicating acute or subacute tympanomastoiditis is characterized by severe vertigo, ataxia, nystagmus, total loss of hearing, and fever. This complication calls for an immediate mastoidectomy and intensive antibiotic treatment because it is the forerunner of meningitis. Permanent loss of inner ear function is to be expected. If the condition of the patient is not much improved within 2 days, the ear may have to undergo a second operation, a labyrinthotomy, to drain the inner ear infection.

5. **Sigmoid sinus thrombophlebitis** occurs when the mastoid infection enters the sigmoid venous sinus. The patient has aural pain and a septicemic fever with chills. The classic picket-fence fever chart may be masked by antibiotic treatment. The condition is diagnosed from the patient's clinical course and the disappearance of mastoid air cells overlying the sigmoid sinus plate. As soon as septicemia is detected, blood should be drawn for culture, and the patient should be treated with intensive intravenous antibiotics. The patient must be carefully observed for the possible development of cavernous sinus thrombophlebitis and orbital manifestations. Once the patient's condition is stable, one must perform an open-cavity mas-

toidectomy, with packing of the sigmoid sinus and extraction of the infected clot from the lumen of the sinus. If the clot cannot be extracted because of adherence to the walls of the sinus or because of inferior extension, the internal jugular vein may have to be ligated in the neck to prevent embolization to the heart.

6. **Extradural abscess** should be suspected in a patient with mastoiditis who has intense headache, superior or posterior to the ear. At the time of the mastoidectomy, one should expose the dura mater, both of the temporal lobe and of the cerebellum. If an extradural abscess is discovered, the dura mater should be exposed until normal dura tissue is seen, to avoid leaving a loculated focus of pus.

7. **Meningitis** may complicate tympanomastoiditis and may become apparent when the patient is tested for stiff neck and Brudzinski's sign. In most instances, the infection responds to intensive intravenous antibiotic therapy. A mastoidectomy is sometimes required.

8. **Otitic hydrocephalus,** an uncommon complication of acute otitis media, is characterized by the onset of severe headaches, usually in a child or adolescent, which begin a few weeks after recovery from the otitis. The characteristic findings include the following: papilledema; marked elevation of cerebrospinal fluid (CSF) pressure; absence of cells and normal protein content in the CSF; ventricular dilatation and no mass effect on computed tomographic (CT) scanning; and lateral rectus muscle paralysis from compression of the abducent nerve by the diffuse intracranial hypertension manifested by diplopia. This self-limiting disorder may result from a temporary impairment of CSF absorption caused by the otitis media. It is managed by applying measures to reduce the intracranial hypertension, that is, repeated lumbar punctures or possibly corticosteroids. For the comfort of the patient, a patch may be used to cover the eye with a lateral rectus paralysis, to eliminate the annoying diplopia.

9. **Petrositis** is caused by the entrapment of residue of coalescent mastoiditis in the air cells of the tip of the petrous apex. The two cardinal manifestations of petrositis are pain and persistent ear discharge after simple mastoidectomy for coalescent mastoiditis. A variant of petrositis is **Gradenigo's syndrome,** characterized by the triad of orbital pain, diplopia, and persistent otorrhea. Petrositis must also be suspected when a patient with acute otitis media in the absence of labyrinthitis or a major pathologic finding in the mastoid develops meningitis. The diagnosis is made from the patient's medical history, from the clinical findings, and from evidence of a destructive inflammatory process, as demonstrated in Stenver's and base views of the petrous pyramid and tip or by CT scanning. The initial

treatment of petrositis is intensive intravenous antibiotic therapy, with drugs chosen according to culture and in vitro sensitivity studies. When this regimen fails, the patient must undergo a petrosectomy, which is actually a medial extension of a mastoidectomy with the creation of a drainage tract around the bony labyrinth to allow the infection trapped at the apex to drain into the middle ear or the mastoid process. The procedure is a petrosotomy, rather than a petrosectomy.

III. CHRONIC INFECTIONS OF THE MIDDLE EAR AND MASTOID PROCESS

A. Chronic Tympanomastoiditis without Complications

The disorder usually called "chronic otitis media" or "chronic tympanomastoiditis" should be subdivided into "recurrent chronic otitis media" and "continuous chronic otitis media." "Recurrent chronic otitis media" signifies an inflammatory condition of the middle ear and mastoid with a perforation of the drumhead, accompanied by discrete episodes of suppuration separated by intervals asymptomatic except for some hearing loss due to the perforation, ossicular degeneration, or possibly cochlear damage due to previous clinical or subclinical labyrinthitis. By contrast, in "continuous chronic otitis media," the ear continues to suppurate, despite every form of nonsurgical treatment.

1. **Recurrent chronic otitis media** is usually characterized by a central or "benign" type of perforation; no otoscopic evidence of cholesteatoma is present. Occasionally, the perforation is marginal, but without apparent cholesteatoma. Episodes of drainage are often caused by upper respiratory tract infections or contamination of the ear with water. The drainage is usually free of offensive odor and is mucoid. This type of chronic otitis media is well managed by cleaning of the ear by suction or irrigation with aluminum subacetate solution, by the instillation of a combined antibiotic-corticosteroid ear solution, and sometimes by the administration of an oral antibiotic, according to culture and in vitro sensitivity studies. An occasional patient may be allergic to one of the ingredients of the ear drops, especially neomycin, so an increase in ear drainage may indicate the need to prescribe a different ear solution. An alternative is to teach the patient to insufflate boric acid powder into the ear several times a day, to dry the ear canal and middle ear. When this type of recurrent drainage is easily stopped with such medications and when mastoid roentgenograms show no occult destructive inflammatory process or cholesteatoma, and if the patient can tolerate occasional episodes of drainage, it is reasonable not to prescribe surgical treatment. The patient should be instructed to report immediately any symptoms of complications such as headache, ear pain, vertigo, or facial weakness. As long as no major problem exists, periodic ex-

aminations of the ear by the otolaryngologist should suffice. Tympanoplasty or tympanomastoidectomy does not usually eliminate benign recurrent drainage, probably because of the ill-functioning eustachian tubes of these patients.

2. **Continuous chronic otitis media** must be treated surgically, but only after specific causes of chronic otitis media have been excluded. These specific causes include tuberculous otitis, fungal otitis, noncholesteatomatous otitis media caused by a gram-negative organism, chronic ear suppuration in an immunocompromised patient, chronic suppurative otitis media as an unrecognized sign of Wegener's granuloma, neoplasia of the middle ear and mastoid manifesting as a persistent suppuration, and histiocytosis X of the temporal bone. These specific causes of chronic ear suppuration must be diagnosed by appropriate and complete evaluation of the patient, careful bacterial studies, radiographs, and perhaps even biopsy. Treatment should be dictated by the precise cause of the suppuration. The type of surgical procedure applicable to chronic nonspecific tympanomastoiditis, with or without cholesteatoma, is some form of mastoidectomy coupled with a tympanoplasty. It is beyond the scope of this discussion to consider the various types of surgical procedures.

B. Chronic Tympanomastoiditis with Complications

Some of the complications of chronic suppurative otitis media are similar to those of acute otitis media, and others occur more commonly in patients with chronic infections of the ear. The complications of chronic suppurative otitis media are listed in Table 9–3. For the most part, these complications are life-threatening and must be managed aggressively. When one complication occurs, the chances are high that more will follow.

1. Complications within the temporal bone

a. ***Facial paralysis*** in the presence of chronic otitis media

TABLE 9–3

Complications of Chronic Suppurative Otitis Media

1. Complications within the temporal bone
   a. Facial paralysis
   b. Labyrinthitis (serous, suppurative, or horizontal canal)
   c. Petrositis
   d. Perisinus abscess
   e. Conductive or mixed hearing loss
2. Extratemporal bone complications
   a. Extradural abscess
   b. Brain abscess
   c. Localized otitic meningitis
   d. Generalized otitic meningitis
   e. Otitic hydrocephalus
   f. Lateral sinus thrombophlebitis

requires prompt surgical intervention. The operation may be a mastoidectomy alone or a mastoidectomy with decompression of the bony facial canal, depending on perioperative findings.

b. ***Labyrinthitis*** Serous labyrinthitis should be regarded as a warning that the infection itself will soon invade the labyrinth. The condition requires a mastoidectomy with or without tympanoplasty, depending on the type of diseased tissue found in the ear at the time of operation. Suppurative labyrinthitis is a serious complication wherein the inner ear is immediately and irreversibly destroyed, and intracranial sepsis becomes imminent. The condition requires intensive presurgical treatment with intravenous antibiotics chosen according to culture and sensitivity studies. The patient must undergo a radical mastoidectomy and labyrinthectomy, with the widest possible drainage of the vestibular and cochlear compartments. A horizontal semicircular canal fistula is usually caused by a cholesteatoma that has eroded the bony covering of the horizontal semicircular canal. It is recognized by a positive fistula test result in a patient with chronic otitis media and may be confirmed by anteroposterior polytomographic radiographs of the temporal bone. The situation requires an open-cavity mastoidectomy (modified radical or radical mastoidectomy), depending on the condition of the middle ear. Whether the bony defect in the semicircular canal should be covered with a soft tissue graft or a bony graft remains controversial. Simple exterioration of the canal without violating the endosteum is usually successful in treating vertigo.

c. ***Petrositis*** Because chronic otitis media usually occurs in hypocellular temporal bones, and because petrositis is a trapped infection in the cells of the apex of the temporal bone, the condition is most often a complication of acute coalescent mastoiditis rather than of chronic otitis media. Petrositis occurring in a chronically infected ear must be treated in a similar manner, that is, by mastoidectomy and petrosectomy.

d. ***Perisinus abscess*** may complicate chronic as well as acute mastoiditis and is often an unexpected finding at the time of mastoidectomy. This condition is sometimes diagnosed preoperatively, by noting an area of bone destruction adjacent to the sigmoid groove. It represents an accumulation of pus and granulation tissue on the wall of the exposed sigmoid sinus. Such an abscess is significant because it represents a springboard for rapid septic invasion of the lumen of the venous sinus with subsequent sigmoid sinus thrombophlebitis. If recognized radiologically, this entity signals immediate open-cavity mastoidectomy.

e. ***Conductive or mixed hearing loss*** Chronic suppurative otitis media results not only in a perforated drumhead, but also in various types of ossicular fixation or destruction. Additionally, it is common for such patients to manifest varying degrees of sensorineural hearing loss, possibly from subclinical recurrent labyrinthitis by the round window or oval window membranes. The conductive, but not the sensorineural, component of the overall hearing loss may be corrected by tympanic membrane grafting and ossiculoplasty. The overall rate of improvement in hearing in middle ear disease more extensive than type I (drumhead perforation alone) is not satisfactory. Only under unusual circumstances should improvement in hearing be an indication for tympanomastoidectomy in chronic suppurative otitis media.

2. **Extratemporal bone complications**

a. ***Extradural abscess,*** which is similar to perisinus abscess, consists of a collection of pus against the dura mater of either the temporal bone or the cerebellum, with prior erosion of the tegmen or cerebellar plate (Trautmann's triangle). Sometimes, such an abscess occurs without bony erosion because the infection gains entry intracranially through small perforating veins. This condition should be suspected when a previously dormant chronic otitis media becomes intensely painful, although it is most often a chance finding at the time of operation. This type of abscess may escape diagnosis on radiographs, although destruction of the tegmen may be suggestive. Occasionally, extradural abscess results by thrombophlebitic extension of the mastoid infection through an intact bony dural plate. This complication, which should be suspected when a patient has had more than the usual amount of ear and head pain, dictates surgical exposure of the dura mater, even though the bony plate is intact at the time of operation. The significance of an extradural abscess is the imminent invasion of the dura mater, with a consequent subdural abscess, leptomeningitis, or brain abscess. An extradural abscess is an absolute indication for an immediate open-cavity mastoidectomy.

b. ***Brain abscess,*** most commonly seen in the temporal lobe or in the cerebellum, complicates chronic tympanomastoiditis and, occasionally, acute otitis media. The complication passes through the three clinical pathologic phases of localized encephalitis, localization, and enlargement of the abscess. During the first phase, symptoms may be mild and may include chills, a slight fever, headache and vomiting. The patient may be irritable and may experience a convulsion. In a few days, the patient enters a latent or quiescent stage, with few striking symptoms or findings, perhaps including malaise, listlessness, and irritability. One to 3 weeks later, the third stage begins, caused by an expanding abscess. At first, the findings are consistent with a general increase in intracranial pressure, that is, papilledema, headaches, bradycardia, projectile vomiting, and apathy. This phase is followed by focal symptoms and signs that depend on the location of the abscess within the brain. In cerebellar abscess, the common findings are ipsilateral cerebellar ataxia, ipsilateral hypotonia and weakness, ataxic gait, spontaneous nystagmus, and rapid emaciation. The most common findings in temporal lobe abscess are nominal aphasia, progressive contralateral hemiparesis, and visual field defects. The diagnosis of brain abscess is made from the patient's medical history, the evolution of the symptoms, and by the electroencephalographic and CT findings. Treatment is surgical and calls for drainage or excision of the abscess by a neurosurgeon. Once the condition of the patient is stable, a radical mastoidectomy must be performed on the chronically infected ear.

c. ***Localized otitic meningitis*** is an irritative reaction of the dura mater and arachnoid to a contiguous infectious process. Most commonly, this infection is an extradural abscess. It may be a reaction to an infected sigmoid thrombophlebitis, suppurative labyrinthitis, osteomyelitis of the petrous tip, or a brain abscess with secondary meningeal irritation. Symptoms are headache and fever. Irritability, drowsiness, vomiting, and, in infants, convulsions may occur. Signs may be absent, or they may include nuchal rigidity, a positive Kernig's sign, and other evidence of meningeal irritation. Spinal fluid may be normal, or it may contain lymphocytes with normal sugar levels and negative cultures. When this complication occurs in patients during the first week of a case of acute otitis media, myringotomy for culture and drainage and intensive parenteral antibiotic treatment may suffice. When localized meningitis occurs in a patient with chronic otitis media or 1 to 2 weeks after an episode of acute otitis media, the patient should be admitted for an urgent mastoidectomy. At the time of operation, it is imperative to explore the dura mater of the temporal lobe and, if nothing is found, that of the cerebellum. If an area of dural infection is found, the bony plate should be removed until normal dura mater is exposed. If no extradural infection is found on the temporal lobe or the cerebellum, the cell tracks to the petrous apex should be explored. Patients with localized meningitis related to purulent labyrinthitis require a labyrinthectomy with wide drainage of the labyrinth and cochlea.

d. ***Generalized otitis meningitis*** is discussed previously in this chapter, in the section on acute otitis media with complications.

e. ***Otitic hydrocephalus*** is discussed previously in this chapter in the section on acute otitis media with complications.

f. ***Lateral sinus thrombophlebitis*** usually follows chronic mastoiditis. Earache and mastoid tenderness are followed by generalized headache and papilledema after a period of days to a few weeks. Other neurologic signs are uncommon. Treatment is as for sigmoid sinus thrombophlebitis, which is previously discussed in this chapter.

10

VERTIGO

ARNOLD E. KATZ

I. GENERAL PRINCIPLES

Vertigo as a chief complaint is encountered as often as duodenal ulcer, pneumonia, or acute appendicitis. It presents a challenging diagnostic problem, and probably no other symptom strikes as much anxiety in the heart of the resident physician as the dizzy patient. Such need not be; most conditions can be diagnosed from the patient's medical history, and many patients are grateful once their condition has been explained to them, their prognosis outlined, and therapy instituted. Vertigo can also be the initial symptom of life-threatening disease that can be averted if appropriately diagnosed and treated early.

A. Definition

Vertigo is a hallucination of movement. The senses are deceived, and the patient believes that he is moving or is seeing abnormal movement of surroundings. The patient may act to counteract this perceived motion and may lose his equilibrium. The term vertigo is not a synonym for faintness, weakness, syncope, or nausea. Occasionally, patients use the term dizziness to describe nonvertiginous states, and this possibility must be fully evaluated in the medical history.

B. Balance Theory

Although the vestibular system has diffuse connections with the central nervous system, it is most helpful to think of the vestibular apparatus as two systems, right and left, in constant dynamic balance. The interaction of these two peripheral systems with the central nervous system informs the organism of movements and allows the body to adjust to new conditions. The right and left vestibular systems work as a team, constantly checking each other. When an inconsistency exists in the information derived from one or the other vestibular system, that is, a pathologic diminution in function of one vestibular system without a corresponding reflection of that activity in the other system, a crisis develops. The cerebral cortex interprets this inconsistent balance information as a condition of constant motion and leads to the hallucination of movement or vertigo. Along with the hallucination of movement, nystagmus, ataxia, and, usually, nausea and vomiting occur. In response to this crisis, the cerebellum is able to suppress the electrical activity of the vestibular nuclei, and repair and compensation may proceed. This repair process usually occurs within days and possibly weeks. This information provides us with two clinical axioms.

1. **Peripheral vestibular origin** Vertigo resulting from peripheral vestibular malfunction must always be associated with nystagmus.
2. **Central origin** If symptoms are nonepisodic and continuous for more than 2 or 3 weeks, the cause is not peripheral.

C. Central versus Peripheral Vertigo

Nearly 80% of patients with vertigo have peripheral vestibular dysfunction; however, a major effort should be expended to rule out the possibility of a central cause. Most causes of peripheral vertigo are not life-threatening, whereas symptoms of central vertigo may herald the presence of a small, treatable acoustic neuroma. We now have the ability to diagnose minute tumors largely limited to the internal auditory canal. One must be aware of the possibility of this disease and use the available diagnostic techniques.

II. EVALUATION

A. Medical History

In the search for the cause of vertigo, the patient's medical history is of paramount importance. Initially, it is essential for the patient to describe his symptoms; one should ask general questions such as, "What do you mean when you say you are dizzy?" Patients are frequently distraught over this frightening symptom and may become tangential in their descriptions. One must first allow the patient to describe associated symptoms; then, however, the physician must become specific in questioning. It is most helpful to have patients describe the initial spell in minute detail. The following questions are of critical importance.

1. **How long did the spell last?** Although it may be difficult for the patient to estimate time, especially if nausea and vomiting accompany the vertigo, it is essential to obtain an estimate of the duration of the spell. Ménière's disease spells last between 20 minutes and 2 hours, whereas vestibular neuronitis usually

lasts from several days to 2 to 3 weeks. Spells associated with cupulolithiasis usually just last minutes.

2. **What were you doing at the time of onset?** Whether the patient had been lying in bed and had rolled over or whether he had been probing the ear with instruments is of interest in establishing the origin of the spells.

3. **What time of the day was it?** Could this vertigo be related to an episode of hypoglycemia, or could it be related to chemical exposure in the work environment?

4. **During the spell, did you notice any decreased hearing, ringing in your ears, or fullness in either ear?** One would expect these accompanying symptoms to be present in a patient with endolymphatic hydrops.

5. **Did you have any nausea, vomiting, or sweating?** Peripheral vertigo is usually associated with these vegetative symptoms, whereas vertigo of central origin seems to cause much less distress.

6. **Did you lose consciousness?** If the patient lost consciousness, one should suspect a central cause.

7. **Did position affect the spell?** If so, this would be further evidence of a peripheral cause, but it certainly would not rule out a central disorder.

8. **Have you had any recent trauma?**

9. **Do you have drainage from your ears?** Such drainage suggests a chronic suppurative otitis media.

10. **Do you notice any decrease in your hearing?** One of the most important symptoms of an acoustic neuroma is a unilateral, progressive, sensorineural hearing loss. If a dizzy patient has such a hearing loss, every effort must be made to rule out the presence of an acoustic neuroma.

11. **Do you have or have you had any venereal diseases?** Endolymphatic hydrops can result from syphilis, and in children, congenital lues should be considered.

12. **Do you or does anyone in your family have diabetes mellitus?** The first sign of early diabetes may be reactive hypoglycemia, and these patients may have "dizziness" 3 to 5 hours after a meal.

13. **Did your spell occur after a major intake of salt?** Excessive salt intake, such as at a party while eating peanuts or popcorn can exacerbate endolymphatic hydrops.

14. **Is any history of hypothyroidism present, or do you have any symptoms of that disease?** Cerebellar ataxia, episodic vertigo, and sensorineural hearing loss can occur in patients with hypothyroidism.

B. Physical Examination

Although the physical examination is important, it is usually disappointingly normal. A complete physical examination is required, including careful study of the eyes for nystagmus and the ears for middle ear disease, as well as a detailed neurologic examination. One should especially search for any cerebellar function abnormalities. Finger-to-nose testing, gait testing, and the Romberg test should be performed. Neurologic consultation is also reasonable in this group of patients.

C. Audiometric Evaluation

All patients evaluated for vertigo should receive an audiometric evaluation including, at least, pure tone testing and tests of discrimination, tone decay, and recruitment. Békésy audiometry and evoked-response audiometry may be helpful if these tests are available. Any hearing loss in a patient complaining of vertigo must be evaluated, to determine whether the hearing loss is conductive or sensorineural. Once the hearing loss has been documented as sensorineural, it should be further studied, to ascertain whether it is a sensory hearing loss resulting from damage to the cochlea or a neural hearing loss resulting from damage to the more central hearing nerve, midbrain, or cortex. See Chapter 11.

1. **Pure tone testing** This type of testing enables one to determine whether a hearing loss is conductive or sensorineural. A conductive hearing loss may result from chronic suppurative otitis media with erosion of the ossicles, perforation of the tympanic membrane, or the presence of cholesteatoma. Conductive hearing loss in a vertiginous patient may be caused by otosclerosis.

2. **Discrimination** is a valuable test in distinguishing between sensory and neural hearing losses. This distinction is important because neural hearing losses in a vertiginous patient suggest the presence of an acoustic neuroma. When the pure tone thresholds have been obtained, words are spoken through the earphones at about 40 db louder than the patient's threshold. Even in patients with a moderate sensory hearing loss, discrimination scores should range around 70% or higher. In patients with slight neural hearing losses, however, discrimination scores may be 0 to 5%. Such a finding suggests an acoustic neuroma.

3. **Tests of recruitment** Many tests can demonstrate the presence of recruitment. Recruitment is found in patients with sensory hearing losses, in which the cochlea itself is damaged. Functionally defined, recruitment is an abnormal sensitivity to increases in loudness. The Short Increment Sensitivity Index (SISI) is designed to detect the presence of recruitment. A patient with recruitment probably has a sensory hearing loss and not an acoustic neuroma.

4. **Tone decay** Testing for tone decay is important in distinguishing between sensory and neural hearing losses because patients with sensory hearing losses can hear a tone for as long as it is presented. Patients with acoustic neuromas, however, experience a rapid diminution of the sound, even when presented at the same volume. Such tone decay is strong evidence for the presence of an acoustic neuroma.

D. Electronystagmography

Together with the simple caloric test, this technique can be helpful in determining the cause of vertigo.

1. **Simple caloric testing** is accomplished with the supine patient's head and neck elevated 30°, so the horizontal semicircular canal is vertically placed. Cold or warm water can then be used to induce nystagmus, the duration of which can be measured with a stopwatch. Depression of response on one side may suggest a central lesion, as may direction-changing nystagmus (Ann. Otol. Rhinol. Laryngol., *61*:987, 1952).
2. **Electronystagmographic technique** Because of the difference in electrical potential between the positively charged cornea and the negatively charged retina of the eye, eye movements in patients with nystagmus may produce changes that can be electronically recorded. The nystagmus can then be analyzed both qualitatively and quantitatively. The tracing of these movements, called an electronystagmogram, accurately measures the speed of the nystagmus as determined by the slow phase velocity, and a sensitive diagnosis of hypofunctioning or hyperfunctioning of one of the paired vestibular organs can thereby be made. Caloric tests performed during electronystagmographic examination provide much more information than one is able to obtain with Frenzel glasses and a stopwatch. Moreover, the electronystagmogram itself can give additional information. Abnormal pendulum tracking, calibration overshoot, and an abnormal ocular fixation index are additional indications of vertigo of central origin (Paparela, M.M., and Shumrick, D.A.: Otolaryngology. Vol. 1. Philadelphia, W.B. Saunders, 1980, p. 250).

E. Radiologic Evaluation

Every patient evaluated for vertigo should receive noninvasive radiographic analysis of the internal auditory canals to rule out the presence of an acoustic neuroma. Computed tomographic (CT) scanning of the internal auditory canal is at present the most sensitive noninvasive radiographic technique, although polytomographic studies of the internal auditory canals are often adequate. If any of the previous evaluation suggests an acoustic neuroma, air-contrast CT scanning should be performed because up to 20% of acoustic neuromas have no polytomographic evidence of internal auditory canal disorder. Radiologic evaluation is necessary in every patient evaluated for vertigo; this author has diagnosed acoustic neuromas in patients with normal hearing and in one patient with congenital lues.

III. PERIPHERAL CAUSES OF VERTIGO

It is important to differentiate peripheral or end-organ vertigo from vertigo caused by a disorder of the central nervous system. Although few peripheral causes of vertigo are life-threatening, vertigo of central origin frequently represents a serious illness. If the vertigo is not associated with nystagmus or if it persists longer than 3 weeks, a central cause must be suspected. Vertigo associated with severe nausea, vomiting, and sweating is much more likely to be associated with peripheral disease than vertigo not associated with vegetative symptoms. Vertigo associated with loss of consciousness or seizures suggests central involvement. Direction-changing nystagmus also suggests central involvement, as do several of the audiologic and electronystagmographic changes previously described. Almost 80% of patients with vertigo have peripheral disease, however, and one is usually able to make a diagnosis from their medical history.

A. Ménière's Disease

The patient with Ménière's disease has severe vertiginous spells that last from 20 minutes to 24 hours. They are abrupt in onset and more severe than the spells induced by caloric testing. These spells have no neurologic accompaniments or sequelae. Patients are

TABLE 10–1

Peripheral Causes of Vertigo

A. Ménière's disease
B. Benign paroxysmal positional vertigo
C. Viral labyrinthitis
D. Toxic labyrinthitis
E. Serous labyrinthitis
F. Acute suppurative labyrinthitis
G. Labyrinthine fistula
H. Disequilibrium of aging
    1. Cupulolithiasis of aging
    2. Ampullary disequilibrium of aging
    3. Macular disequilibrium of aging
    4. Vestibular ataxia of aging
I. Trauma
    1. Perilymph fistula
    2. Temporal bone fracture
    3. Acute acoustic trauma
    4. Barotrauma
J. Otosclerotic inner ear syndrome
K. Acute alcoholism
L. Syphilis of the inner ear
M. Motion sickness
N. Cogan's Syndrome

completely conscious and oriented during the entire episode and usually experience nausea, vomiting, and sweating. Audiologic evaluation reveals no evidence of central disease, and an electronystagmogram, if taken between spells, is usually of little help. Although Ménière's disease has no cure, 80 to 90% of patients improve in time because their spells become less frequent and less severe. Some patients have long remissions between episodes, with or without therapy, and most patients report an aura before the spell that consists of tinnitus or aural fullness. This aura allows most patients to be able to drive by enabling them to pull over to the side of the road before the spell becomes incapacitating. Medical treatment varies and may include anticholinergics, vasodilators, and sedatives. It is difficult to establish the effectiveness of any of these treatments because the spells are unpredictable, and the disease usually improves spontaneously. The following treatment plan is helpful.

1. **Diuretics** have been the mainstay of treatment. Chlorthalidone, 100 mg every morning, chlorothiazide, 500 mg every day, or hydrochlorothiazide, 25 mg 2 to 3 times a day, is commonly prescribed.
2. **A salt-restricted diet** of under 1000 mg/day should be recommended. Some patients mention that spells are experienced soon after partaking of salted peanuts or salted popcorn.
3. **Streptomycin** is sometimes used to destroy the labyrinth while preserving hearing in the unusual bilateral, incapacitating case. Treatment should be continued until the patient has no response to caloric irrigation of either ear.
4. **Surgical treatment** is occasionally necessary, and many procedures have been described. In general, the more destructive the operation to the labyrinth, the more likely it is to induce permanent cessation of vertiginous episodes. These procedures usually impair hearing, and because Ménière's disease is bilateral in about 10% of patients, the surgical approach should be considered only when all else has failed.

B. Benign Paroxysmal Positional Vertigo

This condition is easily distinguished from Ménière's disease because the vertiginous episodes only occur with positional changes, usually when the patient assumes a supine position and turns the involved ear downward. In about 5 seconds, the patient notices symptoms of vertigo and nausea. The attacks usually last less than a minute, and the patient usually demonstrates a rotatory nystagmus toward the involved ear. In most instances, the condition is self-limited; however, some patients do need surgical intervention. Recovery may be hastened by asking the patient to perform deliberate dizziness therapy (DDT). The patient is asked to assume several times a day the positions that bring on the spells (Laryngoscope,

80:1429, 1970). Although most positional vertigo is benign, central disease, such as cerebellar tumors, tumors of the fourth ventricle or temporal lobe, multiple sclerosis, or even cerebrospinal fluid hypertension, may cause positional vertigo. The electronystagmogram is helpful in detecting central causes. If the patient has no latent period, and the nystagmus does not fatigue, a central cause should be suspected. Another clue to centrally induced positional vertigo is direction-changing nystagmus.

C. Acute Viral Labyrinthitis

This disorder has a catastrophic onset including vertigo, nausea, and vomiting lasting from a few days to 2 or 3 weeks. The incapacitated patient frequently either has or is recovering from a viral infection. These spells are not episodic, and the patient usually does not have auditory involvement. It is a disease of young adults and may be seen in epidemic form. The nystagmus occurs away from the involved ear and is therefore destructive in nature. Patients frequently need to be admitted to the hospital for treatment with a vestibular suppressant, such as diazepam (Valium). In a week or so, the severe vertigo is gone; however, some disequilibrium may persist for months. Patients may notice some imbalance when stressed, such as while playing tennis or during any other vigorous physical activity. Because most of these patients are young, healthy adults, they compensate well.

D. Toxic Labyrinthitis

Although labyrinthitis caused by lead, arsenic, zinc, or quinine is seldom seen today, the physician must be aware of this type of unsteadiness due to the direct effects of ototoxic antibiotics. Streptomycin, dihydrostreptomycin, gentamicin, neomycin, paromomycin, all of which belong to the aminoglycoside group, may induce ototoxicity. As new antibiotics are developed, potential ototoxicity must remain a concern, especially if these agents are similar to the aminoglycosides. Diuretics, such as ethacrynic acid, also cause vestibular toxicity. Vertigo may occur alone, or it may be accompanied by tinnitus and hearing loss with many of these drugs. Treatment consists of an awareness of potential toxicity and discontinuance of the drugs at the first sign of any deleterious effect. Although the labyrinthitis is generally dose related, and although prescription of these drugs within safe limits of dosage results in no frank toxicity, idiosyncratic responses may cause damage without warning.

E. Serous Labyrinthitis

This sterile inflammation of the inner ear is usually caused by trauma or by a neighboring infection. The classic example of serous labyrinthitis is vestibular irritation following stapedectomy, although the disorder may accompany acute serous otitis media. Nystagmus may be present in either direction and usually lasts from several hours to several days. Hearing is usually unimpaired, and the entire episode is most often completely reversible. It is important to rule out the presence of acute suppurative labyrinthitis.

F. Acute Suppurative Labyrinthitis

This condition is usually a sequela of chronic suppurative mastoiditis. The symptoms, which are sudden in onset, generally occur in an ear that has been draining for many years. These symptoms include marked vertigo, nystagmus, nausea, and vomiting. The patient's hearing is not destroyed initially, but it may be reduced. The nystagmus initially has a quick component toward the infected ear for the first several hours, and then, if the disease progresses, it starts to beat to the opposite or normal ear. At this time, hearing in the diseased ear is totally lost, and vestibular function is completely absent. The situation is a surgical emergency, and after a brief period of intensive antibiotic therapy, labyrinthectomy should be performed to prevent the development of meningitis. Nystagmus persists for 2 to 3 weeks, until the patient compensates for the loss of that labyrinth.

G. Labyrinthine Fistula

This condition, usually seen in an ear that has been draining on a long-term basis, indicates erosion of a discrete portion of the bony labyrinth by infection or cholesteatoma, without extension of the infection throughout the membranous labyrinth. Although this disorder is usually caused by cholesteatoma, it may also occur in patients with congenital syphilis, glomus jugulare tumors, or other granulomatous or osteolytic lesions, such as histiocytosis X, osteogenesis imperfecta, or Paget's disease. The diagnosis of labyrinthine fistula is made by raising the pressure in the external ear canal with a pneumatic otoscope. When the air pressure in the canal is elevated, one should note a conjugate deviation of the eyes to the opposite side, and if the application of high pressure is continued, nystagmus will result (Ann. Otol. Rhinol. Laryngol., *86*:402, 1977). On diagnosis of the fistula, the physician must attempt to remove the infection or cholesteatoma as soon as possible, to prevent the development of acute suppurative labyrinthitis.

H. Disequilibrium of Aging

This type of dizziness is frequently seen in elderly patients. This condition should be viewed as the vestibular counterpart of presbycusis because age causes pathologic changes in the vestibular sense organs or neuropathways or both (Schuknecht, H.F.: Pathology of the Ear. Cambridge, Harvard University Press, 1974).

1. **Cupulolithiasis of aging** is caused by a degeneration of the utricle and the anterior and lateral semicircular canals that can result in calculus deposition on the cupula of the posterior semicircular canal. This disorder is manifested by severe, short-lived vertiginous episodes precipitated by certain hand positions and occasionally causing the patient to fall. The syndrome is sometimes self-limiting, but it may persist throughout the patient's life. If this disease has been brought on by head

trauma, it is much more likely to be self-limited. Surgical intervention is sometimes helpful.

2. **Ampullary disequilibrium of aging** is caused by degenerative changes in the ampullary mechanism of the semicircular canals. Patients experience the sensation of rotatory movement when they turn quickly to either side or when they flex or extend the neck. Nystagmus is fleeting and is difficult to observe. Once the sensation of disequilibrium has passed, a feeling of unsteadiness may persist for several hours.

3. **Macular disequilibrium of aging** is precipitated by change of head position relative to gravity after a protracted period in another position. This condition is most common in a bedridden patient who has long remained supine and who attempts to arise. The vertigo can be severe enough to allow the patient to reach a sitting position only in stages. The condition can and should be differentiated from orthostatic hypotension by the absence of visual blackouts or other signs of intracranial ischemia.

4. **Vestibular ataxia of aging** is central in origin, with the pathologic process probably located in the vestibular nerves, in the medial, lateral, or descending vestibular nuclei, in the descending medial, longitudinal fasciculi, or in the vestibulospinal tracts. These patients experience a constant sensation of disequilibrium during ambulation. Although they are comfortable when sitting or standing, these patients are unable to control their center of gravity while walking. Such patients walk hesitantly and take frequent sideways steps. Most persons thus affected are in their seventies and eighties, and the disorder persists for the remainder of their lives. Treatment for this group of unfortunate patients is usually unsatisfactory.

I. Trauma

Trauma to the head can induce certain types of positional vertigo.

1. **Perilymph fistula** Membrane ruptures of the oval or round window may result from trauma induced by physical stress. Hearing loss and vertigo may occur simultaneously or separately. The vertigo is usually incapacitating and is accompanied by nausea, vomiting, sweating, and nystagmus. These membranes may heal spontaneously with bed rest; however, surgical intervention may be necessary.

2. **Temporal bone fractures** Transverse fractures of the temporal bone involve the labyrinth more frequently than longitudinal fractures. Severe vertigo with total hearing loss is common and is discussed in Chapter 3.

3. **Acute acoustic trauma** Severe impulse acoustic trauma, such as produced by explosives, can instantaneously cause major hearing losses accompanied by severe vertigo. Ruptured tympanic membranes with dislocations of the ossicles are also seen

following blast injury. The diagnosis should be suggested by the patient's medical history, and treatment depends on the type of damage. Compensation should occur within 3 weeks and may be stimulated by labyrinthine exercises (Laryngoscope, *80*:1429, 1970).

4. **Barotrauma** may result from gradual changes in ambient pressure during air travel or deep-sea diving. Pressure changes should be uneventful during ascent in an airplane, when entering an area of decreased pressure, because air rushes out through the eustachian tube. Eustachian tube dysfunction may occur on landing of the aircraft, when it may be difficult for air to enter the middle ear through the eustachian tube. At this time, autoinsufflation is important. Even commercial airlines are only pressurized to about 5000 feet, and pressure changes between 0 and 5000 feet are significant. Similarly, the descent during a deep-sea dive should be more difficult in equilibrating middle ear pressure than the ascent, because the air within the middle ear space is expanding during ascent and should be able to escape through the eustachian tube. If one is unable to equilibrate the pressure within the middle ear, the tympanic membrane may rupture or the mucosal vessels may hemorrhage. Vertigo may become severe when one is unable to equilibrate pressure within the middle ear. Systemic and intranasal decongestants should be used; however, prevention of the condition is much more desirable. Flying or diving when one has a cold or during severe allergic episodes should be discouraged.

J. Otosclerotic Inner Ear Syndrome

Otosclerosis may be associated with vertigo because both diseases are common. Ménière's disease may be seen in conjunction with otosclerosis, and postural vertigo may also occur in patients with this disease. A third variety of dizziness, termed otosclerotic inner ear syndrome, has been described in which spells last from 20 minutes to 6 hours and are usually experienced as a vague floating or semifainting sensation. The caloric test on the infected ear qualitatively reproduces a spell, whereas in Ménière's disease, the caloric test produces vertigo that is usually less intense than that occurring during a Ménière's spell. Stapedectomy in these patients sometimes relieves the vertigo.

K. Acute Alcoholism

Alcohol commonly produces vertigo in the acute and chronic stages of intoxication. The effects are related to the time it takes for alcohol to dissolve in the endolymph and the tissues of the inner ear. By altering the specific gravity of these structures, a positional nystagmus is produced. Long-term alcohol ingestion causes vertigo of a more central origin; lesions have been documented in the hypothalamus, the third ventricle, and the periaqueductal gray matter. Wernicke's encephalopathy is also frequently associated with nystagmus, vertigo, and ataxia.

L. Syphilis of the Inner Ear

A syndrome similar to Ménière's disease can be seen in patients with either congenital or acquired syphilis of the inner ear. This author has also, however, witnessed the removal of a small acoustic neuroma from a patient under treatment for congenital lues. If such a lesion had not been discovered and removed early, the result would not have been so favorable.

M. Motion Sickness

This condition, the most common disorder of the inner ear, manifests as sea sickness, air sickness, and car sickness. Car sickness is usually increased when the patient is not driving and is in the back seat. Indeed, fighter pilots, who do not suffer from air sickness even after the most difficult maneuvers, can develop nausea, sweating, and unsteadiness when riding in the back seat of an automobile. Asymmetric congenital vestibular responses are influenced by constitutional or psychogenic factors. Combinations of scopolamine and amphetamine are effective in the treatment of this disorder. Other medications frequently prescribed are hyoscine, cyclizine, diphenhydramine, promethazine, and meclizine.

N. Cogan's Syndrome

This autoimmune disease is characterized by interstitial keratitis, episodic vertigo, and hearing loss. This uncommon disease occurs primarily in young adults, and the pathologic findings are of a systemic necrotizing angiitis of the polyarteritis type. Endolymphatic hydrops has been reported in polyarteritis nodosa and, less frequently, in Wegner's granulomatosis. These differential diagnoses should be considered in treating a patient with a systemic disease.

IV. DISORDERS CENTRAL TO THE VESTIBULAR END ORGAN

Although the cause of vertigo is central less than 20% of the time, one must identify central involvement because vertigo originating in the central nervous system is much more likely to herald life-threatening disease than that originating in the peripheral vestibular system.

A. Acoustic Neuroma

This disorder accounts for more than half of all tumors of the cerebellar pontine angle and usually produces signs and symptoms between the ages of 30 and 40 years. Acoustic neuromas have been reported in children as young as 7 years old, however. In any patient evaluated for vertigo, one should assume the presence of an acoustic neuroma until it is ruled out by audiologic, electronystagmographic, and radiologic testing, as previously described. A small

TABLE 10–2

Central Causes of Vertigo
A. Acoustic neuroma
B. Vestibular neuronitis
C. Tumors of the cerebellum, midbrain, or cerebral hemispheres
D. Multiple sclerosis
E. Epilepsy (temporal lobe seizures)
F. Vertebrobasilar migraine
G. Trauma
1. Head trauma
2. Cervicogenic vertigo
H. Herpes zoster oticus
I. Vascular insufficiency
1. Vertebrobasilar artery insufficiency
2. Lateral medullary (Wallenberg's) syndrome
3. Thrombosis of the internal auditory artery
J. Medications
K. Systemic disorders
L. Syringobulbia
M. Arnold-Chiari deformity with hydrocephalus
N. Lermoyez syndrome
O. "Illusory" vertigo

acoustic neuroma can be removed with little mortality or morbidity. Removal of large acoustic neuromas is much more frequently accompanied by facial paralysis, central nervous system deficits, or death.

B. Vestibular Neuronitis

This term has been applied to patients with viral labyrinthitis. Evidence suggests that the catastrophic event occurs within the labyrinth, although the nerve fibers themselves certainly may be involved. Diagnosis and treatment are as for viral labyrinthitis.

C. Tumors of the Cerebellum, Midbrain, or Cerebral Hemispheres

Such tumors may cause a chronic vertigo, but it is rarely true rotatory vertigo. More commonly, it is a lightheaded or unsteady feeling. Cerebral and pontine gliomas are more often seen in the young, whereas in the elderly, tumors in this area are usually metastatic. Gliomas cause various cerebellar signs, depending on their location, and about one-third cause a nystagmus that is coarse and well sustained. Brain stem lesions may also cause diplopia, dysarthria, dysphagia, and a crossed type of sensory and motor loss. Frequently, these tumors display central signs on audiometric testing and on electronystagmographic evaluation. CT scanning is helpful in the diagnosis of these lesions.

D. Multiple Sclerosis

Mild vertigo is frequently an early symptom of multiple sclerosis, a disease with many and varied symptoms. Even the classic triad of nystagmus, intention tremor, and scanning speech is by no means constant. Nystagmus is seen in only 70% of the patients. This idiopathic demyelination usually affects young adults and is characterized by remissions and exacerbations. The steady, slow, and downhill course results in sensory and vestibular disturbances, bladder dysfunction, and coordination problems. Once the disease has been diagnosed, steroids are frequently given. Other types of diffuse sclerosis, such as Schilder's disease, are often associated with vertigo and deafness. This type of sclerosis usually begins in childhood and adolescence and is associated with dementia, spasticity, and other neurologic symptoms. Death may occur within several years of the onset of symptoms, and no known treatment exists.

E. Epilepsy (Temporal Lobe Seizures)

Vertigo is seen in patients with epilepsy, especially in those with temporal lobe seizures. The vertigo may be simultaneous with the aura preceding the seizure; however, if the patient does not lose consciousness, the vertiginous episode may occur alone. Diagnosis may be difficult in these patients. In patients who lose consciousness, diagnosis should be much more apparent. An electroencephalogram may only be abnormal during the episode, which occasionally must be induced by hyperventilation, sleep deprivation, hypoglycemia, or barbiturate administration. In patients with posttraumatic or essential epilepsy, treatment with anticonvulsant agents is indicated.

F. Vertebrobasilar Migraine

Vertebrobasilar artery symptoms are frequently part of the migraine syndrome and may cause severe vertigo. Migraine headaches are preceded by an aura, the nature of which depends on the region most affected by ischemia during the vasoconstrictive phase. The clinical features of vertebrobasilar migraine arise from impairment of circulation to the brain stem. Any of the following symptoms may be apparent: vertigo, dysarthria, ataxia, paresthesias, diplopia, or visual field disturbances. Loss of consciousness may occur with involvement of the midbrain or reticular formation. One should suspect this condition when the vertigo is followed by a throbbing or occipital headache. The headache is frequently accompanied by vomiting, and the patient usually passes into a normal sleep. The episode has no neurologic or otologic sequelae, but the patient usually has a history of classic hemicranial migraine headaches and a family history of migraine. Therapy for this condition is difficult, and a neurologist should be consulted for this and other neurologic causes of vertigo.

G. Trauma

1. **Head injury** and trauma to the ear and temporal bone are discussed in Section I of this book and previously in this chapter, under benign paroxysmal positional vertigo. The vertigo following head trauma is usually of a positional type; however, small hemorrhages are found within the brain stem and vestibular nuclei in fatal cases of brain concussion. The differential pressures after severe head trauma are most pronounced in the brain stem and probably account for the frequency of posttraumatic dizziness when no peripheral abnormalities are demonstrable.
2. **Cervicogenic vertigo** The mechanism of vertigo caused by cervical trauma is not clear. The musculotendinous structures of the neck affect the vestibular nuclei complex through the spinovestibular tracts. Pain, spasm, and inflammation of these structures can result in strong asymmetric spinovestibular impulses, which, in turn, may produce sensations of dizziness and disequilibrium that may be increased by movement of the neck. Cervicogenic vertigo may also be caused by compression of the vertebral artery from osteoarthritis. Therapy includes application of local heat and administration of muscle relaxants and analgesics. Although immobilization in a cervical collar may be helpful, symptoms may persist for months.

H. Herpes Zoster Oticus

The Ramsay Hunt syndrome characteristically causes facial paralysis and a vesicular rash of the auricle. Occasionally, however, this disorder is associated with other neurologic symptoms, such as loss of facial sensation, tinnitus, hearing loss, and vertigo. The patient has unilateral, excruciating ear pain, as well as the other symptoms to a varying degree. The facial paralysis and the inner ear symptoms occur either simultaneously with the appearance of the vesicles or 7 to 10 days later. Treatment is controversial, but a short course of prednisone may decrease the edema of the cranial nerves. The patient may be given prednisone, 60 mg a day for 2 days, with the dose gradually reduced over a 2- to 3-week period. If the symptoms worsen, treatment may be extended for 4 to 6 weeks.

I. Vascular Insufficiency

This disorder must be considered in the differential diagnosis of vertigo, especially in patients over 50 years of age. This process may be important even in younger patients with diabetes, hypertension, or one of the hyperlipidemias. The presence of intrinsic cardiac disease, such as congestive heart failure or cardiac arrhythmias, must also be determined. Orthostatic or postural hypotension must be considered, especially if symptoms occur on arising after eating a meal. When the viscosity of the blood is too great, as in polycythemia vera or secondary polycythemias, vertebrobasilar artery insufficiency is common, with secondary vertigo and tinnitus.

1. **Vertebrobasilar artery insufficiency** Intermittent vertebrobasilar artery insufficiency may produce vertigo lasting from several minutes to several hours. Although vertigo may appear alone, it is frequently accompanied by visual disturbances, dysphagia, and dysarthria. Loss of consciousness and sensory or motor-function impairment may also be present. Compression of the vertebral artery may be at fault, or the disorder may result from the subclavian steal syndrome, in which the subclavian artery is occluded proximal to the origin of the vertebral artery. Flow may then reverse in the vertebral artery to produce symptoms of vertigo, diplopia, dysarthria, or syncope. One should search for a loud bruit or a palpable thrill in the supraclavicular fossa and a difference in the systolic blood pressure in the two arms.
2. **Lateral medullary syndrome of Wallenburg** also has vertigo as a prominent symptom. This syndrome is caused by infarction of the lateral portion of the medulla as a result of occlusion of the posterior inferior cerebellar artery. Symptoms include vertigo, nausea, vomiting, and nystagmus. The patient experiences ataxia and falls to the side of the infarction. The patient also notes a loss of pain and temperature sensation on the same side of the face and on the opposite side of the body. Dysphagia, ipsilateral paralysis of the palate and vocal cord, and ipsilateral Horner's syndrome complete the picture. Horner's syndrome consists of ptosis, myosis, and an ipsilateral decrease in facial sweating.
3. **Thrombosis of the internal auditory artery** Vascular occlusion of the internal auditory artery produces sudden hearing loss and loss of vestibular function. Initial symptoms may include vertigo, hearing loss, or tinnitus, whether alone or in combination. The symptoms appear suddenly and usually persist for days or weeks. The vertigo may be incapacitating until central compensation occurs.

J. Medications

The peripheral ototoxic effect of various drugs is described earlier in this chapter. A number of medications also induce vertigo through the central nervous system. Chronic ingestion of alcohol may induce vestibular disturbances, and lesions have been documented in the hypothalamus as well as in the neighborhood of the third ventricle and periaqueductal gray matter. Other medications affecting the auditory vestibular system at central levels include meperidine, morphine, mephenesin, barbiturates, antihistamines, phenytoin, trimethadione, indomethacin, sulfonamides, mercury, and gold. Although these effects are usually temporary, they may persist for extended periods. Spontaneous or positional nystagmus is frequently seen, especially after barbiturate ingestion. Hypervitaminosis D has been associated with vertigo, headache, and memory deficit. Vitamin deficiencies have also been associated with vertigo, the most common of which are deficiencies of vitamin B_1 (thiamine) and nicotinic acid.

K. Systemic Disorders

Thyroid dysfunction is known to induce deafness and ataxia. Hypoglycemia may also lead to vertigo. Vertigo has also been noted in patients with diabetic or carcinomatous neuropathy.

L. Syringobulbia

This condition is seen in patients with enlarging cavity formation within the medulla oblongata and frequently occurs in association with syringomyelia, which is a widening of the central canal within the spinal cord. The patient has a segmental sensory loss or dissociation (loss of pain and temperature sense and preservation of sense of touch) over the neck, shoulders, and arms. Thoracic scoliosis is also present. Symptoms usually begin in adult life; however, they may be seen in late childhood or adolescence. The symptoms progress irregularly and are often arrested for long periods. Treatment is far from satisfactory, and radiotherapy, formerly recommended, is probably worthless unless the patient has an underlying tumor.

M. Arnold-Chiari Malformation

This condition, in which the medulla and inferoposterior portions of the cerebellar hemispheres project through the foramen magnum, frequently results in obstructive hydrocephalus. It may occur in patients with syringomyelia and is usually associated with a spinal meningocele or myelomeningocele. The symptoms of hydrocephalus dominate the clinical picture in infants. In addition, a second type of Arnold-Chiari malformation may occur in patients who have no meningomyelocele. The clinical manifestations are varied. If the hydrocephalus is severe, however, the cranial sutures are widely separated and the anterior fontanelle much enlarged. The veins of the scalp are congested, and the frontal region bulges forward. These children seem little troubled by headache; however, convulsions are common, anosmia is present, and otic atrophy may also occur. Nystagmus is seen, along with limb weakness and incoordination.

N. Lermoyez's Syndrome

This rare variant of Ménière's disease is characterized by dramatic improvement in hearing, following a typical vertiginous spell.

O. "Illusory" Vertigo

This term can be used to describe the symptoms of patients who may have vertigo of psychiatric origin or who may be malingering. It is probably impossible to distinguish between the two because no test exists by which to determine whether the patient's unsteadiness or vertiginous spells are a result of some unresolved psychiatric conflict or whether they are inspired by secondary gain. Suspicion should arise if the audiogram is inconsistent, if the affect is inappropriate, or if secondary gain is achieved from the symptoms. Evasiveness and tangentiality are common in patients with vertigo; however, grossly inconsistent reports suggest "illusory" vertigo. If one suspects that the vertiginous episodes are a result of either psychiatric problems or malingering, appropriate psychiatric or psychologic referral should be made in a sympathetic manner, in the hope that this evaluation will be the first step to a resolution of the patient's symptoms.

11

AUDIOLOGY

HUBERT L. GERSTMAN

The objective of diagnostic audiology is threefold. First, it provides assistance in locating the site or sites of lesion. Second, it enables one to analyze the ability of patients to function in everyday communication and in special situations necessary to vocational and social adequacy. Third, it plays a role in rehabilitation, in which medical or surgical therapies are augmented by such techniques as hearing amplification and counseling. When medical and surgical procedures are inappropriate, the audiologist must manage the rehabilitation effort. It is not the object of this chapter to explain fully the branching logic related to test procedures. Readers must appreciate the tests described and resultant conclusions as generated by fully qualified independent professional workers.

I. AUDIOGRAMS

A. Hearing Sensitivity

The audiogram is a graphic representation designed to provide information for those who treat patients with hearing impairment. The baseline "0," rather than appearing at the lower part of the graph as is more common, appears in the upper portion, so most of the space of the graph is devoted to a "picture" of the pattern of hearing loss (Fig. 11–1). Because of various physical factors of resonance fluid mechanics, physical mechanics, and the reflecting, absorbing, and filtering properties of the ear, thresholds of acuity at various frequencies are not identical and follow a curvilinear path (Fig. 11–2). In audiometry, the "0" depicts the average, normal hearing at each frequency. Thus, the clinical audiogram is a third-level abstraction and does not present a "real" picture of

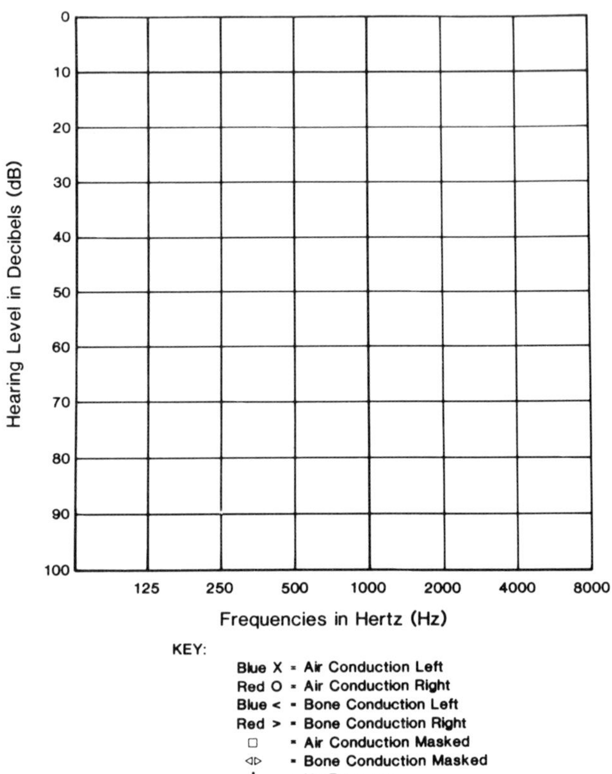

Fig. 11–1. The audiogram.

auditory function. Many clinics now use digital equipment that produces a digital audiogram, rather than the graph.

B. Masking

When measuring hearing, it is frequently necessary to introduce a noise into one ear while testing the other ear. This procedure is referred to as masking. The object of masking is to hold constant the effects of the testing situation, to enable one to determine which ear is being tested. Audiologists may mask with calibrated intensities, and it is thereby possible in electronic hearing tests to measure the amount of noise necessary to mask a sound in the opposite ear.

C. Hearing Impairment

Table 11–1 gives the degree of clinical hearing impairment associated with various audiometric scores.

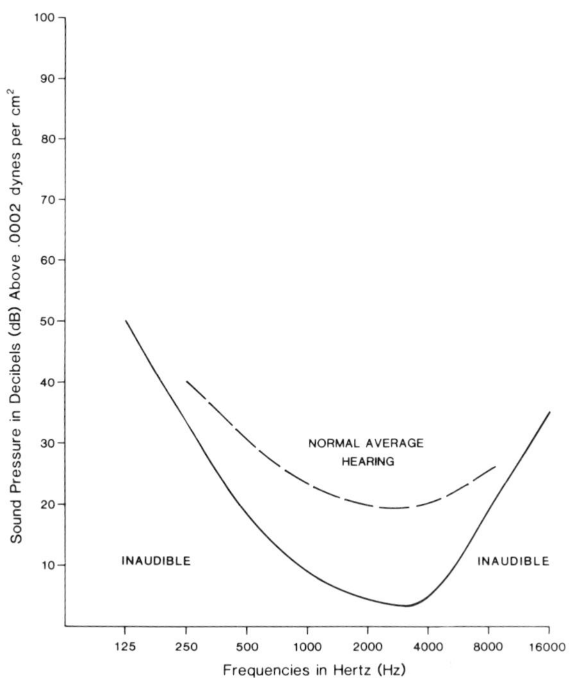

Fig. 11–2. Sensitivity of the human ear.

II. TESTS OF AUDITORY FUNCTION

A. Tuning Fork Tests

These tests are descriptive in nature, whereas audiometrics are aimed at more refined measurement. Tuning forks, in their pure-tone state, measure only low-frequency sound and depend on the nature of the mechanical energy applied for appropriate interpre-

TABLE 11–1

Description of Auditory Impairment Based on Pure-Tone Analysis

db HL*	Narrative descriptors
0–25	Range of normal hearing
26–30	Borderline hearing loss
31–40	Mild hearing loss
41–60	Moderate hearing loss
61–70	Moderately severe hearing loss
71–90	Severe hearing loss
90 to audiometric limits	Profound hearing loss

*db, Decibels; HL, hearing level (reference: average normal hearing)

tation. Overstriking of the forks yields numerous higher-frequency overtones that may or may not add to the sophisticated judgment necessary to interpretation. The commercially available Bárány noise boxes, frequently battery driven, are often too loud for necessary masking and may also be misleading, particularly to the inexperienced otologist, in patients with "dead ears" or significant unilateral hearing loss. To set a tuning fork into motion, the tines should be pinched, rather than struck. If struck, they should be struck lightly on the elbow or knee. The reliability of tuning fork testing depends on the ability of the user to pinch or to strike each fork with the same degree of force each time. Of course, this technique is difficult, and as a consequence, tuning fork tests may not be reliable. See Chapter 7.

B. Pure-Tone Audiometrics

1. **Pure-tone air-conduction audiometry,** through earphones, yields a measurement of the overall acuity of the patient's hearing. This basic measurement of auditory ability provides an audiogram that represents the pattern of hearing acuity in each ear.
2. **Pure-tone bone conduction audiometry** yields information on sensorineural reserve in each ear. A difference between bone conduction, stimulating the cochlea directly, and air conduction, through the external and middle ear, allows one to distinguish between conductive and sensorineural disorders. An air-bone gap of 10 decibels (db) or greater indicates the presence of a middle ear problem. When air- and bone-conducted patterns yield thresholds that are essentially the same, the sensorineural component is considered to be primary.

C. Tympanometry

Impedance, immittance, and tympanometry are terms used almost interchangeably in the discussion of this procedure. These tests deal with the area of compliance of the tympanic membrane and provide measures of stiffness, mass, and friction. The term immittance has developed as the generic term in the research literature. Clinically, one more frequently hears the term tympanometry applied to these procedures. At one level, tympanometry may be considered to be electronic, pneumatic otoscopy, although tympanometric measures yield far more information than that provided by otoscopy; we are interested in more than the mobility of the tympanic membrane itself. The reading is determined by the compliance of the tympanic membrane and the volume of the external canal. The normal tympanogram demonstrates that the tympanic membrane is maximally compliant at a state of zero air pressure, usually measured in mm H_2O, popularly referred to as millimhos. The tympanogram is analyzed in terms of location of the peak or point of maximum compliance, the shape of the graph, and the amplitude or height of the peak. The negative-pressure tympanogram indicates a retracted eardrum with essentially normal mobility and can be seen in a partial-effusion state.

D. Acoustic Reflex

This reflex may be elicited by ipsilateral or contralateral stimulation. Most current machines elicit contralateral reflex (sound stimulus in the side opposite to the test ear). The reflex is elicited by a loud sound. The benefit of a four-way reflex analysis, including both sides ipsilaterally and both sides contralaterally, is useful in determining the site of a lesion. Reflex responses vary from individual to individual and from frequency to frequency. In general, the acoustic reflex threshold is considered normal from about 70 to 100 db; reference: average normal hearing. Reflexes are usually reported to be within normal limits, elevated, or absent. On occasion, a reflex is elicited at much lower thresholds than normal, such as at thresholds lower than 70 db. This finding is usually associated with a cochlear disorder and is related to tolerance or recruitment. When retrocochlear lesions are suspected, the reflex-decay test should be administered.

E. Special Tests

1. **Adaptation and decay** The unimpaired auditory system is capable of processing the acoustic signal at a variety of amplitudes over a modestly sustained period. For instance, most pure tones may be processed at threshold for 60 sec without any interruption in the auditory function. A patient with a cochlear disorder may require an increase of some 5 to 15 db over threshold to maintain such a sound for 1 min. On the other hand, a patient with a retrocochlear disorder may adapt completely and may sustain no sounds for more than a few seconds, even though the sounds may reach high intensities at suprathreshold levels. A variety of modifications of the tone-decay tests have been proposed. Most audiologists use as a criterion a 1-min presentation while sustaining the tone between a 0- and a 20-db sensation level (patient's own threshold) for 60 sec. A similar test may be used in fixed-frequency Békésy audiometry, in which the patient tracks his own threshold on a self-recording audiometric device. Other forms of Békésy audiometry include sweep-frequency continuous versus pulsed-tone audiometry. Adaptation is also seen in this technique.

2. **Cochlear abnormality** One frequent behavioral consequence of cochlear loss is a reduced tolerance for loud sounds. This feature, in turn, is associated with the ability of the patient with cochlear impairment to sense smaller differences at moderate suprathreshold levels. The ear with cochlear damage relates to loudness values differently from the normal ear. The disorder relates in some manner to the propensity for the outer rows of hair cells to suffer more damage than the more pro-

tected inner row, as well as to the occasional occurrence of incomplete hair-cell damage to the cochlea. Whatever the exact physiologic cause, one is able to quantify cochlear damage with some specific tests.

a. ***Békésy audiometry,*** on a continuous trace basis, shows a narrower excursion between the just-noticeable-difference (JND) point and the just-not-noticeable-difference (JNND) point on the tracing.

b. ***Alternate binaural loudness balance (ABLB) testing*** requires the testing of a normal ear at the same frequency at which a patient has cochlear damage in the contralateral ear. One is then able to trace the abnormal increase in loudness and to document the cochlear disorder.

c. ***Short increment sensitivity index (SISI)*** If one runs a steady-state tone at a 20-db sensation level for a normal ear, the normal ear will detect 5-db intensity increases on that base tone. One is even able to detect 3-db increases of this sort. Only the abnormal cochlear ear detects 1-db increases consistently, however. This phenomenon only occurs at a lower, 20-db, sensation level. At higher levels, normal subjects become "sensitive." The SISI test usually involves 20 presentations of 1-db increments. A score of 70 to 100% is considered positive for cochlear impairment.

d. ***Tolerance tests*** The patient with cochlear impairment usually reacts to loud speech, masking noise, or other stimuli. A variety of loudness listening tests may be presented. For hearing aid use, we are interested in the most comfortable listening level (MCL), as well as in the uncomfortable listening level (UCL). This uncomfortable level indicates the need to modify the hearing aid in some way, to maintain the patient's comfort. This reduced tolerance is associated with the abnormal increase in loudness phenomena and explains the common complaint that some sounds are not loud enough and others too loud. The reduced "dynamic range" plays an important role in the rehabilitation of patients in need of sound amplification.

3. Speech Tests

a. ***Speech reception threshold (SRT) testing*** is similar in concept to pure-tone threshold testing, except it is for the lowest level at which speech is not only detected, but understood. The SRT should generally compare favorably with the best 2 of 3 frequency averages of pure-tone determinations at 500, 1000, and 2000 Hz. This pure-tone average comparison with SRT is frequently used to test the reliability of the patient or of the test conditions. The SRT serves as the sensation level for a variety of other speech tests, particularly the discrimination test.

b. ***Discrimination testing*** A variety of discrimination tests are available for estimating the amount (percentage) of what the patient typically hears and understands in continuous ongoing speech communication. Many of these tests involve word lists that are attempted to be phonetically balanced, to represent a loading of the various sounds and their frequency of occurrence in the language tested. The score is reported as a percentage of those words appropriately identified, that is, discriminated. The intelligibility function of the ear and the auditory system provides valuable behavioral information for both diagnostic and rehabilitative purposes. A person with normal sensory reserve and a conductive disorder generally discriminates 100% when the sounds are loud enough to overcome the disorder. In the patient with sensorineural hearing loss, intelligibility depends on a variety of factors; however, modestly reduced discrimination, allowing for intelligibility of 75 to 80%, is generally associated with cochlear disorders. Poor or absent functioning is usually associated with neural disorders. Other factors, such as the status of the cortex after a stroke, may influence the ability of the patient to perform this particular test exercise. Moreover, a variety of signal-to-noise conditions may influence the patient's ability to perceive speech. As a consequence, most clinics now present discrimination testing in both quiet and noisy backgrounds, varying from straightforward broadband white noise to speech-babble tapes. Some tests include cafeteria noise or speech babble. This procedure allows the measurement of behavioral function under "real" conditions. A variety of competing signal-type tests are included in the so-called central test battery, used to evaluate the ability of the auditory system on either side or on both sides when the competing messages are such that the processing system is tested, or when the cortical interpreting system is tested. Competing signals may be presented on the same side or on the contralateral side, or, as with the staggered spondaic word test (SSW), the noncompeting and competing activities are developed within the same test framework. Another variety of test, called filtered speech testing, falls into the same essential rubric. In filtered speech testing, one may filter out all the low-frequency sounds on one side and all the high-frequency sounds on the other side, to test the ability of the brain stem to fuse the impulses and to forward them to the brain.

F. Brain Stem Audiometry

Physiologic testing of the brain stem through evoked-response audiometry has been called by a variety of names in the literature, such as brain stem auditory evoked-response (BAER), brain stem evoked-response audiometry (BSER), and auditory brain stem response (ABR). ABR appears to be the most commonly accepted term at this time. Five waves are commonly generated, although more recent reports have discussed the sixth wave, and current research is investigating later waves as well. Waves after the sixth are commonly thought to be related to cognitive activity, whereas the first five waves are reliable and appear in essentially the same form in infants as in adults. Indeed, the indexes are so strong that they are now used in some intensive care units as measures of "brain death." It is thought that the ABR follows the ascending neurologic path, but a perfect one-to-one correspondence has not been established. Clinically, clicks are the most common stimuli, and latencies of specific waves and interwave latencies are the major parameters for determining abnormality. The procedure is typically applied to those who cannot respond to voluntary audiometry, such as infants and nonvocal children or adults. The procedure is also used in patients with suspected nonorganic impairment and for those with a suspected neurologic hearing disorder.

G. Nonorganic Hearing Loss

The audiologist may use many tests in patients with suspected functional nonorganic disorders or in suspected malingerers. The scope of this chapter does not allow a complete discussion of these procedures. However, it should be noted that a number of reflexive and physiologic conditions are correlated with various types of behavior that cannot be easily or reliably controlled by the patient, but can be measured and may be used to determine auditory thresholds.

III. HEARING AIDS AND AURAL REHABILITATION

A. Candidates for Amplification

Patients in need of amplification require the positive support of all those involved in the process. The United States Food and Drug Administration (FDA) now requires that all children who are candidates for hearing aid use be cleared by a physician. The FDA also recommends that all adults be similarly cleared, but the agency allows adults to sign a waiver if they so choose. The otolaryngologist is usually the physician who provides this clearance. The older literature indicated that patients with "perceptive" or "neurologic" hearing impairment were poor candidates for hearing aids. It is now time to put that shibboleth to rest because few people with impaired hearing do not benefit from amplification. Some benefit much more than others; however, modern electronics, miniaturization, and knowledge of acoustics of the ear and the hearing aid, as well as knowledge of the ear mold, now allow us to provide amplification to most patients. Certainly, the benefits are limited under a variety of conditions and situations, but analogously, one does not benefit from eyeglasses in a steamroom. Situations in which the normal auditor cannot hear because of the presence of noise are not usually corrected, for patients with hearing impairment, by the wearing of a hearing aid.

B. Types of Hearing Aids

Hearing aids come in several different styles, such as in-the-ear-canal models, all-in-the ear devices, behind-the-ear models, body-worn hearing aids, devices attached to the eyeglasses (eyeglass temples), and bone conduction oscillators, requiring either a separate oscillator piece or eyeglasses. Hearing aids are usually worn on the ipsilateral side of the damage. In patients with binaural hearing loss, one hearing aid is often fitted to each ear; these devices are called binaural hearing aids. In some cases, such as in patients with unilateral damage, the microphone is fitted to the side with hearing impairment, and the signal is routed to the amplifier on the side with normal hearing. The difference in the time of arrival of the signal, among other factors, is interpreted by the brain as "two-sided" hearing (contralateral routing of signal [CROS]). The so-called BICROS (bilateral-contralateral routing of signal) instrument routes the signal from the poorer ear to the better ear, but because the better ear also receives amplification, both signals come through the better side, and both are amplified. In unusual patients who require a considerable amount of power, the signal may be crossed, to separate the microphone from the receiver and thus to avoid false signals caused by feedback.

C. Determinants of Successful Hearing Aid Selection

1. **Clarity of signal** If we consider an impaired ear as one that has "noise" in the circuitry, then any hearing aid that adds to the noise becomes annoying, if not debilitating. Thus, the hearing aid should be internally "clean" and fitted to minimize noises generated by the body. One consideration in body-worn instruments is the amount of clothing noise, for instance. Assuming that the hearing aid is free from self-generated or internal noises, the next step is to attend to its microphone placement. The microphone should be placed to reduce the pickup of external noise and to "find" the signal on which the candidate is to focus. A recent device has a microphone embedded in its mold in the ear canal, to take full advantage of the pinna, which absorbs and reflects various sounds and performs a preliminary analysis on the incoming signal. Other advances include so-called directional microphones on behind-the-ear hearing aids. This phenomenon may also explain the popularity of the all-in-the-ear hearing aid, which imbeds all the amplification, electronics as well as the microphone, right at ear level. Currently, over 40% of sales are for all-in-the-ear or ear-canal instruments. The normal auditor has two ears; one function of the two-eared system is to separate signal from noise. Thus, if one may be fitted with binaural amplification, the success of this fitting may be attributed to the candidate's ability to separate signal from noise.
2. **Increased discriminatory ability** Most patients who have sensorineural hearing impairment sufficient to desire a hearing aid have a concomitant reduction in their ability to dis-

criminate among sounds. Increased discriminatory ability, when needed, should be a constant factor in the fitting of a hearing aid. Testing of the hearing aid candidate for noise discrimination is standard practice. An improvement in the patient's ability to discriminate noise from words distinguishes a satisfactory fitting from a poor fitting.

3. **Tinnitus** may be a consideration in the fitting of a hearing aid. The hearing aid itself may "mask" internal tinnitus sounds and may satisfactorily solve more than one problem at once. In some cases, the tinnitus is loud and annoying enough to be wholly debilitating. In such extreme cases, fitting of a tinnitus-masking hearing aid may be indicated. Such a hearing aid has continuously generated broad- or narrow-band white noise, depending on the nature of the tinnitus. A tinnitus masker may be combined with a hearing aid to alleviate both poor reception of speech and continuous tinnitus.

4. **Conductive hearing loss** When the conductive pathologic condition is inactive and a surgical procedure is not indicated, a hearing aid may be satisfactorily fitted. The limitations of such amplification affect only the sensorineural mechanism. When the sensorineural reserve approaches normal limits, the hearing aid selection is based primarily on the degree of gain needed.

5. **Infection** On occasion, the external or middle ear has an active infection that prohibits the fitting of an endaural insert. In such cases, a bone-conduction vibrator is fitted, and, as in pure-tone bone-conduction audiometry, the middle ear mechanism is thereby bypassed, and sound is directed to the inner ear. It is generally less desirable to use this fitting because of the amount of power needed to overcome the additional impedance offered by the skull and the additional power needed to drive the bone-conduction oscillator (on the order of 35 db). For the patient with sensorineural hearing loss, hearing aids may be satisfactorily selected from a dealer's stock, or they may be custom manufactured.

6. **Gain** is an important consideration that, among other things, determines whether a hearing aid may be worn at ear level or on the body, separating the microphone from the receiving elements and thereby eliminating feedback (squeal).

7. **Mechanical limitations** include frequency response, frequency emphasis, power limiting (control of maximum output), and the type of ear mold to be worn. Thus, patients with a high-frequency sensorineural hearing loss may be "brought into balance" with a hearing aid that improves their ability to perceive high frequencies. If the loss is severe enough, such patients may be offered a CROS aid. Patients with a tolerance or recruitment problem may be offered a hearing aid that

allows them satisfactory listening while controlling the degree of intensity that reaches the ear.

8. **Central difficulties** Although it is rare to find a person who cannot be helped by amplification, some patients have discriminatory abilities that are so reduced that amplification may be "unwarranted." Such patients most often have an eighth-nerve lesion, wherein discrimination is reduced and tone decay is present. In other patients, however, the effects of amplification are worth while, even when the effects are limited to the transmittal of background noise to the ear and nervous system.

9. **Hereditary, congenital or early childhood profound hearing loss** In such patients, the fitting of a hearing aid assumes an important role. In patients with the most profound hearing loss, one can generate some response to intense auditory stimulation, even if the response is a result of stimulation of the tactile sense. In fitting a hearing aid to a preverbal child or an infant, one hopes to deliver usable portions of the sound spectrum to the ear. In the absence of this possibility, one hopes to deliver some sensation that allows perception of the rhythm and stress patterns of speech and language as added cues to learning and understanding. Any auditory or quasiauditory experience can help in the training of the peripherally deaf child. Such fittings also contribute to the ongoing diagnostic process of ruling out other disorders that resemble deafness, such as psychologic disturbance, mental deficiency, and disorders of the central nervous system. **No child is ever too young for auditory evaluation or amplification.** Each individual patient's needs must be assessed. The patient must participate in the process of diagnosis and hearing-aid-selection because the patient provides information relative to factors such as comfort, ease of use, perceived benefits, and maintenance of the instrument. To overcome the patient's reluctance to adapt to hearing aid use, the team of specialists must be reassuring. Much of "aural rehabilitation" is counseling rather than teaching, treating, or directing.

IV. HEARING AID COUNSELING

A. Expectations of the Patient

The process of hearing aid selection must be integrated with the task of eliciting a positive response to the idea of wearing a hearing aid while educating the patient in the various limitations of amplification. As in most other clinical settings, the patient is typically seeking a "magic pink pill" to cure the ailment. Indeed, the most difficult patients frequently have worn hearing aids for many years and are still seeking an instrument that will restore their hearing to "normal."

B. Adaptation

The characteristic frequency response of a hearing aid produces a sound of low fidelity, often described by the wearer as "tinny." The reason for this reaction lies not only in the hearing aid itself, but also in the user's own acoustic system. The coupling may merely emphasize the degree of the hearing loss. Because the hearing aid has no curative powers as such, the individual's system does not improve. Any improvement occurs because of the patient's own ability to adapt, sometimes in spite of the hearing aid and its fitting.

C. Trial-and-Error Process

For learning to take place, time must pass; therefore, the hearing aid user must be convinced of the need to become accustomed to the device and must be forewarned not to expect immediate success in the new experience. The success of an aural rehabilitation program depends on the development of "the experimental attitude;" that is, the patient must be willing to engage in trial-and-error learning and must be encouraged to view the "misses" not as mistakes but as a learning experience.

D. Mechanical Considerations

The patient with a hearing aid must obviously be introduced to the mechanical elements of the instrument. One must learn to recognize when the battery has worn down and when the ear mold is dirty. The patient must also become familiar with the various adjustments, such as the telephone induction coil, the frequency-response switch, and the volume control wheel. These elements may not be as simple as they sound, but with practice, the patient should be able to adapt to the techniques required for his own particular needs. If possible, the audiologist should be available to the patient during the early period of adjustment to the hearing aid, to determine, for example, whether the battery is upside down or whether a malfunction actually exists, and thereby to prevent a "failure experience."

E. Hints for the Patient

1. **Try not to become overtired.**
2. **Use your eyes.**
3. **Begin with easier situations,** especially few people in quiet surroundings.
4. **Learn to concentrate.**
5. **Ask for help in following conversations,** especially the general topic under discussion.
6. **Maintain a comfortable volume level.**

F. Hints for the Patient's Family

1. **Face the person and speak distinctly.**
2. **Keep the room well lit,** especially so that your face can be easily seen.
3. **Do not shout.**
4. **Do not talk from another room.**
5. **Speak at eye level to the wearer of a hearing aid.**
6. **Do not smoke, chew, or cover your lips while speaking.**
7. **Tell the person the subject of the conversation.**
8. **Reduce background noise,** whether from open car windows, radio, television, or running water.
9. **Be patient.** The message may not be heard as you said it.
10. **Follow up with a written note,** for important messages.

III

NOSE AND SINUS

12

OLFACTION

ROBERT H. GILMAN

I. GENERAL PRINCIPLES

Smell and taste are the least understood of the special senses. Smell is a long-range system. The source of the stimulus may be at a considerable distance from the individual receiving the stimulus. In man, unlike in lower mammals, smell plays a small role in survival. Smell does contribute to the individual's perception of the environment, however. Disturbances of this sense may jeopardize both physical and emotional adaptation to this environment. The olfactory receptors, the most direct extension of the central nervous system in the body, are the only peripheral sensory receptors that are also first-order neurons. They have multiple higher and lower central nervous system connections, and their function may be affected by a variety of central disorders.

II. ANATOMIC AND PHYSIOLOGIC CONSIDERATIONS

A. Olfactory Threshold

The olfactory epithelium is located on the superior concha, the upper nasal septum, and the roof of the nose between them. Reception depends on the air flow's reaching the receptor areas. Olfactory threshold depends on the number of molecules of odorant per unit of time that reach the receptors. Therefore, **any mechanism that prevents the flow of air to the receptor area increases the olfactory threshold.** Sniffing decreases the olfactory threshold.

B. Adaptation

This term refers to the loss of perception for a continuously presented stimulus. The rate of adaptation is directly proportional to the strength of the odor. Perception of certain odors depends on trigeminal as well as olfactory nervous stimulation. For example, the smell of coffee is almost purely olfactory, whereas that of ammonia is considered almost purely sensory.

C. Localization

The ability to localize smell is poor in man, and what localization does exist is related more to the sensory than to the olfactory quality of the substance. For this reason, unilateral anosmia is seldom recognized by the patient and is easily missed by the physician.

D. Mechanism of Olfaction

"Hematogenous olfaction" is a misnomer. Some olfactory perception can be secondary to the excretion of the substance by the lungs; the substance then reaches the olfactory receptors by the exhalation of air. No direct odor perception exists from the vascular space.

E. Relation of Taste to Smell

Taste and smell are intimately related. Taste is less sensitive and more limited than smell; smell is of greater necessity for taste than taste is for smell. Hence, patients with smell disturbances often complain of decreased taste.

III. OLFACTORY TESTING

A. Definitions

1. **Minimum perceptible odor (MPO)** is the minimum concentration of odorant needed for individuals to recognize that they are smelling. Tests designed to measure this ability are tests of threshold.
2. **Minimum recognizable odor (MRO)** is the minimum concentration of odorant needed for individuals to recognize what they are smelling. Tests designed to measure this ability are tests of identification. MPO is more objective than MRO; MRO is also culturally and geographically dependent.
3. **Combined testing** In evaluating patients, most centers combine a test for threshold with a test for identification. Tests based on pupillary, cardiovascular, respiratory, cyclogalvanic, or electroencephalographic recording are available, but they are not practical for clinical use.

B. Methods and Apparatus

1. **Ehlsberg olfactometers** have been around since the 1930s and are simple to make and an easy way to measure olfactory threshold for MPO. The olfactometer is used to deliver a measured volume of specific odorant to each nostril separately to determine threshold. The apparatus consists of a 500-ml Erlenmeyer flask plugged with a foil-wrapped, 2-hole rubber stopper containing inlet and outlet glass tubing that projects

just inside of the container. The outlet tube is connected to a nosepiece. The inlet tube is connected to a 3-way stopcock with a 30-ml syringe attached. The flask is filled with 30 ml phenylethyl alcohol. To conduct the test, the 3-way stopcock is turned to prevent escape of the odorant from the bottle, and the syringe is then filled with air. The stopcock is then turned to close the air intake; one places the air-filled syringe in direct connection with the inlet tube. The patient holds his breath and occludes one nostril. The nosepiece on the outlet tube is then placed in the nonoccluded nostril. The examiner then blasts 2-ml odorant and asks the patient if he perceives the odor. If the patient cannot perceive the odor, the blast is increased by 2-ml increments until the patient's olfactory threshold is identified. The procedure is repeated 3 to 6 times until the average threshold is obtained. The procedure is then repeated for the opposite side of the nose. Thresholds increase with age; the mean threshold for perception in adults is about 11 ml.

2. **Doty smell identification test** The MRO is most easily tested clinically using the Doty smell identification test (DOT-SIT). This test uses a commercial microfragrance label with an accompanying multiple-choice questionnaire. The patient is asked to scratch the label, and thereby to release the odor, and to identify the odor from a list of possibilities. The portability and ease of administration of this test make it the best available for smell identification. The test manual explains the administration of the test and its interpretation and is available commercially.

IV. DISTURBANCES IN OLFACTION

These disorders are outlined in Table 12–1.

V. TREATMENT OF OLFACTORY DISORDERS

The treatment is, whenever possible, directed at the cause of the disturbance, which, most commonly, is nasal obstruction. Treatment may include the removal of obstructing nasal lesions, allergic desensitization, or the replacement of estrogens, steroids or vitamin A in those deficiency states. See Chapter 13.

A. Medical Treatment

Some patients in the postinfluenza and idiopathic group (see Table 12–1) seem to respond to medical treatment with one of the following regimens:

1. **Vitamin A** 100,000 U intramuscularly once per week for 6 weeks, followed by 50,000 U orally per day for 12 weeks. Alternately, one may give vitamin A, 100,000 U orally once per

TABLE 12–1

Disturbances in Olfaction

I. Hyperosmia: increased acuity of smell
   A. Causes of lower thresholds
      1. Hunger
      2. Nausea
      3. Obesity
      4. Occupation (wine tasters, perfumers)
      5. Cystic fibrosis
      6. Addison's disease (untreated; relieved with steroids)
      7. Strychnine poisoning
      8. Virilizing nonhypertensive congenital gonadal hyperplasia
   B. Olfaction appears sharpest with intermediate nasal swelling and with increased temperature and humidity
   C. Women show greater olfactory acuity than men; olfactory acuity lowest at ovulation

II. Parosmia: abnormal smell (dysosmia)
   A. Cacosmia: unpleasant smell
   B. Causes of parosmia
      1. Streptomycin
      2. Skull fracture
      3. Uncus injury
      4. Impending anosmia
      5. Recovering anosmia
      6. Influenza sequela
      7. Sinusitis

III. Phantosmia: hallucination of smell
   A. Schizophrenia
   B. Temporal lobe seizures
      1. Lesions of the hippocampus, uncinate gyrus, or amygdala
      2. Often likened to the odor of burning flesh

IV. Hyposmia: decreased smell acuity (higher thresholds)
   A. Presbyosmia: age-related hyposmia
   B. Hypogonadism (female; relieved with estrogens)
   C. Tobacco (reversible)
   D. Upper respiratory infection (reversible)
   E. Radiation therapy (reversible)
   F. Olfactory membrane removal
   G. Pregnancy (especially the second and third trimesters)
   H. Diabetes
   I. Vitamin A deficiencies

TABLE 12–1 (Continued)

V. Anosmia: complete loss of smell
  A. Intranasal
    1. Airway obstruction (most common cause)
      a. Vasomotor rhinitis
      b. Allergic rhinitis and polyps
      c. Ethmoid sinusitis
      d. Nasal tumor
      e. Nasopharyngeal tumor
      f. Choanal atresia
    2. End-organ disease
      a. Atrophic rhinitis, ozena
      b. Exposure to industrial (alkaline battery) fumes
      c. Nutritional deficiencies (vitamin A, zinc, copper)
  B. Intracranial
    1. Traumatic (7.5% of head injuries)
      a. Shearing of olfactory nerve
      b. Contusion of the olfactory bulbs
      c. Hemorrhage at the base of the frontal lobes
      d. Fracture of the cribriform plate (LeFort II or III, frontoethmoid)
    2. Infectious
      a. Influenzal sequela
      b. Osteomyelitis of the frontoethmoid area
      c. Brain abscess of the frontal lobe
      d. Meningitis of the frontal lobes
      e. Syphilis of the olfactory nerves or meninges
    3. Tumor-related
      a. Frontal-lobe tumor
      b. Meningioma of the olfactory groove or sphenoidal ridge
      c. Vascular tumor of the floor of the anterior fossa
      d. Pituitary or parasellar tumor
      e. Esthesioneuroblastoma
    4. Vascular
      a. Arteriosclerosis of the anterior cerebral artery
      b. Cerebrovascular accidents
    5. Other
      a. Iatrogenic (postlaryngectomy)
      b. Epilepsy
      c. Diabetes mellitus
      d. Pernicious anemia
      e. Lead poisoning
      f. Cadmium poisoning
      g. Amphetamine toxicity
      h. Pseudohypoparathyroidism
  C. Congenital
    1. Congenital hypogonadal eunuchoidism
    2. Familial dysautonomia
    3. Turner's syndrome
    4. Kallmann's syndrome
  D. Hysterical

day for 2 weeks, followed by 50,000 U once daily for 6 to 12 weeks.

2. **Zinc sulfate,** 220 mg orally 3 times daily.
3. **Prednisone,** 60 mg a day for 3 days, followed by 40 mg a day for the next 3 days, 20 mg a day for the next 3 days, 10 mg a day for 2 days, and 5 mg on the last day.
4. **Cocaine,** applied topically and repeatedly to the olfactory epithelium, with 2 drops of 10% cocaine once daily for a month and then discontinued for a month; the process should be repeated again for a month. This regimen should be continued for an additional 2 months if successful. If unsuccessful, alternate-month treatment can be continued for up to a year. The topical anesthetic tetracaine has been used in place of cocaine.
5. **Other medications** that have been recommended at various times in the past include strychnine, vitamin B complex, and vitamin E.

B. Nonmedical Treatment

Some nonmedical methods for aiding patients with olfactory dysfunction have also been advocated. Because individuals with a decreased ability to smell often lose their enthusiasm for eating, it is important to try to stimulate the patient's appetite, to encourage proper nutrition. The addition of commercially available simulated food odors during cooking has been advocated to make foods more palatable to patients with olfactory dysfunction. Odor-amplified foods seem to be preferred by persons with hyposmia. Another technique is simply the encouragement of individuals with hyposmia to chew their food longer because the further masticatory breakdown of food allows the release of more molecules of odorant to interact with the smell receptors. Moreover, rapid alternation among various foods on one's plate lessens the degree of adaptation to any one food type and maximizes the amount of odor in a meal. Finally, attention to the textural quality and variety of food can help to compensate for losses in olfactory acuity and may stimulate an interest in foods. Consultation with a registered dietitian can be of great benefit.

13

NASAL OBSTRUCTION

JULIUS DAMION

I. MEDICAL HISTORY AND PHYSICAL EXAMINATION

A. Medical History

Nasal obstruction is one of the most common complaints in otolaryngology. Numerous local and systemic causes of nasal disease may result in nasal obstruction, and its evaluation is based on medical history, physical examination, roentgenograms, and laboratory tests. A diagnosis of allergic, vasomotor, or drug-induced obstruction is frequently made by the patient's medical history. Previous surgical intervention or trauma should suggest the possibility of perforations, scarring, or synechiae. The patient should be questioned about the time of onset and duration of the symptoms, their laterality, and whether they are constant or intermittent. Mucosal changes usually produce bilateral obstruction, whereas structural anomalies may cause either unilateral or bilateral obstruction. Constant obstruction usually indicates an anatomic problem; seasonal obstruction is associated with allergic disorders. The association of nasal obstruction with environmental irritants or food should be noted, and one should record all topical and systemic medications used, including over-the-counter nasal sprays. Metabolic or endocrine alterations, as in hypothyroidism, diabetes mellitus, or pregnancy, may contribute to nasal obstruction. A variety of nonnasal complaints may result from mechanical obstruction of the nose or of the structures opening into it, such as the sinuses, the lacrimal system, and the middle ear. Thus, the patient may complain of a dry tongue, halitosis, sore throat, postnasal drip, snoring, sinus headache, nasal discharge, resonance changes, toothache, tearing, fullness of the ears, and hearing loss.

B. Assessment of the Whole Patient

The mannerisms of a patient or the unusual importance attributed to certain features of the nose may indicate a psychologic or emotional disturbance superimposed on any nasal problem. A patient's habits or breathing patterns may offer clues to the nature of the problem; for example, a collapsing nasal valve is suggested by a patient who pushes the ipsilateral cheek up and away from the nose to improve nasal patency.

C. External Nose Assessment

The shape of the nose is a limiting factor in the size of the nasal airway. A nose that is narrow, either because of heredity or as a sequela of rhinoplasty, is likely to have a compromised nasal airway. The external nose may be evaluated by considering each of its components: the bony pyramid, the cartilaginous pyramid, and the tip. Deviation, depression, or other deformities of any of these structures may indicate the cause of the nasal airway obstruction.

D. Internal Nose Assessment

The internal and external nose should be considered as two parts of a unit, structurally and functionally related. The initial examination of the internal nose is made by examining the relationship among the nares, columella, septum, and lateral walls with a strong light source, but without a potentially distorting nasal speculum. This method may be the most productive way of examining the internal nose of a small child. The nasal speculum is then used to examine the deeper intranasal structures, including the septum, the turbinate bones, and the mucosa. One should note the character of the mucosa and the presence of crusts, blood, odor, and discharge. The nasal examination is then repeated following topical vasoconstriction and anesthesia, if necessary. This technique aids in visualizing structures hidden by mucosal congestion, and the degree of improvement in the patency of the nasal airway helps one to determine how much of the obstruction is caused by congestion and how much by structural anomalies. Palpation of intranasal structures helps in their characterization and identification.

E. Nasopharyngeal Assessment

Despite the availability of flexible fiberoptic endoscopes, the best instruments for examining the nasopharynx remain a head mirror, a light source, and a nasopharyngeal mirror. Topical anesthesia of the orpharynx is often necessary during prolonged observation. Relaxation of the soft palate is promoted when the patient says "ah-haa" or when the patient breathes nasally throughout the examination.

II. SPECIAL DIAGNOSTIC TESTS

A. Culture and Sensitivity Tests

These tests should be performed when a patient has any purulent discharge.

B. Nasal Smears

These tests are useful for distinguishing allergy, which is characterized by eosinophil predominance, from infection, which is characterized by neutrophil predominance.

C. Skin or Radioallergosorbent (RAST) Tests

These tests are useful in identifying inhalant or food allergies.

D. Sinus Roentgenograms

Mucosal thickening is associated with allergies, whereas sinus opacity and air-fluid levels suggest infection.

E. Polytomographic and Computed Tomographic (CT) Scans

These studies allow one to delineate the extent of neoplasms.

F. Other Tests

Other useful diagnostic measures include glucose tolerance and thyroid function tests.

III. MUCOSAL CHANGES

A. Physiologic Changes

1. **Nasal cycle** Eighty percent of the population experience the physiologic alternation of congestion and decongestion of the nasal turbinates that is termed the "nasal cycle." The alternation occurs, on the average, every 2.5 hours, and this physiologic activity decreases with age. Because the total nasal airway resistance remains constant throughout the normal nasal cycle, the patient usually does not complain unless the congestive phase is abnormally long or unless an underlying obstruction is present. An increased awareness of the characteristics of the normal cycle may prompt the patient to report that the obstruction alternates between one nasal passage and the other, however.
2. **Positional obstruction** of the nasal airway is another normal physiologic occurrence. While the patient is lying on either side, the dependent side of the nose becomes obstructed, with congestion of the turbinate occurring in 20 minutes. Persons with a pre-existing obstruction of the nasal airway usually sleep on the side of the obstruction because placement of the open nasal passage in the dependent position promotes bilateral obstruction.

B. Pathologic Changes

1. **Metabolic and endocrine alterations** that cause nasal obstruction include pregnancy and the menstrual cycle (most common), hypothyroidism, and diabetes mellitus. Congested, edematous mucosa often produces nasal obstruction in the second and third trimesters of pregnancy. Nasal stuffiness and polyposis have been associated with diabetes mellitus. A diagnostic workup for these underlying causes should include a glucose tolerance test and thyroid function tests, with endocrinologic consultation for treatment as indicated.

2. **Allergic rhinitis** In this disorder, an antigen stimulates a sensitive nasal epithelium to produce IgE, which reacts with receptor sites on mast cells and basophilic leukocytes. The subsequent release of histamine and other pharmacologic mediators produces vascular dilation, glandular secretion, and smooth muscle contraction and results in the mucosal edema, rhinorrhea, sneezing, and itching of the eyes and nose characteristic of allergic rhinitis. Seasonal allergic rhinitis is usually caused by inhalants and involves sneezing, lacrimation, and a watery nasal discharge. Perennial allergic rhinitis is caused by dusts, molds, and danders, is worse in the heating season, and is characterized by persistent mucoid drainage. Foods have also been implicated, in particular eggs, citrus fruits, corn, wheat, and other grains. A family history of allergic rhinitis is common. Examination discloses a bluish or pale nasal mucosa with a thin, watery discharge. A purulent discharge is produced by secondary infection. Nasal polyps are commonly associated with allergic rhinitis. Lacrimation, conjunctivitis, chemosis, and a transverse nasal crease from a child's "allergic salute" may be present.

   Diagnosis is made on the basis of the patient's symptoms, in association with exposure to possible allergens, and is supported by the presence of eosinophils or mast cells on a nasal smear, positive results on RAST or intradermal tests, and a total peripheral eosinophil count greater than 600 or an elevated serum IgE level. The initial treatment for allergic rhinitis is avoidance of the allergen. Medical management for prophylaxis and symptomatic relief includes the following:

   a. ***Sympathomimetic agents*** counteract the effects of vasoactive mediators; examples are epinephrine, pseudoephedrine, and phenylpropanolamine.
   b. ***Antihistamines*** are most effective when given prophylactically (competitive inhibitors); examples are diphenhydramine (Benadryl), chlorpheniramine maleate (Chlor-trimeton), and dexchlorpheniramine maleate (Polaramine). Antihistamines are also available in combination with sympathomimetic agents; examples are Actifed, Dimetapp, and Drixoral.
   c. ***Cromolyn*** blocks mediator release from mast cells.

d. ***Topical corticosteroids*** may be helpful, but prolonged use is not advised because of systemic absorption; examples are dexamethasone and beclomethasone.
e. ***Systemic corticosteroids*** may be indicated in the short-term treatment of severe symptoms; a typical regimen is prednisone, 50 mg orally, once a day for 2 days.
f. ***Intranasal corticosteroid injection*** may give excellent results, but blindness has been reported following intravascular injection.
g. ***Immunotherapy*** is indicated when avoidance of the allergen is impractical and when medical management does not control the symptoms.

3. **Atrophic rhinitis** Atrophy of the nasal mucosa and turbinates may be a result of aging or of nasal trauma, or it may be idiopathic. Although nasal airway resistance is decreased, patients paradoxically complain of nasal obstruction. Mucopurulent, malodorous crusts are present in the nasal passages. Therapy is aimed at debridement of crusts and restoration of normal nasal mucosa; this goal is promoted by douching the affected area with saline solution.

4. **Bacterial rhinitis** The hallmark of bacterial rhinitis is mucopurulent discharge, usually produced by a gram-positive organism. Coagulase-positive staphylococci are a common cause of this disorder and often colonize the nares and nasopharynx of hospital personnel. Streptococci may also produce rhinitis, but with accompanying pharyngitis and systemic symptoms. Gram-negative organisms capable of producing rhinitis include Haemophilus influenzae, Escherichia coli, and salmonellae. Treatment involves the administration of appropriate antibiotics. Material for culture should be obtained from a patient who is seriously ill or who is not responding to conventional treatment. By using a head mirror with adequate lighting, one may find that the discharge emanates from a sinus ostium. See Chapter 15.

5. **Fungal rhinitis** As opportunistic pathogens, fungi are most likely to be found in patients with underlying systemic disorders such as leukemia or diabetes, or in those treated with immunosuppressive agents or radiation. The most likely organisms are candida, aspergillus, nocardia, cryptococcus, and phycomycetes. Infection is characterized by purulent nasal discharge and may involve necrosis of the septum,palate, orbit, and sinuses. Treatment is directed against the underlying disorder as well as against the fungus. See Chapter 15.

6. **Drug-induced rhinitis (rhinitis medicamentosa)** The prolonged use of topical nasal decongestants causes a rebound congestion of the nasal mucosa. This disorder may encourage further use of the decongestant, with a resulting rhinitis medicamentosa. Systemic medications, such as rauwolfia derivatives

for hypertension, may also cause nasal congestion (see Table 13–1). Intranasal examination reveals a red, hypertrophied, and granular-appearing mucosa. Treatment consists of discontinuing all topical nasal preparations and the suspect systemic medications. A steroid spray may be substituted for topical decongestants. Such a spray will help restore a more normal airway; however, the patient must avoid the temptation of reinstituting topical nasal decongestants. The nasal mucosa usually recovers slowly; the patient should be re-examined to confirm the absence of an underlying structural abnormality.

7. **Vasomotor rhinitis** is excessive engorgement of the nasal mucosa and profuse watery rhinorrhea secondary to autonomic dysfunction and characterized by a cholinergic discharge. The disorder is triggered by chemical irritants, changes in weather or humidity, or by stress. The obstruction is of greater degree and duration than the normal congestion-decongestion reflex and occurs in the absence of allergy. Examination reveals pale,

TABLE 13–1

Drugs Causing Nasal Obstruction

Agent	*Effect*
Alcohol	Engorgement of nasal membranes
Antithyroid drugs	Nasal congestion
Aspirin	Activation of peripheral chemoreceptors that control the vascular bed of the respiratory tract, with consequent nasal stuffiness
Cocaine	Local vasoconstriction and paralysis of sensory nerves
Ephedrine	Destruction of cilia; production of squamous metaplasia; vasodilation; sclerosis; vasoconstriction
Epinephrine	Vasoconstriction followed by congestion secondary to reactive hyperemia and vasodilation
Estrogen, progestins	Engorgement of nasal mucosa
Hashish, marijuana	Irritation of the respiratory tract with consequent nasal congestion
Iodides	Increase of mucous secretion
Lycopodium (used as a coating for pills)	Nasal obstruction
Rauwolfia serpentina (reserpine)	Nasal congestion and rhinitis by cholinergic action
Tobacco	Irritation of mucous membranes and impairment of ciliary action

(Adapted from Blue, J.A.: Overmedication of nasal mucosa. Mod. Med., *37*:90, 1969.)

swollen, polypoid turbinates. Eosinophils are rarely found on nasal smears, and allergic skin testing is negative.

Symptomatic treatment includes the use of oral decongestants and antihistamine preparations. Topical corticosteroids may be beneficial. Surgical management of intractable cases includes electrocautery or cryocautery of turbinate mucosa, submucous resection of the turbinates, or vidian neurectomy.

8. **Viral rhinitis** Acute viral rhinitis or the "common cold" is the most common cause of nasal obstruction. Other symptoms include the acute onset of malaise, sore throat, serous or seromucous nasal discharge, and irritation that produces sneezing. A nasal smear demonstrates the predominance of neutrophils. Because this disease is self-limited, treatment is symptomatic and consists of rest, ingestion of fluids, humidification, and administration of analgesics and topical decongestants. Antibiotics are reserved for the complication of bacterial infection of the upper respiratory tract.

IV. STRUCTURAL CHANGES

A. Cartilaginous and Bony Changes

1. **Septal anomalies**
   a. ***Deviation*** of the cartilaginous or bony septum, with resulting nasal obstruction, is usually caused by trauma. Associated bony spurs may add to the obstruction and may predispose the patient to epistaxis. Those with long-standing septal deviation have a compensatory hypertrophy of the turbinate on the concave side. Submucous resection of the nasal septum or septoplasty may be employed to improve the nasal airway.
   b. ***Hematoma or abscess*** The most common cause of septal hematoma, which is a collection of blood between the mucoperichondrium and the septal cartilage, is surgical or nonsurgical trauma to the nose. Diagnosis is made by identifying a widened septum that is soft on palpation. Treatment includes topical application of cocaine to the nasal mucosa, incision and drainage of the hematoma, and packing of the nose to prevent reaccumulation of fluid. Failure to drain a septal hematoma may lead to pressure necrosis of the septal cartilage, with loss of nasal support, or to formation of a septal abscess. Such an abscess may be diagnosed by a history of nasal trauma in the presence of a tender, warm, erythematous, fluctuant mass representing a collection deep to the mucoperichondrium of the nasal septum. Treatment includes incision and drainage and the administration of intravenous penicillin. Failure to treat a septal abscess may result in rapid septal destruction, with a risk of cavernous sinus thrombosis.

c. ***Perforation*** Trauma is the most common cause of septal perforation. Nonsurgical trauma includes digital injury, cocaine abuse, inhalation of chemicals, inflammatory conditions, such as septal abscess, tuberculosis, and syphilis, and granulomatous disorders, such as Wegener's granulomatosis and sarcoidosis. Symptoms include recurrent epistaxis, crusting, whistling, and nasal obstruction. Diagnosis is easily made on examination of the septum after careful removal of crusts. Initial management consists of humidification and application of petroleum jelly or antibiotic ointment, to control crusting and epistaxis. Further treatment may include surgical or nonsurgical closure, with the insertion of a Silastic button.

2. **Collapse of alar cartilage** is caused by prior trauma, cartilaginous resorption, loss of cartilaginous resilience, or hereditary factors. Diagnosis is made by observing the approximation of the ala nasi to the columella on inspiration and the consequent obstruction of the inflow of air. Definitive management is surgical.

3. **Valving** The nasal valve is a 10 to 15° angle between the caudal end of the upper lateral cartilage and the nasal septum. If the valve is unusually narrow or if it is collapsible, the patient will have a sensation of nasal obstruction on inspiration. Diagnosis is made by confirming the presence of a narrow valve on intranasal examination, by observing the external nose on deep inspiration, and by noting an improvement of the nasal airway on insertion of a speculum or on lateral traction on the cheek. The treatment for severe cases is surgical.

4. **Bony turbinate hypertrophy** A prominent bony inferior turbinate may touch the septum and may shrink minimally when vasoconstrictors are applied. Differentiation between soft tissue engorgement and bony hypertrophy is made by palpation. Treatment consists of submucous resection of the obstructing portion of the bony turbinate.

B. Soft Tissue Changes

1. **Adenoidal hypertrophy** Hypertrophy of the adenoids is a common cause of nasal obstruction in children. Mouth breathing, snoring, sleep disturbance, and a history of frequent upper respiratory infections are characteristics of this disorder. These patients may have "adenoid facies" and middle ear effusions. Excessive adenoidal tissue is seen on mirror examination of the nasopharynx or directly through the nares after vasoconstriction. The presence of such excessive tissue may be confirmed by lateral neck radiography. If the disorder is sufficiently symptomatic, the patient may need an adenoidectomy; otherwise, the adenoidal tissue is expected to regress with time.

2. **Nasal and choanal polyps** **Nasal polyps** are composed of

edematous, hyperplastic mucosa, they occur bilaterally in clusters, and they involve the ethmoid sinuses. Patients have nasal obstruction, sinusitis, and in some severe cases, a widened midface. These polyps are common in persons with allergic or vasomotor rhinitis and are also seen in children with cystic fibrosis. Therefore, it is essential that any child with nasal polyps undergo a sweat test. Such polyps also occur as part of the "asthma triad": intrinsic asthma, aspirin sensitivity, and nasal polyposis. Topical corticosteroid sprays may be tried if the polyps are small and few. If this regimen is not successful or if the polyps are well established, nasal polypectomy is the treatment of choice. When preoperative sinus roentgenograms indicate involvement of the maxillary, ethmoid, and sphenoid sinuses, intranasal or external ethmoidectomy, maxillary antrotomy, and sphenoidotomy may be indicated to remove the diseased mucosa. Topical beclomethasone spray may decrease the incidence of postoperative recurrence. By contrast, a **choanal polyp** is a large, single mass that originates in the maxillary sinus and is treated by surgical removal, with a maxillary antrotomy.

3. **Neoplasms** of the nasal cavities and sinuses are uncommon. They are characterized by progressive, unilateral nasal obstruction, purulent rhinorrhea, and epistaxis. Biopsy for tissue diagnosis may be performed either in the office or the operating room. **Papillomas** are benign, wart-like tumors found on the septum or the lateral wall of the nose. Treatment involves excision by electrocautery. **Inverting papillomas** occur concomitantly with nasal polyps, usually on the lateral wall of the nose. Unlike ordinary papillomas, these lesions are unilateral and are locally invasive. Advanced cases show bony destruction. Treatment is by wide excision with lateral rhinotomy. A 30% recurrence rate and 10 to 15% rate of malignant degeneration have been reported. Other benign tumors of the nasal cavities are **osteomas, adenomas,** and **mixed salivary tumors.** Nasal obstruction with facial pain, paresthesias, and epistaxis should alert the physician to the possibility of a malignant tumor of the nasal passages or nasopharynx. **Squamous cell carcinoma** of the septum is seen as an ulcerative, friable lesion. Squamous cell carcinoma of the sinuses is insidious and may grow to a substantial size before detection. Other malignant lesions of the nasal cavities and nasopharynx include **adenocystic carcinoma, melanoma, basal cell carcinoma,** and **sarcoma.** Unilateral or bilateral nasal obstruction with epistaxis in an adolescent male is suggestive of a **juvenile nasopharyngeal angiofibroma.** Diagnosis is made on inspection of the nasopharynx visually and radiographically. Biopsy should not be performed in the office because of the vascularity of the tumor. Embolization may be performed prior to surgical excision. **Nasopharyngeal carcinoma** is common in southern Chinese pop-

ulations and is uncommon in Caucasians. It becomes manifest most commonly as a unilateral serous otitis media in the adult and may have associated posterior cervical adenopathy and cranial nerve palsies. Because of its location, primary treatment is usually by radiotherapy.

4. **Wegener's granulomatosis** affects both sexes, most frequently in the fourth or fifth decades of life. It causes acute necrotizing lesions of the upper respiratory tract, glomerulonephritis, and acute, focal necrotizing vasculitis. Signs and symptoms include nasal obstruction, bloody nasal discharge, and distortion of facial contour. Treatment consists of cyclophosphamide with corticosteroids. Remissions occur in 95% of patients.

C. Traumatic Changes

1. **Postsurgical obstruction** Nasal obstruction may be caused by an undercorrected septal deformity or by an overzealous removal of septal cartilage that results in nasal collapse. The apposition of two raw surfaces within the nose, whether the result of surgical or blunt trauma to the nose or of the difficult passage of a nasogastric tube, may cause the formation of synechiae, scars, and stenosis. These changes produce nasal obstruction, easily diagnosed by intranasal inspection. Treatment is by surgical excision.

2. **Blunt trauma** Acute injury to the nose may produce airway obstruction from a septal dislocation, a septal hematoma, or a displaced nasal fracture. Reduction of traumatic nasal deformities in infants is generally easy because of the largely cartilaginous composition of the nose. Dislocation that produces nasal airway obstruction in children should be reduced as soon as possible; otherwise, a delayed functional or cosmetic abnormality may result. In an unco-operative child, it may be necessary to examine and reduce such a dislocation under general anesthesia. Nasal and facial bone roentgenograms are obtained for medicolegal purposes and usually add only incidental information to the clinical examination. Immediate intranasal examination is necessary to identify a septal hematoma, a deviation, or a mucosal laceration. If a patient with nasal trauma is seen prior to the development of edema and ecchymosis, one may reduce a fracture or dislocation immediately. Otherwise, the patient should be re-evaluated in 5 days for possible reduction of the fracture or dislocation. Septorhinoplasty may be indicated if closed reduction of traumatic nasal deformities is unsuccessful.

D. Congenital Disorders

1. **Midline nasal mass** in a young patient who has had meningitis should raise the suspicion of a nasal encephalocele, a glioma, or dermoid cyst. Each may be associated with bony cranial

defects, intracranial anomalies, and leakage of cerebrospinal fluid. An **encephalocele,** a protrusion of part of the cranial contents through a defect in the skull, may be seen as an external or an intranasal mass. It is typically blue, soft, compressible, and may be transilluminated. The ability to pass a probe lateral, but not medial, to an intranasal encephalocele differentiates it from a polyp. The mass is pulsatile and expands with compression of the jugular veins (positive Furstenberg test). A **glioma** is an encephalocele that has lost its intracranial connection. It may occur as an external or intranasal red, noncompressible mass that does not transilluminate. The Furstenberg test is negative. A **dermoid,** which is an ectodermal cyst containing dermal appendages, is an external or intranasal firm, noncompressible, nonpulsatile mass, associated with a pit on the nasal dorsum. Until the absence of an intracranial connection has been confirmed, manipulation of the midline nasal mass is to be avoided. If radiologic evaluation demonstrates intracranial attachments, neurosurgical consultation should be obtained, and intracranial exploration and resection should be performed. Extracranial resection of the remaining mass may be accomplished either then or later.

2. **Choanal atresia** is the failure of the bucconasal membrane to rupture at the seventh to eighth week of gestation. The atresia may be unilateral, bilateral, membranous, or bony. Unilateral atresia may be unsuspected in infancy. The patient has unilateral nasal obstruction and mucoid discharge. Diagnosis is made by the inability to pass a catheter through the nose into the pharynx or by the failure of radiopaque dye to pass from the nasal cavity into the nasopharynx. Treatment is by surgical correction. Bilateral atresia is an airway emergency in the newborn because newborns are obligate nose breathers. Respiratory distress and cyanosis are present and are relieved by crying. A bilateral nasal discharge is seen. Diagnosis is made by the inability to pass a catheter into the pharynx through either nasal cavity. A McGovern nipple taped to the mouth secures an oral airway prior to surgical correction.
3. **Congenital atresia,** a rare cause of nasal obstruction, is associated with a severe external nasal deformity, as well as with other midface and cranial anomalies.

V. OBSTRUCTION BY FOREIGN BODY

Unilateral nasal obstruction with a foul-smelling discharge in a child or a mentally disturbed person is suggestive of an intranasal foreign body. If mucosal ulceration has occurred, epistaxis may be present. Treatment is immobilization of the patient, application of topical vasoconstrictors and anesthetics, suctioning to find the foreign body, and removal of the foreign body. General anesthesia may be required for unco-operative patients. A rhinolith begins as an intranasal foreign body, which eventually becomes encrusted and calcified. Symptoms are those of an intranasal foreign body, and treatment is by removal.

14

EPISTAXIS

VICTOR E. CALCATERRA

I. ETIOLOGIC FACTORS

The search for a predisposing cause is an essential component in the treatment of epistaxis.

A. Local Factors

Such factors should not be overlooked.

1. **Broken blood vessels** The most common cause of epistaxis is the spontaneous and unexpected break or erosion of a superficial blood vessel, usually on the septum.
2. **Dryness of the nasal mucosa,** more common during the winter, in elderly individuals, and in patients taking medication that reduces mucus output, is a frequent cause of spontaneous nasal bleeding.
3. **Abnormal anatomic features,** such as septal deviations or spurs, cause eddy currents of airflow that result in localized dryness and crusting and lead to bleeding.
4. **Factitious ulceration and excoriation** must be considered.
5. **Nasal trauma** is frequently accompanied by epistaxis, but the bleeding usually subsides or is easily controlled.
6. **Nasal infections,** usually viral, produce an increase in epistaxis that does not usually require medical management.
7. **Neoplasms** The nasal bleeding associated with neoplasia is usually scant and intermittent, sometimes characterized by blood-stained mucus alone.

8. **Other causes** include septal perforations, foreign bodies, and intranasal adhesions.

B. Systemic Factors

Systemic disorders must be considered in the management of patients with epistaxis.

1. **Coagulopathy** underlying epistaxis is often obvious from the patient's medical history. Many patients, however, present with epistaxis and no history of coagulation abnormalities. Tests for coagulation function should nevertheless be done to rule out mild dysfunction. The recent use of aspirin or aspirin-containing medications should be considered.
2. **Hypertension** appears to promote epistaxis, and the patient's blood pressure should be measured.
3. **Chemotherapy,** affecting either coagulation or vascular integrity, often underlies problematic epistaxis.
4. **Generalized debilitating diseases** promote nasal bleeding by causing vascular and mucosal fragility.
5. **Arteriosclerosis** is probably a common cause of epistaxis in elderly patients, although the association is difficult to prove.
6. **Other causes** include hereditary hemorrhagic telangiectasia and vitamin C deficiency.

II. VASCULAR ANATOMIC FEATURES

The blood supply to the nasal cavity is derived from both the external and internal carotid arterial systems.

A. External Carotid Artery

The external carotid artery provides the major blood supply to the nasal cavity.

1. **The sphenopalatine artery,** the terminal branch of the maxillary artery as it passes through the sphenopalatine foramen, supplies the posterior three-quarters of the septum and lateral nasal wall.
2. **The descending palatine artery** gives rise to the greater palatine artery, which passes through the incisive canal of the hard palate and supplies the inferoanterior portion of the nasal septum.
3. **The superior labial branch of the facial artery** sends a branch into the vestibule of the nose and supplies the anteroinferior portion of the nasal septum.

B. Internal Carotid Artery

The internal carotid artery supplies the anterior and posterior ethmoid arteries by the ophthalmic artery.

1. **The larger anterior ethmoid artery** supplies the superior por-

tion and the anterior third of both the septum and the lateral nasal wall.

2. **The posterior ethmoid artery** is distributed to the superior concha and the corresponding area of the septum.

III. SITES OF BLEEDING

A. Anterior Septum

The anterior septum (Kiesselbach's or Little's area) is the site of bleeding in over 90% of cases. The feeding vessels are usually the distal portion of the greater palatine artery, which passes through the incisive canal, the anterior ethmoidal artery, and the distal branch of the superior labial artery.

B. Lateral Nasal Wall

Bleeding from the lateral nasal wall is less common and may be derived either from the sphenopalatine artery posteriorly or the anterior ethmoidal artery anteriorly.

C. Posterior and Superior Nasal Cavity

Bleeding from the posterior and superior nasal cavity is common in difficult cases because of the inaccessibility of the site. It often occurs in older patients and is not easily visualized by anterior or posterior rhinoscopy. Even though the exact site cannot be clearly identified, the general location of the bleeding source should be established. If superior, the bleeding vessel is likely to be one of the ethmoidal arteries; if inferior, it is likely to be the sphenopalatine artery.

IV. EVALUATION

The pattern of nasal bleeding determines which examinations and tests are necessary. Patients with recurrent epistaxis or chronic bloody nasal discharge require a diagnostic focus different from that in patients with acute active epistaxis in whom the top priority is control of the bleeding.

A. Anterior Rhinoscopy

This essential study is the mainstay of the evaluation. Using a head mirror or a headlight, a nasal speculum, and a suction apparatus, one may determine the site of bleeding. Visualization of the nasal cavities may be enhanced by spraying the nose with vasoconstrictors. If no active bleeding is seen at the time of rhinoscopy, wiping of a suspicious area of the septum or other part of the nose with a cotton-tipped applicator may reactivate the bleeding and may thereby enable one to identify the site of origin. Application of a topical anesthetic permits more thorough intranasal manipulation with instruments such as suction tips and forceps, to aid in the search for the bleeding point. Subsequent procedures to control the bleeding, such as cautery or packing, can then be performed with less discomfort to the patient.

B. Posterior Rhinoscopy

Nasopharyngeal examination by posterior rhinoscopy is essential in patients with recurrent epistaxis and chronic bloody nasal discharge, to rule out neoplasia.

C. Blood Pressure Determination

The patient's blood pressure should be measured, to exclude a diagnosis of hypertension.

D. Sinus Roentgenograms

Roentgenograms of the sinuses are necessary for recognizing neoplasia or infections.

E. Screening for Coagulopathies

Appropriate tests include serum prothrombin time, partial thromboplastin time, platelet count, and bleeding time.

F. Medical History

A thorough medical history may uncover any medical problems that underlie the epistaxis.

V. MANAGEMENT

A. Acute Active Epistaxis

1. **Blood volume replacement** Although control of the bleeding is usually the first priority, in patients with massive blood loss, severe hypotension may require emergency assessment of the cardiovascular status and replacement of blood volume.
2. **Compression of the nostrils** Pinching of the nostrils presses the lateral walls of the nose against the septum, tamponades the bleeding site, and thereby controls most active nose bleeds. Tilting the head back and lying down are to be avoided. The insertion into the nose of cotton soaked with a vasoconstrictor, followed by compression of the nostrils, may be helpful.
3. **Anterior nasal packing** is useful if compressing the nostrils does not stop the bleeding. The bleeding point should be identified with a headlight or a head mirror, nasal speculum, a suction apparatus, and topical anesthesia if necessary.
   a. ***Hemostatic agents,*** such as absorbable gelatin sponge (Gelfoam), are helpful because they provide both tamponade and promotion of clot formation. These agents are inserted with bayonet forceps, but may not require removal because they dissolve with time.
   b. ***Microfibrillar collagen hemostat (MCH)*** The topical application of MCH (Avitene) has enjoyed increasing popularity in the treatment of epistaxis. Its light and fluffy

texture, however, makes it difficult for packing or topical application. To overcome this problem, one may fill a 3-ml plastic syringe with MCH, cut off the tip of the syringe, and "inject" the compressed agent onto the site of bleeding. Because MCH eventually dissolves, removal is unnecessary.

c. ***Petrolatum gauze*** inserted in horizontal layers with bayonet forceps is a reliable and time-tested method for controlling nasal bleeding. The packing should be removed in 5 days. This should not be used in any patient with an underlying coagulopathy. Removal of the packing will cause increased bleeding.

4. **Cautery** may be used rather than packing, but it is difficult to perform when bleeding is profuse and is less reliable because the resulting necrosis may not be sufficient to seal a bleeding vessel. On the other hand, cautery is more comfortable for the patient than packing. If a bleeding point is identified and is temporarily controlled, one should cauterize around the site to prevent dislodgement of the clot. Widespread and indiscriminate use of cautery is to be avoided.
   a. ***Chemical cautery*** may be performed with several different agents. Silver nitrate on a wooden stick applicator is most common. Chromic acid, fashioned into a bead by dipping a heated wire applicator tip into the crystals, and trichloroacetic acid impregnated into a small cotton pledget on a wire applicator are more caustic than silver nitrate and are therefore more effective. These agents must be used with caution, and never on both sides of the septum simultaneously since this may lead to septal perforations.
   b. ***Electrocautery*** employs either thermal or high-frequency current (fulguration).

5. **Nasal balloon placement** for hemostasis is an alternative to packing or cautery. Some such apparatus consist of a single balloon designed to tamponade only the nasal cavity; others consist of two balloons for the nasal cavity and nasopharynx. Although it is not as reliable as nasal packing, this method is quicker and less traumatic for the patient. The insertion of nasal balloons requires no special instruments or skill; therefore, it is useful for physicians who are not specialists in otolaryngology.

6. **Posterior nasal packing** is used when all the previously discussed methods of management fail and when the bleeding site appears to be in the posterior nose or the nasopharynx (usually, the bleeding site cannot be identified exactly). One method is to use a Foley catheter by passing its tip through the nasal cavity to the nasopharynx and inflating the balloon to fill the nasopharynx. Packing is then inserted anteriorly against the occluded nasopharynx. A more reliable method is

the conventional posterior pack made from gauze. With the posterior pack in place, the anterior nasal cavities usually require packing with petrolatum gauze. The posterior pack must be secured by tethering it anteriorly to a piece of gauze at the nostril's rim. Patients with a posterior pack require hospitalization. Close observation, with blood-gas determinations, is important because of the possibility of hypoxia. Patients may experience considerable discomfort, especially with swallowing, and they may require intravenous fluids. The use of prophylactic antibiotics for possible otitis media and sinusitis is recommended. The posterior pack is left in place for 5 days, depending on the severity of epistaxis. Pack removal is performed in stages, first by loosening the strings of the posterior pack, then by removing the anterior packing, and finally by withdrawing the posterior pack. If bleeding recurs after the first 2 steps, then hemostasis can be achieved again without repeating the entire process of posterior pack insertion.

7. **Arterial ligation** is necessary if bleeding cannot be controlled by appropriate packing or if bleeding recurs after removal of the posterior pack. The appropriate vessel to ligate is determined by the location of the bleeding point.
   a. ***Transantral maxillary artery ligation*** is most common and should control epistaxis from the nasopharynx, the posterior nasal cavities, the septum, and the inferolateral nasal walls.
   b. ***Anteroposterior ethmoid artery ligation,*** through a Lynch incision, is performed when the site of bleeding is located in the superior portion of the nasal cavity. This procedure is often required when a maxillary artery ligation fails to control the bleeding.
   c. ***External carotid artery ligation*** is uncommon because it is less successful in controlling epistaxis than the former two procedures. Because the point of ligation is so proximal relative to the bleeding site, collateral vessels may maintain vigorous perfusion of the bleeding vessel and make a recurrence of the epistaxis more likely.
8. **Carotid arteriography** When bleeding persists following vessel ligation, selective carotid arteriography of the external or internal carotid system is helpful in localizing the responsible vessel. This technique is particularly useful in identifying collateral sources of bleeding or failure of a previous ligation. The extravasation of blood into the nasal cavity can frequently be demonstrated if the procedure is performed while the patient is actively bleeding. If the identified bleeding vessel is surgically accessible, ligation can be performed again. Otherwise, with the catheter already in place for arteriographic study, the bleeding artery can be embolized using plugs of absorbable gelatin sponge. Embolization of anterior or posterior ethmoid arteries is not possible because they are part of the internal carotid arterial system.

B. Recurrent Epistaxis

Patients often complain of controllable, but annoying, recurrent nosebleeds. In such cases, one must determine the cause, to ascertain the appropriate method of management.

1. **Moisturization** with petroleum jelly, xipamide (Aquaphor), or mineral oil softens dry nasal mucous membranes. Humidification of the home is also helpful.
2. **Surgical correction of septal deviation or spurs,** which often result in bleeding because of associated dryness of the mucous membranes, should be considered.
3. **Cautery** is helpful in eliminating a solitary superficial vessel that bleeds intermittently. A clue to such a diagnosis is recurrent bleeding from only one nostril.
4. **Scraping and scarification of mucous membranes** at the bleeding site are occasionally indicated in patients with recurrent epistaxis that is refractory to other measures.
5. **Surgical transection of the distal portion of the greater palatine artery,** after it passes through the incisive canal, can be performed in patients with recurrent anterior septal epistaxis. If one uses a small intranasal incision, the procedure will be simple and suitable for an outpatient operating room.
6. **Treatment of underlying systemic disorders,** such as hypertension or bleeding disorders, is essential.

C. Chronic or Intermittent Bloody Nasal Discharge

Small intranasal hemorrhages may occur but may remain unrecognized by the patient until blowing the nose yields blood or blood-stained mucus. Alternately, small hemorrhages may be carried posteriorly by mucociliary flow to the nasopharynx or into the oropharynx or hypopharynx, to be expelled by "coughing," spitting, or nasopharyngeal aspiration.

1. **Treatment methods for recurrent epistaxis** are often appropriate; see the preceding section of this chapter.
2. **Treatment of an underlying nasal or sinus infection** may correct the problem.
3. **Exclusion of a diagnosis of neoplasm** A careful examination including roentgenograms of the nasopharynx and sinuses should be performed to rule out an occult neoplasm.

15

SINUS DISORDERS

ROGER L. HYBELS

I. INFLAMMATORY DISEASES

A. Acute Suppurative Sinusitis

This form of sinusitis, which is an active bacterial infection of recent onset in a sinus cavity, may be the first infection that has occurred in the sinus, or it may be an exacerbation of a chronically diseased sinus. Viral sinusitis occurs with each upper respiratory infection, is self-limited, and does not carry the surgical implications of bacterial infection. Fungal infections are considered separately in this chapter.

1. **Etiologic factors** Several underlying conditions can lead to acute sinusitis, many of which may interact in any given patient. Viral upper respiratory infection leads to necrosis of mucosal epithelium, edema with transudation of fluid, ciliary dysfunction, and at times, edematous occlusion of the sinus ostium. This condition provides a culture medium for bacteria in the sinus. An allergic response of the sinus mucosa may have the same effect. The spread of infection into the maxillary sinuses from diseased tooth roots is possible and should be suspected when the other sinuses are normal. Diving or swimming can allow contaminated water to be forced into a sinus, often the frontal sinus. Impaired drainage through the natural ostium for any reason results in stasis of normal secretions followed by infection. Factors that affect drainage may be mechanical, such as cicatricial stenosis, presence of foreign bodies, polyps, or neoplasms, or they may include ciliary loss or dysfunction or lymphatic engorgement.

2. **Diagnosis**

a. ***Symptoms and signs*** Acute sinusitis, essentially an empyema, is the only form of sinus disease causing appreciable pain. Before headache or facial pain is attributed to sinusitis, the patient's medical history should be reviewed carefully for consistency, specificity, and conformity to the typical and expected clinical course of this entity. Vague symptoms that are migratory in location and chronic are unlikely to be caused by sinus disease. The discomfort is typically localized over the involved sinuses, especially those in proximity to the skin, that is, the frontal maxillary and anterior ethmoid sinuses. Pain originating in sinuses located deeper anatomically may be ill defined or retro-orbital. Commonly, the patient with maxillary sinusitis feels pain in several anterior teeth that causes him to consult a dentist. The patient may complain of a foul discharge, either anteriorly or posteriorly. Anterior rhinoscopic examination reveals inflammation in the area of the involved sinus. Pus emanates from the direction of the natural ostium; this pus often streams in the direction of natural ciliary flow toward the posterior choana and is seen in the pharynx. Percussion or pressure over the sinus elicits tenderness; however, the examiner must attempt to distinguish a true positive response from the reaction of an individual who recoils from most aspects of an examination. Unfortunately, atypical forms of facial pain are common in such patients. Transillumination of the maxillary and frontal sinuses is sometimes helpful and usually further confirms the examiner's impression. Systemic effects are typically of low grade, with malaise, minor temperature elevation, and normal white blood cell count. During the physical examination, one should seek definitive evidence of the sinus disorder. If such evidence is not found, the probability of acute sinusitis will decrease.

b. ***Radiographic studies*** Radiographs should be ordered when acute sinusitis is suspected. Four views are necessary and should be learned: (1) Waters; (2) Caldwell; (3) lateral; and (4) base. Sinusitis is manifested by an air-fluid level or by complete opacification. The clinician should review the radiographs because radiologists interpret many findings as "sinusitis." The otolaryngologist is better able to place radiographic findings in perspective and is familiar with the patient's medical history and examination, as well as being experienced in the pathophysiologic features and surgical treatment of sinusitis. At birth, only the maxillary antra are present; the ethmoid cells appear shortly thereafter. The frontal sinus begins to develop at 1 year of age, and the sphenoid sinus at 3 to 4 years. In 5% of the population, one or both frontal sinuses may fail to develop, and this anomaly should not be interpreted as opacification. See Chapter 33.

c. ***Bacteriologic factors*** Cultures are not routinely necessary, but they should be performed if no response to treatment is evident. Gram-positive cocci are the usual offending bacteria. These organisms include streptococci, staphylococci, and pneumococci. Anaerobic or microaerophilic streptococci or Haemophilus influenzae are also seen. The compromised host may have more esoteric infecting organisms.

3. **Treatment** Initial measures are medical and include administration of antibiotics, mucosal shrinkage with topical agents to encourage drainage from the sinuses, application of local warm compresses, and administration of analgesics. Amoxicillin or erythromycin are reasonable first choices of antibiotics. When sinusitis fails to resolve medically, further therapy becomes necessary; the treatment of specific sinuses is considered next.

   a. ***Maxillary sinusitis*** The patient should be seen 2 to 3 weeks after initiation of medical treatment, and if the sinusitis is not resolved, the sinus should be irrigated by puncture through the inferior meatus. Material should be obtained for culture, and the sinus should be cleaned of bacteria, fluid, and inflammatory cells. Whether irrigation should be performed earlier in the course of the infection is unresolved. Antibiotics may have rendered obsolete the axiom against violating bone during an acute infection. Fortunately, irrigation is unnecessary in most patients. Infections that do not clear after a single irrigation may require repeated attempts; some of these infections become chronic.

   b. ***Frontal sinusitis*** If the infection is not caused by swimming, the patient may have a demonstrable abnormality that affects the functioning of the nasofrontal duct, such as an ethmoid disorder, an old fracture, or an osteoma. It is necessary to treat this underlying problem when the acute infection has been resolved. The medical methods previously described are instituted. Trephination of the frontal sinus is rarely indicated, but it may be necessary in the following instances: when the pain is severe and is unrelieved by analgesics, when the patient fails to respond to antibiotics within 48 hours, when no drainage can be demonstrated through the natural duct, and when a complication occurs.

   c. ***Ethmoid sinusitis*** Disease in the ethmoid sinuses is unusual, but it may occur as a recurrence of chronic sinusitis or in association with a mucocele or obstruction by a mass such as a foreign body, polyps, or a neoplasm. Treatment is the same as for other forms of sinusitis. Acute "ethmoiditis," which occurs in infancy, is a misnomer. In actuality, it is a maxillary sinusitis, but the maxillary primordia are located at the level approximating the ethmoid sinuses in the adult.

d. ***Sphenoid sinusitis*** is rare; drainage must be established if medical treatment fails.

B. Subacute Suppurative Sinusitis

This form of sinusitis can be thought of as an unresolved acute sinusitis, perhaps caused by neglect, inadequate or inappropriate therapy, or an unexpected organism. At times, normal ciliary mechanisms are incapable of removing thick mucopus after treatment of an acute infection. Patients with allergies are more likely to have this problem than other persons. The primary symptom is a persistent, purulent, foul-smelling discharge localized to a specific side. Discomfort is minimal, and symptoms may be vague. Culture is indicated because the most usual infecting organisms cannot be assumed to be present. The culture should be obtained from a definite stream of mucopus, or in maxillary infection, lavage is possible. Irrigation can be performed on more than one occasion. Treatment with an appropriate antibiotic and with a topical decongestant usually clears the infection.

C. Chronic Suppurative Sinusitis

This disorder is associated with irreversible mucosal changes or inadequate drainage, or both. The mucosal disorder consists of hypertrophy, submucosal fibrosis, ciliary dysfunction, and microabscesses.

1. **Etiologic factors** A common cause of mucosal change is repeated bacterial insults to the sinus. The drainage through the natural ostium may be affected by the mucosal disease itself or by any of the factors enumerated for acute sinusitis. Occasionally, a single acute infection leads to a chronic state when treatment has been ineffective. In maxillary sinusitis, a dental origin should be sought. The commonest contributing factor in multisinus disease is atopy of the mucosa, which should be suspected in all patients. In some allergic individuals, massive hyperplasia of the mucosa occurs under the stimulus of bacterial infection and is referred to as hyperplastic sinusitis. Chronic sinusitis is a problem of adults; if the disorder is seen in children, one should look for an underlying disease, such as cystic fibrosis, immune disorders, wasting diseases, or developmental anomalies. In part, this association with age is explained by the incomplete development of the sinuses in childhood.

2. **Symptoms and signs** Chronic sinusitis is manifested by a foul discharge of long duration and consistent location. Exacerbations may be acute and symptoms may be similar to those of acute sinusitis, including pain; otherwise, pain is not a fea-

ture of the chronic disease. The physician must be suspicious of the patient with "sinus headaches," which are more or less constant and of long duration. Sinus disease causing this type of pain is usually the result of a complication or an underlying neoplasm. See Chapter 25.

3. **Treatment** Surgical treatment is indicated for symptomatic patients, such as those with a chronic discharge or acute exacerbations of increasing frequency or duration, and for patients with complications of sinusitis. Medical treatment provides only temporary benefits because the underlying disorder is not corrected. Radiographic studies should be performed to confirm the clinical impression and to guide the surgeon. Thickened mucosa lining a sinus is not itself symptomatic nor does it indicate active disease. This radiologic finding is often interpreted as "sinusitis" by the inexperienced physician when evaluating a patient with sinus pain or postnasal drip. A sinus previously operated on may be opacified permanently on radiographs. When a clouded sinus is seen radiographically and the diagnosis is obscure, irrigation may resolve the dilemma. The goal of any surgical procedure is to provide dependent drainage or to eliminate the sinus, either by obliteration or by making it continuous with the nasal cavity. As a rule, one should perform the most conservative procedure possible. When multisinus disease is present, therapy should be directed first at the antra. The remaining sinuses should be observed, to assess the effect of eliminating disease in the antra. Intranasal disease, such as abnormalities of the septum or polyps, and allergy should be corrected early. If simple measures fail, more extensive procedures may be necessary. These measures should be taken in a careful and logical manner.

D. Barotrauma

An improperly aerated sinus can undergo trauma similar to that occurring in the middle ear when subjected to changes in environmental pressure. This injury occurs during transit to positions of higher pressure. Under normal conditions, pressure inside a sinus equals that of the surrounding atmosphere. When a position of higher ambient pressure is reached, as in diving or in descent in an aircraft, air must enter the sinus to equalize pressures. If the ostium is blocked, this equalization process may not be possible. Hemorrhage and inflammation can occur when the pressure gradient is high, and severe pain may result. Barotrauma usually resolves spontaneously, but nasal mucosal decongestants may be helpful. Egress of air from a sinus at a pressure higher than ambient does not usually cause trauma; therefore, ascent during diving or flying is not a problem.

E. Mycotic Infections

Fungi are generally harmless to a healthy individual, but they may become invasive in an immunologically compromised or metabolically susceptible host. The usual underlying factors are debilitation secondary to neoplasms or their treatment, immunosuppressive therapy, antibiotic therapy, and brittle diabetes.

1. **Phycomycetes** These fungi infect vessels, mainly those in the brain, lungs, and less often, the abdomen. This class of fungus contains mucor and rhizopus. The sinuses provide a portal of entry to the brain by the retro-orbital route. The commonest associated factor is diabetes. Examination often reveals a black (necrotic) turbinate and total ophthalmoplegia. The maxilla may be involved extensively. Because these fungi are common inhabitants of the upper aerodigestive tract, a diagnosis can only be made if a biopsy shows a fungus characterized by nonseptate hyphae invading tissue. This condition is life-threatening, and vigorous debridement, administration of amphotericin B, and control of the diabetes must be instituted.
2. **Aspergillus** Probably more common than generally thought, aspergillus is of low pathogenicity and typically remains localized. In fact, it often becomes pathogenic in areas of compromised local resistance, such as an obstructed sinus with poor aeration. This fungus is frequently found incidentally during exploration of a chronically opacified sinus and may have a green appearance. Drainage is adequate treatment.

II. COMPLICATIONS OF SUPPURATIVE SINUSITIS

A. Bone Infection

Osteitis or osteomyelitis of the skull or facial bones has become rare since the development of antibiotics. The usual organisms are Staphylococcus aureus, streptococci, pneumococci, and anaerobic streptococci.

1. **Frontal bone** This bone is the most commonly affected, and infection occurs secondary to acute frontal sinusitis, trauma, or operation. This disorder is frequently seen after diving, when contaminated water is forced into the sinus. Because young children do not have developed frontal sinuses, osteomyelitis of the frontal bone in children is hematogenous, if not traumatic. This complication occurs secondary to thrombophlebitis of the veins that communicate the infected mucosa to the cancellous portions of the surrounding bone. The infection is most often confined to the frontal bone by cranial sutures and remains of low grade and chronic. The major symptoms are local pain, a doughy edema on palpation, persistent low-grade fever, and at times, fistulization. A more fulminating form involves rapid progression to high fever, sys-

temic toxicity, local pain and tenderness, edema of the forehead (Pott's puffy tumor), and edema of the upper eyelid. Venous channels also exist between the sinus and both tables of the bone and lead to either subpericranial or epidural abscesses. An epidural abscess may have severe intracranial complications. Radiographic features may be misleading because visible bony changes lag behind the disease process itself. Treatment consists of drainage of pus, including trephination of the sinus, and high doses of intravenously administered antibiotics. Antibacterial therapy should be continued for an extended period. The sinus may need definitive surgical treatment at a later date if the disease becomes chronic or if drainage remains inadequate.

2. **Maxilla** Historically, infection of the maxilla follows the trauma of lavage or operation. The commonest cause now may be dental disease. Along with the typical symptoms of sinusitis, the patient has marked swelling of the cheek. Orbital complications and fistulization are possible. High-dose antibiotic regimens and drainage of the antrum constitute treatment.

3. **Sphenoid bone** Infection of the sphenoid bone is a complication of suppurative disease in the sphenoid sinus or the petrous pyramid. The diagnosis may be difficult; ill-defined, deep, or retro-orbital pain may be the major symptom.

B. Orbital Complications

Orbital complications occur by direct extension or by venous thrombosis from contiguous sinuses. The most common origin is the ethmoid and then the frontal sinuses. Orbital infections, as well as cavernous sinus thrombosis, may be difficult to differentiate because of similarities in presentation. Computerized tomography (CT) or ultrasonography is helpful in proper diagnosis. Ophthalmologic consultation should be obtained because emergency operation may be necessary when vision is threatened by compromise to the central retinal vessels.

1. **Cellulitis** is a diffuse process involving the loose areolar tissues and is manifested by edema of the upper eyelid, straightforward proptosis, conjunctival chemosis, restricted motion of the globe, pain, and fever. Therapy includes the administration of intravenous antibiotics and appropriate treatment of the affected sinus, usually the ethmoid sinus.

2. **Orbital abscess** The presenting symptoms of an abscess are similar to those of cellulitis, but more of a mass effect occurs. The direction of proptosis may depend on the position of the abscess, and toxicity may be greater than with cellulitis. Pressure to move the globe in a posterior direction is likely to be met by resistance. Vision is more likely to be affected than in cellulitis. Treatment is similar to that for cellulitis, with the additional necessity of drainage of the abscess.

3. **Periorbital abscess** results when the bony wall is penetrated, but the periorbita is not. This localized collection of pus produces a less severe symptom complex than the abscess previously described. The eye is displaced opposite from the abscess. Chemosis is unlikely, and edema of the eyelid is localized. The abscess should be drained, and the sinus should be treated.
4. **Superior orbital fissure syndrome** results from an infection or a mass in the sphenoid sinus that affects the contents of the superior orbital fissure. Cranial nerves III, IV, VI, the ophthalmic branch of V, and the sympathetic nerve to Müller's muscle in the eyelid are affected. Ophthalmic vein compromise is discernible on retinal examination. The inflammatory involvement of the eyelids and conjunctiva and the proptosis seen in other syndromes are absent. Treatment is directed against the sinus disease.

C. Central Nervous System Complications

The whole spectrum of intracranial bacterial complications can result from primary acute sinusitis or from an acute exacerbation of chronic sinus disease. As might be expected, the organisms are the same as in sinusitis. Any sinus may serve as the source, but the frontal is the most common and the maxillary the least common. Infection may spread from the sinus to the cranium by diverse pathways. These tracts may be created by bony defects, whether traumatic or congenital, by bone absorption through infection, by thrombophlebitis, either in directly communicating veins or through diploetic veins, secondarily through the orbit, and along the cranial nerves (olfactory). The life-threatening central nervous system complication must be addressed before the sinus is definitively treated. The sinus must not be ignored, however, because the problem may recur.

1. **Meningitis** The clinical picture is the same with a sinus focus as with any cause. If meningeal signs occur in a patient with acute sinusitis, immediate lumbar puncture and prompt treatment are indicated.
2. **Brain abscess** Frontal lobe abscess occurs most commonly secondary to frontal sinusitis. The symptoms are fever, headache, nausea and vomiting, and personality changes. Increased intracranial pressure and convulsions may occur in patients with advanced disease. Temporal lobe abscess originates in the sphenoid sinus or is secondary to cavernous sinus thrombosis. Brain abscesses may be clinically silent until a mass effect occurs.
3. **Epidural abscess** may be clinically silent and undiagnosed until brain abscess or meningitis results. The major symptom is persistent pain. Treatment involves removal of bone underlying the abscess until normal bone is exposed in all directions.
4. **Cavernous sinus thrombosis** occurs by septic thrombophle-

bitis through direct venous channels, which exist between it and the frontal (supraorbital and ophthalmic veins) and maxillary (pterygoid plexus) sinuses. The connection from the sphenoid sinus is direct. Orbital suppuration may be the immediate focus of infection. Infection of facial skin and subcutaneous tissues through the facial and ophthalmic veins and of the ear through the petrosal sinuses is another possible source. The onset of severe symptoms is abrupt, with the rapid development of spiking fever and chills. Pain is deep seated and may be accompanied by stiffness of the neck, vomiting, and changes in mental activity. Retinal veins are congested, and edema of the optic disc is present. These signs, which suggest central nervous system manifestations, may precede or may overshadow the changes in the periorbital tisues; this feature helps one to distinguish this entity from those of suppuration in the orbit itself. The orbital signs include periorbital edema, proptosis, and external and internal ophthalmoplegia. The cranial nerves can be affected individually and sequentially, whereas in orbital cellulitis, they are usually involved concurrently. Furthermore, both eyes are eventually affected when the cavernous sinus is infected. Treatment is with antibiotics and anticoagulants once lumbar puncture and blood cultures have been performed.

D. Mucocele

A mucocele is a cyst occurring in a sinus lined by mucus-secreting epithelium. If the cyst becomes infected, the term "pyocele" is used. The cause is obstruction of the normal outflow of the sinus secondary to tumors, trauma, operation, or infectious complications, sometimes remote. Mucoceles are expansile in nature and have a characteristic radiographic appearance of a smooth, rounded opacification surrounded by thinned bone. They become symptomatic when infected or when expansion is great enough to become visible or to displace normal structures. These lesions most commonly occur in the frontal or ethmoid sinuses. In the frontal sinus, the direction of least resistance is inferiorly into the orbit. Those cysts originating in an ethmoid cell displace or erode through the lamina papyracea. Sphenoid mucoceles may cause the orbital apex syndrome, which is similar to the superior orbital fissure syndrome, with the additional feature of involvement of the contents of the optic foramen. Thus, dilation of the pupil, marked ptosis, papilledema, and loss of vision occur. Treatment is surgical.

III. TUMORS

A. Benign

1. **Mucosal cysts** are nonsecreting lesions confined to the mucosa, although they may become large. Normally, these cysts are incidental radiographic findings characterized by a round, smooth mucosal mass with intact bony walls. They are asymp-

tomatic and require no treatment. Unfortunately, because radiographs of the sinus are taken in patients with symptoms, these cysts are often suspected as the cause.

2. **Polyps** Polyposis is basically a disease of the nose, although the commonest site of origin is the ethmoid sinus. Polyps result from an edematous hypertrophy of the mucosa, typically secondary to an allergic stimulus. Normally, polyps do not develop in atopic individuals until adulthood; when polyposis is seen in children, the diagnosis of cystic fibrosis should be considered. The antrochoanal polyp is a distinct entity arising from the mucosa of the maxillary antrum and projecting through the ostium into the nose and, at times, into the nasopharynx. These polyps appear to follow the normal stream of mucus. Infection may play a role in their formation. Surgical removal of the origin of the polyp in the antrum is necessary because recurrence is common after simple avulsion.

3. **Osseous and fibrous lesions** comprise a confusing assortment of related lesions. All are composed of bone, fibrous tissue, or a mixture of the two. The list of potential entities is extensive, but most are rare and undeserving of special mention.
   a. ***Osteoma*** is one of the most common benign bony lesions and is seen in either the frontal or ethmoid sinuses near their joint suture line. Orbital or intracranial extension is noted infrequently. These lesions are usually small and asymptomatic and can safely be followed for evidence of growth. Pain may occur primary to the osteoma itself or secondary to obstruction of the sinus, and the lesion should then be removed.
   b. ***Fibrous dysplasia*** is a dense, slow-growing fibrous lesion containing particles of bone and appearing early in life. The maxilla is the common focus in the head and neck. The best treatment is the conservative approach of surgical contouring, to maintain an acceptable appearance and function. The growth of these lesions slows with age. Some authorities consider other fibro-osseous entities to be variations of this disease.
   c. ***Ossifying fibroma*** is seen most commonly in the superior maxilla. As its name implies, this lesion is largely a fibroma initially, and then it ossifies. It may be necessary to remove these tumors when function or appearance is affected.
   d. ***Giant cell tumors*** Large, multinucleated cells are commonly found in fibro-osseous lesions; however, three distinct pathologic entities fall into this category. True giant cell neoplasms display expansion and thinning of cortical plates. These tumors should be excised completely because of the possibility of recurrence. Hyperparathyroidism may cause a "brown" tumor in the maxilla. This entity should be ruled out in all patients with giant cell lesions. Giant

cell granuloma may be mistaken for the true neoplasm and requires only simple excision.

4. **Inverting papillomas** have a benign histologic appearance but an aggressive clinical course. They may better be classified as malignant tumors because the incidence of overt epidermoid carcinoma present within the papilloma is significant. This tumor arises from the lateral wall of the nose and secondarily involves the sinuses. Wide local excision is accomplished through a lateral rhinotomy or another appropriate incision. This lesion often appears preoperatively to be a typical allergic polyp, albeit unilateral, and is simply avulsed. In such a case, the surgeon is obligated to perform a second procedure to ensure an adequate resection.

5. **Glandular neoplasms** Any mucosal gland can be the source of adenoma; however, minor salivary glands are the commonest source. Mixed tumor is the most frequent of these neoplasms. The incidence of malignant involvement is high, so one must use great care in their treatment.

6. **Dental cysts and neoplasms** Teeth arise from a primordium containing epithelium and connective tissue. The cysts and neoplasms that originate in the odontogenic apparatus contain either one or both of these tissues. The most common lesions are discussed as follows. See Chapter 18.
   a. ***Radicular cysts*** occur at the root of a diseased, erupted tooth. Radiographic examination fails to reveal a tooth.
   b. ***Dentigerous cysts*** originate in the epithelium of a tooth bud or in the enamel layer of an unerupted tooth. Radiographic study demonstrates a cystic lesion with a bony margin and a tooth contained within it. These cysts possess the ability of neoplastic transformation to ameloblastoma.
   c. ***Ameloblastoma*** This epithelial neoplasm occurs in several variations and, at times, appears cystic radiographically or arises in an odontogenic cyst. Ameloblastomas are locally aggressive and require wide excision; they occur mainly in the third and fourth decades of life.
   d. ***Mesodermal neoplasms*** include fibromas, dentinomas, cementomas, and several others.
   e. ***Odontomas*** are tumors of mixed origin that contain all tooth structures. The tumor is normally discovered in childhood and grows slowly. It is commonly found incidentally on routine radiographic examination. Surgical removal is the recommended treatment. See Chapter 18.

7. **Fusion cysts** are developmental anomalies in which epithelium is trapped between the lines of fusion of the maxilla. The epithelium is usually squamous, but it may be cuboidal or columnar. Several variations occur, depending on their location. Treatment involves removal of the epithelial lining.

B. Malignant

Malignant tumors of the sinuses are rare, even when compared only with tumors of the head and neck, except in patients with unique environmental or occupational factors. They are more common in the sixth or seventh decade in men. Possible etiologic factors are tobacco, alcohol, chronic infection, and the environment created by woodworking.

1. **Types of tumors** Epithelial malignant tumors account for most of these neoplasms; epidermoid carcinoma alone accounts for 67%. Adenoid cystic tumor is the most common adenocarcinoma. The maxillary sinus is the site of origin in 80%; the ethmoid sinus is the next most prevalent site. Overall, the ethmoid and sphenoid sinuses are more likely to be invaded secondarily. Malignant melanoma occurs frequently enough to be considered.

2. **Clinical considerations** Sinus tumors are likely to be advanced when discovered because they are often treated initially as an inflammation and they are typically clinically silent until large. The symptoms and signs depend on which wall or structure is invaded. The clinical presentation is not often a clue to the histologic type because the symptoms are much the same for different tumors. Certain characteristics of malignant tumors of the sinus that may help one distinguish them from inflammatory lesions include the following: constant symptoms of a progressive nature; cranial neuropathies; unilaterality of symptoms; slowly developing mass or displacement of the globe, or both; vague, deep-seated pain; epistaxis; trismus; lack of previous sinusitis; and serous otitis media. Few tumors are confined to the sinus of origin; rather, they invade adjacent sinuses or surrounding tissues. Extension is through natural foramina, along neural or vascular channels, through congenital or traumatic openings or by the lymphatic vessels.

3. **Treatment** Attempts to classify these tumors have not been productive. The important question centers around the resectability of a given lesion. Therefore, each situation must be considered individually, with careful physical examination as well as conventional radiographic and CT techniques. Biopsy must be obtained. Surgical excision is the usual treatment. In most patients, full doses of radiation are given postoperatively. When excision is not possible, a sinus drainage procedure is performed before radiation. Regional nodal metastases are uncommon initially, but appear later, along with distant metastases. Intracranial extension has been considered a contraindication to operation, but successful removal is now possible with combined craniofacial procedures. Surgeons show a certain reluctance to attempt resection of tumors in such a complex anatomic and cosmetically critical area. If cure rates

are to be improved, however, a rigorous course must be pursued.

C. Miscellaneous

The variety of pathologic conditions that may appear in the sinuses is immense. Wegener's granulomatosis and lethal midline granuloma should always be considered. Angiofibroma may invade the sinuses from its origin in the nasopharynx. Many forms of sarcoma, including Ewing's sarcoma and rhabdomyosarcoma, are possible. Reticuloendothelial and histiocytic lesions are reported. The sphenoid sinus, by its unique location, is the site of chordomas, craniopharyngiomas, and pituitary tumors. Eosinophilic granuloma is a punched-out, sharply circumscribed lesion. More often found in the skull, it has been reported in the maxillary and sphenoid sinuses. Plasmacytoma occurs either as a manifestation of multiple myeloma or as an isolated lesion. Paget's disease of the maxilla is possible in the older patient. The sinuses may be host to a metastasis from a distant primary tumor, such as tumors of the kidney, prostate, lung, breast, or pancreas. Lymphomas typically are manifested in the context of a systemic disease, but they may be isolated.

IV.

ORAL CAVITY AND LARYNGOPHARYNX

16

BENIGN LESIONS OF THE ORAL CAVITY

DON B. BLAKESLEE AND M. STUART STRONG

I. VARIANTS OF NORMAL

A. Coated Tongue

1. **Description** Coated tongue or hairy tongue resembles a darkly stained shag carpet overlying the dorsal surface of the tongue. This finding is due to hyperkeratosis and elongation of filiform papillae, often caused by antibiotic use, with an ensuing decrease in the normal flora of the oral cavity. Discoloration is secondary to the overgrowth of pigment-producing bacteria.
2. **Assessment** Antecedent infection, drug administration, or illness should be detailed. If reassurance is not adequate, a biopsy should be performed using local anesthesia. The differential diagnosis should include simple staining from food colorings, nicotine staining, geographic tongue, and systemic diseases such as nutritional deficiencies, general disturbances, syphilis, and fungal infections.
3. **Treatment** Good oral hygiene is recommended; brushing with a soft-bristle toothbrush may help.

B. Fissured Tongue

1. **Description** Fissured tongue or scrotal tongue is a common anomaly that is nonpathologic and asymptomatic. The name aptly describes this normal variant. The fissures are variable

in size and depth and cover the dorsal surface. Usually, no discoloration is present unless debris has collected between the crypts or local inflammation exists. A family history of the condition is common.

2. **Assessment** The patient is often unaware of the anomaly. Reassurance from the examining physician is usually sufficient. If doubt persists, a biopsy can be performed. The differential diagnosis should include bifid tongue.
3. **Treatment** No treatment is necessary unless local inflammation is present; then the patient may cleanse the oral cavity with a 3% solution of hydrogen peroxide.

C. Geographic Tongue

1. **Description** Geographic tongue or benign migratory glossitis has a well-defined margin and is map-like in appearance over the dorsal surface of the tongue. These nonindurated, patchy spots are devoid of filiform papillae and vary in size and location. The cause of the condition is unknown. Stress may be an underlying factor. This variant of normal anatomy occurs frequently in young adults and is twice as common in females than in males. Menses may exacerbate the condition. The patient often complains of a burning or itchy sensation on the surface of the tongue.
2. **Assessment** The condition is easily recognized, and reassurance from the examining physician is paramount. The differential diagnosis should include lichen planus and leukoplakia.
3. **Treatment** No treatment is necessary because the condition is self-limiting. Daily observation is helpful to document the changes characteristic of migratory glossitis. If the burning or itching sensation is significant, diclonine solution (Dyclone) or Chloraseptic mouthwash may be used as needed.

D. Papillae

Papillae represent normal anatomic features of the tongue, and patients frequently inquire about these growths. Four types of papillae are found on the dorsum of the tongue. The large, distinct papillae near the posterior portion of the tongue represent circumvallate papillae, which number from 8 to 12 and demarcate the anterior two-thirds of the tongue from the posterior third base of tongue. These papillae do not undergo atrophic changes in patients with systemic diseases. The fungiform papillae are mushroom-shaped and are scattered over the dorsum of the tongue, especially near the tip and lateral surface. These papillae undergo atrophic changes in patients with systemic diseases. The filiform papillae are hair-like and are the most numerous. These papillae are specialized epithelial structures that undergo atrophic changes as metabolism is interrupted in patients with systemic diseases.

These nonspecific changes indicate the need for a more detailed assessment. An example is glossodynia, which is present in patients with pernicious anemia. Foliate papillae appear as folds along the lateral border of the tongue and the anterior tonsillar pillars. These papillae do not undergo atrophic changes, but often become inflamed because of associated lymphoid tissue. Foliate papillae are involved with taste sensation.

E. Fordyce Spots

1. **Description** Fordyce spots are functioning, hyperplastic, sebaceous glands that are frequently found on the buccal surface of the oral cavity opposite the molar teeth. These spots are common in older patients as the mucous membrane thins and becomes more translucent. Fordyce spots appear as clusters of small, yellow-white, raised lesions. The patient is asymptomatic.
2. **Assessment** These spots are frequently observed during routine examinations of the oral cavity. The differential diagnosis should include amalgam tattooing, which occurs during dental procedures.
3. **Treatment** No treatment is indicated because the patient is asymptomatic. Reassurance is appreciated.

II. DEVELOPMENTAL LESIONS

A. Median Rhomboid Glossitis

1. **Description** This rare finding is due to faulty development. The tuberculum impar is trapped between the two halves of the tongue that normally fuse in embryonic life. The red, smooth, and diamond-shaped lesion is located in the midline of the tongue immediately anterior to the circumvallate papillae. The smoothness is due to the absence of papillae. Median rhomboid glossitis is actually not a glossitis; no pain is associated with the condition unless secondary inflammation exists. Males are predominantly affected.
2. **Assessment** The patient may accidentally find this mass and may bring it to the attention of the physician, who must allay any fears of cancer. Identification is apparent. The differential diagnosis includes thyroglossal duct cyst and aberrant thyroid tissue. If a secondary infection is present, cultures are indicated. A biopsy may calm a patient who suspects cancer.
3. **Treatment** No treatment is necessary. If a secondary infection causes discomfort, then improved oral hygiene and mild analgesics should suffice. A chronically irritated area can be removed if symptoms indicate such a course.

B. Dermoid Cyst

1. **Description** This common lesion is found anteriorly and medially in the oral cavity, primarily in the floor of mouth. It is seen as an opaque cyst, usually posterior to the frenulum or lateral to it; if the lesion is superficial, it appears white. A dermoid cyst may become a large, painless, fluctuant mass that interferes with eating and speaking. This cystic hamartoma originates from varied germinal epithelium trapped during embryonic fusion. The growth of the cyst is slow and progressive and occurs entirely superior to the mylohyoid muscle; it is usually first noticed in young adulthood. Congenital sublingual dermoid cysts are rarely seen in infancy. Oral cavity dermoid cysts account for about 1.6% of all dermoid lesions.
2. **Assessment** The dermoid cyst has all the characteristics of a benign lesion. The best assessment is total excision if the patient is concerned about the growth. It is difficult to differentiate a dermoid cyst from a mucocele or a ranula. A dermoid cyst has skin appendages that distinguish it from other epidermoid cysts. Preoperative evaluation with a thyroid scan and xeroradiograms are often helpful in assessing the lesion.
3. **Treatment** No treatment is needed unless the cyst is large enough to interfere with eating or speaking. If a surgical procedure is planned, the excision should be complete, to preclude recurrence of the lesion.

C. Torus

1. **Description** Torus palatinus is a bony midline exostosis of the hard palate that is variable in size and shape. Torus mandibularis is composed of the same hard cortical bone, but it is located on the lingual surfaces of the inferior alveolus opposite the cuspid-bicuspid region, often bilaterally. Tori are common and occur after puberty in about 20% of the population. The presumed cause is a failure of the palatal or mandibular bone to stop growing after fusion.
2. **Assessment** These bony growths should be easily recognized by their characteristic features. Tori are susceptible to trauma, and over-lying inflammation may confuse the diagnosis. Otherwise, these lesions have no clinical significance unless further growth interferes with the wearing of a dental prosthesis.
3. **Treatment** No treatment is necessary. Surgical excision is indicated only if the tori interfere with denture wearing.

D. Osteoma

1. **Description** Osteomas are benign osteogenic tumors primarily found on the skin or face and, less commonly, in the oral cavity. The oral lesions usually appear at the lingual aspect

of the alveolar ridge near the mandibular angle; they are rarely found at the base of the tongue near the foramen cecum. These tumors are comprised of slow-growing, mature bone that produces painless masses. Although the growth is characterized as benign, osteomas can become large. The diagnosis is usually made in the second or third decade of life, most often in females.

2. **Assessment** The most important point to remember when evaluating a patient with multiple osteomas of the jaw is the relationship to Gardner's syndrome. This dominant hereditary defect in connective tissue consists of polyposis of the large bowel, epidermoid cysts of the skin, and multiple osteomas of the facial bones. The facial osteomas appear early in the course of the disease. The large-bowel polyps appear late, and a 40% incidence of malignant degeneration exists. Osteomas should be differentiated from fibrous dysplasia, sclerosing osteomyelitis, and calcified periosteal hematomas.

3. **Treatment** Osteomas should be treated only if they become symptomatic. If jaw opening is compromised or if facial asymmetry develops, the mass should be surgically removed. Usually, an osteoma is either a well-circumscribed, sclerotic mass within bone or a mass on the surface of bone; excision is thereby facilitated.

E. Hereditary Hemorrhagic Telangiectasia

1. **Description** Hereditary hemorrhagic telangiectasia (Rendu-Osler-Weber-syndrome) is an autosomal dominant familial disease characterized by lesions primarily of the facial skin, oral cavity, fingertips, toes, and nasal septum. Lesions of the oral cavity appear as punctate, bright red, raised spots that increase in size with age. They appear frequently at the mucocutaneous junction of the lip and on the tip and anterior dorsum of the tongue. These small arteriovenous fistulas bleed spontaneously or when traumatized. Recurrent epistaxis is the hallmark of hereditary hemorrhagic telangiectasia. The patient has no disturbance of bleeding or clotting time. The lesion usually appears in the second and third decades of life.

2. **Assessment** The diagnosis is made from the clinical triad of telangiectatic lesions, hereditary incidence, and familial pattern. Histologically, the lesions appear beneath the dermis or mucous membrane, with the characteristic finding of dilated vessels lined with endothelium without elastic or muscular tissue. The lack of contractile support accounts for the bleeding.

3. **Treatment** No effective therapy is known. Cautery or laser coagulation of superficial lesions may postpone recurrent bleeding. If severe hemorrhaging occurs, transfusions are indicated as life-saving measures.

III. OBSTRUCTIVE LESIONS

A. Mucocele

1. **Description** This common lesion of the oral cavity is often located on the lower lip or buccal mucosa. It appears as a raised, painless pale cystic lesion that is formed after rupture of a mucous gland or duct, with extravasation of mucus into tissue. The cause of the rupture may be trauma, inflammation, the presence of suture material, or congenital obstruction.
2. **Assessment** The only way to differentiate a mucocele from other cystic lesions of the oral cavity is by excisional biopsy. The histopathologic study shows a characteristic fibrous capsule with an inflammatory response.
3. **Treatment** No treatment is needed unless the mucocele enlarges sufficiently to become bothersome to the patient; then, surgical excision is indicated.

B. Ranula

1. **Description** A ranula, or mucous retention cyst, is a special type of mucocele. It appears as a translucent, cystic swelling of the floor of the mouth, often lateral to the frenulum. The formation of a ranula is due to an obstruction of a secretory duct of one or both sublingual glands. The cyst may become large and may interfere with speech and deglutition.
2. **Assessment** A ranula is readily distinguished by its location and its translucency. Palpation with the forefinger determines the extension of the mass. A histologic diagnosis can only be made after excision.
3. **Treatment** No treatment is indicated unless the patient is symptomatic. The type of ranula determines the extent of dissection. A simple ranula can be treated by marsupialization; a plunging ranula requires excision. To prevent recurrence, both the cyst and the secreting source must be removed. The cyst wall is easily ruptured during dissection.

C. Calculus

1. **Description** Calculi are commonly found throughout the salivary glands; approximately 80% occur in the submaxillary gland and about 20% in the parotid and sublingual glands. Patients usually complain of swelling and pain triggered by salivation. Calculi arise from the precipitation of foreign material within the ducts secondary to inflammation or other irritation. Calculi are composed of calcium phosphate or carbonate.
2. **Assessment** Palpation of the ducts of the submaxillary gland (Wharton's duct) and of the parotid gland (Stenson's duct) is important. Often, a salivary stone may be felt obstructing the duct. Radiographic study may reveal a stone the radiodensity

of which is due to the high mineral content. Usually, the stones of the submaxillary duct are radiopaque; the stones of the parotid duct, radiolucent. Sialography is also useful in demonstrating obstruction.

3. **Treatment** A single acute episode can be treated by dilatation of the duct and removal of the stone. Chronic sialolithiasis usually leads to surgical removal of the affected gland. Chronic supportive sialadenitis may ensue if an obstruction is not relieved. Sialagogues, hydration, warm packs, gentle massage, and oral antibiotics are then recommended. The infecting organism is often a penicillin-resistant strain of *Staphylococcus aureus*. Intravenous antibiotics are occasionally indicated for a severe infection. Again, an appropriate antistaphylococcal penicillin is indicated. Often, pus may be expressed from an infected duct, and Gram staining with a culture should guide antibiotic use.

IV. REACTIVE LESIONS

A. Linea Alba

1. **Description** Linea alba is a linear, whitish area on the buccal mucosa opposite the occlusal line. The patient usually has no symptoms, but habitual cheek biting or poorly fitted dentures may cause soreness. This reactive lesion is commonly found in elderly patients.

2. **Assessment** A complete medical history often suffices. If further evaluation is necessary, a biopsy will show typical reactive hyperkeratosis and an inflammatory cell infiltrate. The differential diagnosis should include a traumatic ulcer.

3. **Treatment** The patient should be reassured that the lesion is benign. An irritative focus should be eliminated. Improved oral hygiene is also helpful.

B. Hyperplastic Alveolar Mucosa

1. **Description** This reactive lesion is called granuloma fissuratum and appears as multiple curtain-like folds of tissue in the gingivolabial sulcus.

2. **Assessment** The diagnosis can be confirmed by having the patient remove the dentures for 2 weeks or more. The reddened, soft, movable folds of tissue fade away once the irritative source is eliminated. A biopsy of a more bothersome lesion shows fibrous tissue proliferation with overlying hyperplasia of the epithelium.

3. **Treatment** Ill-fitting dentures should be corrected or discarded if suitable replacement is available. Persistence of the tissue folds may require surgical excision, to allow refitting of the dentures.

C. Reparative Granuloma

1. **Description** This benign lesion is soft, glossy red, and pedunculated and is located most often on the labial aspect of the gingiva of the maxilla or mandible. Other possible sites include the mucous membrane of the lips, tongue, and buccal mucosa. If the patient has a history of preceding trauma, then the lesion may appear as a painless ulceration; bleeding can be copious. Frequently, this lesion is referred to as an epulis. The cause is unknown, although hormonal changes are suspected. A pregnancy granuloma or epulis often occurs during the second month of gestation. An infectious agent has not been identified.

2. **Assessment** A pyogenic granuloma is a characteristic lesion easily diagnosed by a careful examination of the oral cavity. The diagnosis is more obvious if the patient is pregnant. The lesion can be difficult to distinguish from hyperplastic alveolar mucosa secondary to irritation from ill-fitting dentures. Biopsy, performed if necessary, reveals parakeratosis with nonkeratinizing epithelium.

3. **Treatment** A pregnancy granuloma should be observed. Often, the benign growth resolves after completion of the pregnancy. In general, pyogenic granulomas can go untreated unless recurrent trauma causes bothersome bleeding; then, excision may be necessary. Recurrence is rare, and malignant transformation is unknown.

D. Leukoplakia

1. **Description** This disease of older persons, more often men, is characterized by a sharply outlined, milky white patch or plaque without induration. It frequently involves the tongue, floor of mouth and soft palate. The cause is varied; smoked tobacco, chewed tobacco, alcohol, or local irritation may be responsible. Most often, leukoplakia is innocuous and represents a benign thickening of oral mucosa that acts as a protective mechanism against local irritation, for example, on the edentulous jaw. When the keratosis is found in the floor of the mouth or the soft palate, especially in the presence of areas of redness (erythroplakia), atypia or carcinoma in situ may be demonstrable on biopsy. These changes are often found adjacent to areas of early invasive carcinoma, and a sequential metamorphosis from one to the other occurs in some individuals (Am. J. Surg., *146*:512, 1983).

2. **Assessment** The only reliable method of diagnosis is biopsy. The key histologic findings are hyperkeratosis, acanthosis, and dyskeratosis. The differential diagnosis includes lichen planus, chemical burns, syphilis, and candidiasis.

3. **Treatment** Local excision is indicated if the lesion fails to resolve after removal of irritative sources. Tobacco and alcohol

use should be discouraged. Cryotherapy is an alternate treatment method. Radiation therapy is contraindicated.

E. Candidiasis

1. **Description** The yeast-like fungus Candida albicans is found readily on the buccal mucosa and tongue and is considered to be a commensal organism that becomes a pathogen under certain circumstances. These predisposing factors include systemic use of antibiotics or corticosteroids, pregnancy, diabetes, Cushing's disease, debilitated states, radiation therapy, and chemotherapy. The lesions of the throat are painful and interfere with swallowing. They appear as soft, white plaques attached to the mucous membrane of the oral cavity. These plaques are easily stripped to reveal an underlying, bleeding surface. This feature is a distinguishing characteristic because other plaque-like lesions such as leukoplakia cannot be stripped. Lesions may extend to the corners of the mouth or into the esophagus. An endotoxin-like substance released by candida organisms accounts for much of the associated inflammation.
2. **Assessment** Direct examination with potassium hydroxide (KOH) reveals branching hyphae that are pathognomonic. On the Gram stain, fungi appear as gram-positive organisms larger than bacteria. Candida albicans grows readily on fungal or bacterial media; specific identification can be obtained by subculturing on chlamydospore agar.
3. **Treatment** Nystatin oral suspension should be gargled 4 times daily for several minutes before swallowing. In patients with difficult or recurrent cases, a 1 or 2% gentian violet solution is most useful, but it is esthetically unappealing.

V. ULCERATIVE LESIONS

A. Necrotizing Sialometaplasia

1. **Description** This benign lesion of salivary tissue is seen clinically as a single, painless ulcer of the hard palate. It is easily confused with malignant lesions, especially mucoepidermoid or squamous cell carcinoma. The ulceration may be spontaneous or reactive, usually in response to injury. The cause of necrotizing sialometaplasia is unknown; however, a local self-strangulation may occur secondary to swelling. The lesion occurs predominantly in males; the male-to-female ratio is 3 to 1. No racial predilection has been observed. An association with smoking and alcohol has been reported.
2. **Assessment** The clinical presentation is paramount. The uninformed physician is startled by the extensive ulceration of the palatal mucosa. A definite diagnosis is established only by microscopic examination of the lesion. Histologic features in-

clude coagulative necrosis of minor salivary glands along with prominent squamous metaplasia of acini and ducts, with pseudoepitheliomatous hyperplasia.

3. **Treatment** Treatment is unnecessary because spontaneous resolution occurs within 12 weeks. A firm diagnosis eliminates the chance of a needless operation.

B. Acute Herpetic Gingivitis

1. **Description** Acute herpetic gingivitis is a painful and disabling primary infection of children usually under 16 months of age. Herpes simplex virus type I is a DNA virus responsible for this nongenital herpetic infection. The incubation period lasts from 3 to 12 days, and the primary infection runs a course of 1 to 3 weeks. Small vesicles appear on the gingiva, buccal mucosa, tongue, or lips. These lesions quickly rupture, to form painful ulcers often covered with grayish desquamating epithelium. Malaise, fever, and lymphadenitis accompany the primary infection.

2. **Assessment** Because the disease is self-limiting, a thorough medical history and an awareness of the problem suffice. If any doubt exists, a skin biopsy or a cytologic smear will be helpful and will show giant cells and inclusion bodies. The lesions of herpes simplex, herpes zoster, and varicella infections have an identical appearance, however. A change in specific neutralizing antibody titer occurs in the primary lesion of herpes simplex, but not in recurrent lesions. The titer peaks at 2 to 3 weeks. If the apparatus are available and if the procedures are indicated, the virus can further be identified by electron microscopy and by fluorescent antibody techniques.

3. **Treatment** The disease is self-limiting; thus, supportive and symptomatic measures are indicated. Currently effective prophylactic therapy is unavailable. Because the primary infection is painful, analgesia is important. Salicylates should be adequate. Cleansing mouthwashes, such as benzalkonium chloride (Zephiran) 1:1000 or tetracycline suspension, soothe the involved mucous membranes and help to decrease secondary bacterial infections. More severe infections may require intravenous fluids and systemic antibiotics, if dehydration and superinfections occur. The healing time of primary stomatitis may be decreased by the use of topical antiviral agents, which interfere with DNA synthesis.

C. Recurrent Herpes Infection

1. **Description** Recurrent herpes simplex infection is distinct from the painful primary infection, although the same type I herpes virus is involved. The recurrent form is the "cold sore" or "fever blister" found at the mucocutaneous junction of the lips. After the primary infection, the ubiquitous herpes virus

is not eliminated, but lies dormant in a sensory ganglion. Periodically, external stimuli such as fever, stress, sunlight, and trauma reactivate the virus, which is conducted by peripheral nerve fibers to the epidermis or mucous membrane of the oral cavity. The sequence involves formation of papules that form vesicles, become purulent, and heal without scars within 7 to 10 days. The infection is self-limiting, except in patients with compromised host responses; such patients are predisposed to widespread and more destructive lesions.

2. **Assessment** The same diagnostic procedures outlined for the primary herpetic infection are applicable for the recurrent form. No change in specific antibody titer is seen, however.

3. **Treatment** Supportive care includes topical anesthetics and mouthwashes. Good nutrition also helps, but efforts may be hindered by swallowing difficulty. One should avoid corticosteroid creams because suppression of an inflammatory response may cause a severe infection.

D. Recurrent Aphthous Stomatitis

1. **Description** This benign lesion is often referred to as a canker sore. It usually appears on the tip and sides of the tongue and on the lip and buccal mucosa. The lesion is a painful, small, round ulcer with a white floor and yellow margins, surrounded by an erythematous areola. The cause of this ulcer is elusive. Two theories are prominent: hypersensitivity to a transitional L-form of an alpha-hemolytic streptococcus or an autoimmune response of the oral epithelium. Other possible causes include herpes simplex infection, food allergy, or emotional stress. Greater than 60% of the United States population will periodically have a canker sore, which lasts 10 or 11 days and is followed by a variable asymptomatic interval.

2. **Assessment** Patients rarely seek a physician for an examination of a canker sore because the problem is common and self-limiting. In the exceptional instance, a careful medical history and examination should confirm any suspicions. A biopsy is rarely indicated.

3. **Treatment** Although aphthous ulcers are self-limiting, they are painful, and patients with persistent lesions require symptomatic care. Initial treatment may include milk of magnesia, diphenhydramine hydrochloride (Benadryl), 2% viscous lidocaine (Xylocaine), or a combination of these agents. An oral suspension of tetracycline may enhance oral hygiene and may soothe painful ulcers. Patients should be advised to restrict food intake for an hour after treatment, to maximize the topical benefit. Levamisole, an antianergic agent intended to restore cell-mediated immunity, may help symptomatically. Orabase, an adrenocorticoid topical dental paste, may also be applied to the oral mucosa to reduce the pain.

E. Benign Pemphigus

1. **Description** This chronic bullous disease of unknown origin occurs primarily on the mucous membrane of the oral cavity of adults. The clinical features are multiphasic and painful. Grayish white collapsed vesicles or bullae with peripheral erythematous zones rupture, leaving a bleeding surface and center. The course of the illness is often protracted, with remissions and exacerbations. Benign pemphigoid lesions must be distinguished from pemphigus vulgaris, which has a high mortality rate if untreated. Pemphigus vulgaris usually begins in the nasal or oral mucosa. In contrast to pemphigoid lesions, the bullae of pemphigus vulgaris are larger and are more easily ruptured, resulting in large, denuded areas. This involvement represents a serious problem in the management of secondary infection and in the maintenance of fluid balance. The disease gradually spreads to other parts of the body.
2. **Assessment** Biopsy of an early vesicle and examination under a light microscope enable one to differentiate between pemphigoid and pemphigus vulgaris. The hallmark of pemphigus vulgaris is massive acantholysis of the epidermis. Acantholysis is absent in pemphigoid. Immunofluorescence also helps differentiate between pemphigus and pemphigoid by detection of IgG antibodies. These antibodies react with a specific intercellular antigen, and the fluorescence occurs precisely at the site of acantholysis in pemphigus. In pemphigoid, the fluorescence occurs at the basement membrane.
3. **Treatment** Systemic corticosteroids are usually adequate for suppression of benign pemphigoid. The dose is usually less than 50 mg/day prednisone, but in unusual instances it may exceed 100 mg/day. Diclonine (Dyclone) gargle alleviates the pain associated with ulcerated lesions. Adequate control of pemphigus vulgaris involves large doses of systemic corticosteroids, often followed by methotrexate therapy for immunosuppression. Azathioprine is also successful in controlling the disease.

F. Erythema Multiforme

1. **Description** Erythema multiforme is considered to be a hypersensitivity syndrome that produces a characteristic response of the skin and mucous membranes. Multiple precipitating factors include drug reactions, viruses, infections, endocrine changes, and underlying malignant disease. In 50% of patients, no cause is ascertained. The skin lesions are variable, but they are often characterized by iris or target lesions favoring the extensor areas of the extremities. This lesion consists of a central vesicle or erythema surrounded by alternating, concentric, pale and red rings. Oral lesions occur on the buccal membrane, lower lip, and tongue, and appear first as blisters that even-

tually form painful superficial ulcers with erythematous borders. These lesions usually heal spontaneously in 2 to 3 weeks. The disorder is frequently recurrent and is most common in winter and early spring in children and young adults. A severe form of erythema multiforme has widespread mucosal involvement and is referred to as Stevens-Johnson syndrome.

2. **Assessment** A detailed medical history is invaluable because the patient can often relate recurrent episodes over several years. Antecedent infections, drug administration, or illnesses should be detailed. A complete workup should include cultures, serologic studies, skin tests, and a chest film. Mycoplasma and deep fungi must be suspected in the search for an underlying infection. If the clinical presentation is atypical, a skin biopsy is worthwhile. The characteristic histopathologic picture is acute lymphohistiocytic inflammatory infiltrate around blood vessels.

3. **Treatment** Symptomatic care should include antihistamines, analgesics, oral hygiene, 3% hydrogen peroxide mouthwash, diclonine (Dyclone) solution, and Chloraseptic mouthwash. Appropriate antibiotics are indicated for any infections specifically identified. For patients with severe involvement, hospitalization and intravenous fluids are recommended. Oral prednisone, 2.5 mg, or intramuscular prednisone, 80 to 120 mg/day, should be given until the patient responds. Systemic corticosteroids are commonly used, but their efficacy has not been proved.

G. Lupus Erythematosus

1. **Description** Systemic lupus erythematosus (SLE) is a disease of unknown origin with multiple and varied systemic manifestations, such as arthritis, nephritis, pleurisy, perichondritis, hemolytic anemia, leukopenia, and thrombocytopenia. Discoid lupus is a chronic skin ailment associated with SLE. A patient with discoid lupus rarely develops SLE; more often, a patient with SLE has the cutaneous lesions of discoid lupus. Oral manifestations are common in both disorders. The lesion is an erythematous, maculopapular eruption often associated with butterfly distribution facial manifestations. Women are more often affected than men, and the age of onset is usually between the second and fifth decades. Survival rates for SLE decrease with renal and central nervous system involvement. The pathogenesis, characteristic of the immune-complex diseases, is related to the immunologic mechanisms of tissue injury.

2. **Assessment** The hallmark of SLE is the presence of antibodies to nuclear components. The level of antinuclear antibodies is characteristically elevated. Other important laboratory tests include a complete blood count, urinalysis, renal

function test, serum albumin-to-serum globulin ratio determination, erythrocyte sedimentation rate, rheumatoid factor, fluorescent treponemal antibody absorption, and complement testing. If a biopsy is performed, the histopathologic findings will include fibrinoid deposits in blood vessels and among collagen fibers; hematoxylin bodies are specific. The differential diagnosis must include rheumatoid arthritis, scleroderma, Sjögren's syndrome, drug ingestion, and syphilis.

3. **Treatment** Although a cure is not available, periodic remissions are common. For systemic problems, corticosteroid treatment is the cornerstone. High doses of prednisone, 60 mg/day for 2 weeks, are recommended. This regimen is slowly tapered to a maintenance dose of approximately 10 mg/day. Azathioprine and cyclophosphamide have been added when prednisone has failed. Severe side effects are frequent, particularly corticosteroid-induced psychosis. Patients with less-severe involvement can be treated with rest, salicylates, and antimalarial agents such as chloroquine. Patients with cutaneous lesions should avoid ultraviolet light.

VI. NEOPLASTIC LESIONS

A. Papilloma

1. **Description** Oral papillomas are the most common of benign neoplasms. Unlike their nasal and laryngeal counterparts, oral papillomas are not locally invasive, and malignant degeneration is rare. These painless lesions are exophytic and cauliflower-shaped, usually located on the palate near the uvula. Other common locations are the lips and buccal mucosa. Papillomas are usually small and solitary, but when found on the palate, they may be multiple. The cause is unknown, but it is almost certainly viral. Oral papillomas occur at any age.

2. **Assessment** Oral papillomas are easily recognized because of their distinguishing characteristics. Excisional biopsy provides a definitive diagnosis and eliminates any question of premalignant status. The histopathologic study shows stratified squamous epithelium, generally in the form of tree-like branchings and with the constant finding of keratosis.

3. **Treatment** Surgical removal is recommended if the patient is concerned about these oral lesions. Excision through the pedicle of a papilloma should be avoided, to prevent recurrence. If extensive growth is found over the palate or other area of the oral cavity, an acrylic splint may be needed to promote healing. A dermal graft or dressing such as zinc oxide or Silvadene may be applied to the splint, and the splint may then be secured over the excised area.

B. Fibroma

1. **Description** Two types of fibromas are present in the oral cavity: a true neoplastic fibroma, which is rare, and a fibroepithelial polyp, which is a common sequel to chronic irritation. These asymptomatic lesions appear as pink, elevated, soft growths that are pedunculated or sessile. They occur anywhere in the oral mucosa, but most frequently in areas that are easily traumatized. All ages and sexes are affected.

2. **Assessment** Fibromas are best identified by light microscopy after local excision or biopsy. Dense, interlacing collagen fibers with occasional nuclei are seen. An epithelial sheath with minimal vascularity is also present. True fibromas are well encapsulated. Other forms of fibromatosis include hereditary gingival fibromatosis, gingival fibromatosis from phenytoin (Dilantin), idiopathic fibrosis, and multiple fibromatosis.

3. **Treatment** True fibromas do not regress, and surgical excision is indicated if growth is significant. Fibroepithelial growths are usually small and asymptomatic. Once the source of trauma is removed, these lesions often regress.

C. Pleomorphic Adenoma

1. **Description** Mixed tumors, or pleomorphic adenomas, of the oral cavity originate primarily from the minor salivary glands of the palate. Other areas include the lip and tongue. These lesions are slow growing and asymptomatic unless traumatized. They appear as smooth, spherical, discrete nodules. Histologically, pleomorphic adenomas contain a mixture of epithelial and variable mesenchymal tissue. Although commonly found in the major salivary glands, mixed tumors are universal in the oral cavity. Males and females are affected equally, and the age of presentation ranges widely.

2. **Assessment** This benign oral cavity lesion must be differentiated from other soft neoplasms because over 50% of minor salivary gland tumors are malignant, and the majority of these occur on the palate. In contrast to those of the major salivary glands, mixed tumors of the minor salivary glands of the oral cavity have a greater cellularity, with a predominant epithelial element. Adenoid cystic carcinoma is the most common malignant derivative of minor salivary tissue.

3. **Treatment** Wide local excision, including periosteum and occasionally bone, is indicated to ensure complete removal. Mixed tumors have pseudocapsules and usually extend beyond their fibrous boundaries.

D. Hemangioma

1. **Description** Two types of hemangiomas are seen in the oral cavity, cavernous and capillary. They may occur intraosseously

or as peripheral lesions. The most frequent location is the tongue, followed by the lip and cheeks. Young children are commonly affected. The lesion is often discovered during the preschool years and undergoes a slow, progressive regression. Clinically, the peripheral lesions vary in size, blanch with pressure, and pulsate because of an arteriovenous shunt. Hemangiomas near the surface are red, and those deeply placed are dark purple or blue. Hemangiomas arise from endothelial cells.

2. **Assessment** The two types of hemangiomas are differentiated by light microscopy. The capillary hemangioma is composed of small, thin-walled vascular spaces lined by plump endothelial cells. The cavernous hemangioma is identical, except the vascular spaces are larger and fewer in number. In the oral cavity, a distinction between granulation tissue with a rich vascular supply and a hemangioma may be impossible.
3. **Treatment** Observation is often the best treatment because hemangiomas may regress. Small peripheral lesions can be safely excised, but larger lesions may require extensive block resection. Central, intraosseous hemangiomas involve complex treatment, and excision or biopsy can be hazardous. Fortunately, these lesions are rare. Sacrificing normal tissue is not justified unless life-threatening hemorrhaging exists. Various treatments with irradiation, cryotherapy, or sclerosing agents are not usually recommended.

E. Lymphangioma

1. **Description** Oral lymphangiomas are common lesions found frequently at birth or early childhood. The three known types are capillary, cavernous, and cystic. The cavernous lymphangioma is the most common type. The principal sites are the anterior two-thirds of the tongue, the cheek, the floor of mouth, and the upper lip. All lymphangiomas are lined with endothelium and have a straw-colored, lymph-like fluid. Lesions located superficially are pale white or pink and fluctuant; deeper lesions are elevated, rubbery masses. Lymphangiomas exhibit a slow, chronic growth, and they rarely regress. Growth may cease at puberty unless infection intervenes.
2. **Assessment** The clinical appearance is characteristic. Microscopically, one sees abundant, endothelium-lined cystic spaces containing either coagulated lymph or blood. If surgical excision is contemplated, an arteriogram will be indicated. The differential diagnosis includes hemangioma, muscular hypertrophy, primary and secondary amyloidosis, and neurofibroma. Cystic hygromas of the neck are often associated with lymphangiomas.
3. **Treatment** Lymphangiomas of the oral cavity run a slow, chronic course. Observation and careful exploration are the

best treatment. If the lesion becomes large enough to interfere with swallowing, articulation, and dental occlusion, then surgical excision will be indicated. Complete eradication is impossible unless the tumor is limited. Radical operations are condemned, and, regardless of the method, the recurrence rate is high. Irradiation should not be used in the treatment of this disorder.

F. Neurofibromatosis

1. **Description** Neurofibromas are benign tumors of peripheral nerves, usually occurring as a solitary lesion or as part of a generalized neurofibromatosis (von Recklinghausen's disease). Although they most frequently are found on the skin, neurofibromas are also found in the mouth; the tongue is the most common site. Clinically, these rare lesions appear as firm, elevated, painless nodules or fusiform swellings that slowly increase in size and number. Men are affected more often than women, and the appearance of these peripheral nerve lesions is usually in the second and third decades of life. Multiple neurofibromatosis, or von Recklinghausen's syndrome, is an autosomal dominant disorder associated with neurologic abnormalities and developmental defects. Café-au-lait spots are the most common physical finding. The majority of patients with this disease have a benign course, but a definite risk exists because approximately 8% of neurofibromas undergo sarcomatous change. The prognosis is poor in patients who develop sarcoma.
2. **Assessment** The diagnosis is confirmed by light microscopy after surgical excision. The neurofibromas arise from the Schwann cell, which is of neuroectodermal origin. Histologically, the lesion is nonencapsulated, with a high concentration of elongated Schwann cells compactly arranged in streams and twists. The differential diagnosis includes other peripheral nerve lesions such as schwannoma, granular cell myoblastoma, neurogenous nevi, and neuroma.
3. **Treatment** Usually, intraoral nodules are asymptomatic; however, chronic irritation and trauma may occur. Mastication, speech, and swallowing may be compromised if the tumor's growth is significant. Surgical removal is then indicated. The neurofibroma is radioresistant.

17

DISORDERS OF TASTE

ROGER L. CRUMLEY

I. GENERAL PRINCIPLES

A. Definitions

1. **Ageusia,** the total loss of the sense of taste, is a rare disorder.
2. **Hypogeusia,** decreased appreciation of the sense of taste, and **dysgeusia,** inappropriate and usually unpleasant taste sensation, are much more common than ageusia.
3. **Cacogeusia** is a taste disorder characterized by an obnoxious taste produced by food.

B. Anatomic Features

The human taste buds are located in the palate, the pharynx, and the papillae of the tongue. The fungiform papillae are concentrated on the anterior portion of the tongue and contain three to five taste buds each. The circumvallate papillae on the posterior tongue surface contain thousands of taste buds with a time-latency sensation longer than that associated with the anterior tongue's taste buds. Another difference is that the anterior taste buds appear to be associated with sweet and salty taste, whereas the circumvallate taste buds have a greater sensitivity to bitter taste. Sweetness is best perceived at the tongue's tip; salty and sour sensitivities are greatest on the lateral borders of the tongue. The taste buds of the anterior two-thirds of the tongue are innervated by taste fibers of the chorda tympani nerve, the cell bodies of which are located in the geniculate ganglion. Taste buds located on the posterior third of the tongue and the pharynx are innervated by the glossopharyngeal and vagus nerve fibers.

C. Physiologic Features

Salty tastes are derived from inorganic compounds that ionize in solution, such as sodium chloride and other chlorides, bromides, and iodides. Sour tastes are generally thought to arise from the hydrogen ion. Hydrochloric, sulfuric, and nitric acids taste the same when made up of equal concentrations, although such is not true of organic acids. Sweet tastes are associated with organic compounds, such as polysaccharides, glycerol, alcohols, and ketones. Bitter-tasting compounds are also organic and frequently belong to the alkaloid family; examples are strychnine, nicotine, quinine, and morphine. Some substances, such as sodium salicylate and magnesium, may give rise to a sweet sensation anteriorly, but a bitter taste when applied to the base of the tongue. The midline region of the oral tongue is apparently insensitive to any chemical taste stimulation. An intimate relationship exists between olfaction and taste, even for tastes that are thought to be nonaromatic. As a result, olfactory testing should be performed in patients with alterations of taste. See Chapter 12.

D. Testing of Taste

1. **The drop technique,** as described by Henkin (JAMA, *217*:434, 1971), is probably the most effective way to test for taste. Sucrose is used for sweet, sodium chloride for salty, hydrochloric acid (HCl) for sour, and urea for bitter tastes. Median recognition thresholds are ascertained and are compared with normal values.
2. **Electrogustometry** has been described as a quantitative taste test, but it has lost most of its credibility because of its excitation of trigeminal (pain and tactile sensation) nerve fibers at threshold levels just above those described for taste bud excitation.
3. **Evalulation of olfaction** It is important to assess olfaction in these patients, as previously mentioned. Techniques for assessing olfaction are discussed in Chapter 12.

II. SPECIFIC DISORDERS

A. Drug-Induced Disturbances

The following drugs may produce taste disturbances, usually hypogeusia or dysgeusia: penicillamine, biguanides (phenformin), griseofulvin, metronidazole, lithium carbonate, and rifampin. Treatment is simply the discontinuance of the offending medication.

B. Postinfluenza-like Hypogeusia and Hyposmia (PIHH)

A syndrome of hypogeusia, with or without dysgeusia, and hyposmia has been described following an influenza-like illness (Ann. Otol. Rhinol. Laryngol., *84*:672, 1975). These patients have an abrupt decrease in taste and smell acuity during an upper respiratory illness. Taste and smell sensations do not return in many cases. On physical examination, these patients have thinning of the usual tenacious nasal mucous blanket and an abnormally wide patency of the nasal airway. Testing of taste by the three-stimulus drop technique demonstrates elevated thresholds in such patients. Treatment of this condition is at present unsatisfactory, although some reports have noted resolution of the disorder following the oral administration of zinc sulfate, 110 mg q.i.d.

C. Trauma

The incidence of taste disturbances following head trauma is unknown. Occipital trauma is more likely to produce loss of smell, and this condition can confuse the identification of pure taste disturbances. Patients may complain of dysgeusia and dysosmia without any objective loss of taste or smell. The difficulty of testing taste sensation contributes to the identification and characterization of the incidence of decreased taste following trauma. Many investigators believe that the most common explanation is that of anosmia produced by tearing of olfactory nerve rootlets in the cribriform area and an apparent loss of taste, which is actually due to the loss of perception of aromatic flavors; salt, sweet, bitter, and sour taste sensations are retained in such patients. Occasionally, normal taste acuity returns spontaneously. That some patients with hypogeusia and hyposmia following head injury exhibit a lowered serum concentration of zinc indicates that alterations in zinc metabolism may contribute to taste disturbances. A trial of zinc therapy is recommended in such patients.

D. Sarcoidosis

Decreased taste sensation has been reported in some patients with olfactory sarcoidosis (Arch. Otolaryngol., *103*:717, 1977).

E. Acute Zinc Loss

The association between zinc serum concentrations and taste sensitivity is well documented. In patients with acute viral hepatitis and zinc deficiency, as well as in those with regional enteritis and similar zinc-depleting disorders, taste sensation is poor. Other malabsorption syndromes, such as chronic alcoholic cirrhosis, may also be associated with taste dysfunction. Histidine may lower serum zinc levels. The return of taste sensation generally parallels the rise of zinc serum levels to normal. In such patients, taste detection and recognition are impaired. The role of zinc in taste is thought to be due to its function as a co-factor in alkaline phosphatase, the most abundant enzyme isolated from the taste bud membrane. The administration of zinc sulfate, 110 mg q.i.d. orally, is the recommended regimen.

F. Chorda Tympani Dysgeusia

Surgical interruption of the chorda tympani nerve produces taste disorders of varying degree and quality (Arch. Otolaryngol., *92*:76,

1970). Because glossopharyngeal nerve fibers remain intact, the ability to sense bitter and sour tastes is preserved. Some authors report that dysgeusia produced by stretching or otherwise traumatizing the chorda tympani nerve is symptomatically more annoying than is ageusia from chordal transection. Whatever the chordal injury, no effective treatment exists for taste disorders so induced.

G. Disturbances Caused by Radiation Therapy

During radiation therapy of the oral cavity, taste buds are affected, as is the rest of the oral mucous membrane. The circumvallate papillae, rich in taste buds, become reddened and inflamed a few days prior to the onset of generalized mucositis. Subjective alterations in irradiated patients vary, however. Suppression of one or more taste sensations may be accompanied by heightened sensitivity to other tastes. Only rarely are all flavors affected. As already noted, the taste buds associated with the circumvallate papillae may be more severely affected by ionizing radiation than those located on the anterior tongue. In fact, the sensation of bitter and sour tastes is more commonly depressed than that of salty and sweet flavors, which are sensed more anteriorly on the lingual surface. The treatment of taste loss following radiotherapy is symptomatic at best. Artificial saliva may help to disperse taste-active modules within the taste bud membrane. A trial of zinc therapy is recommended for patients with continued complaints. Gradual return of taste function over a 12-month period is the usual course (Lancet, *2*:1138, 1959).

18

DENTAL AND PERIODONTAL DISEASE

ROBERT H. GILMAN

This chapter is designed as an overview of the most common disorders associated with the dental and periodontal tissues. Most of these disorders are treated by dental practitioners. Because otolaryngologists and head and neck surgeons examine oral tissues on a daily basis, a basic familiarity with disorders of the dentition and supporting structures is necessary. This chapter is intended to help head and neck surgeons to recognize some of these disorders, to communicate their findings, and to make referrals, when appropriate, to dental colleagues.

I. GENERAL CONSIDERATIONS

The 2 dental arches, the maxillary and the mandibular, each contain 20 primary teeth or 32 permanent teeth. The primary or deciduous teeth include 2 central incisors, 2 lateral incisors, 2 canines, and 4 molars per arch. The permanent teeth consist of 2 central incisors, 2 lateral incisors, 2 canines, 4 premolars, and 6 molars per arch. The anterior teeth are the incisors and the canines; the posterior teeth are the premolars and the molars. Orientation within the arch and for individual teeth is given in Table 18–1.

A. Definitions and Orientation

The Armed Forces and Insurance Notation System is the most widely used set of abbreviations for specific teeth. For permanent teeth, numbering begins with the maxillary right third molar, which is designated number 1, and proceeds across the maxillary arch to the maxillary left third molar, which is number 16. Numbering resumes with the mandibular left third molar, which is number 17,

TABLE 18–1

Terms of Direction Used in Dental Practice

Term	Direction
Direction within the dental arch	
Term	*Direction*
mesial	toward the midline
distal	away from the midline
lingual	toward the tongue (mandibular arch)
palatal	toward the palate (maxillary arch)
buccal	toward the buccal mucosa (posterior teeth)
labial	toward the lips (anterior teeth)
facial	toward the buccal or labial surface of any tooth
Direction with regard to teeth (all arch directions are also applicable to teeth)	
Term	*Direction*
occlusal	toward the tooth surface that meets the opposite arch dentition
incisal	same as occlusal, but for anterior teeth
coronal	toward the crown of the tooth
apical	toward the root of the tooth
cervical	toward the root-crown junction (cervix) of the tooth

and proceeds across the mandibular arch to the mandibular right third molar, which is number 32. The system works the same way for primary teeth, with lower-case letters, beginning with "a" for the maxillary right second molar and ending with "t" for the mandibular right second molar.

B. Ages of Tooth Eruption

See Table 18–2 for specific ages at which deciduous and permanent teeth erupt.

C. Occlusion

All teeth occlude with 2 opposing teeth, except the mandibular central incisors and the maxillary third molars, which occlude with only 1 opposing tooth. The maxillary arch overlaps the mandibular arch both vertically and horizontally. The vertical overlap is referred to as overbite, whereas the horizontal overlap is referred to as overjet. Occlusion is most commonly subdivided by Angle's classification system. Angle's Class I occlusion is present in about 73% of the population and is considered the normal occlusal relationship. In Angle's Class I occlusion, the mesiobuccal cusp of the maxillary first molar is in the buccal groove of the mandibular first molar. Class II occlusion or mandibular retrognathism is present in approximately 24% of the population. In Angle's Class II occlusion, the mesiobuccal cusp of the maxillary first molar is mesial to the buccal groove of the mandibular first molar. Angle's Class II occlusion can be subdivided into Type I, characterized by maxillary anterior protrusion or "buck teeth," and Type II, characterized by a lack of overjet with labioversion of the incisor roots. Angle's Class III, or mandibular prognathism, is present in ap-

TABLE 18–2

Ages of Tooth Eruption

Deciduous teeth	Maxillary (months)	Mandibular (months)
Central incisors (CI)	7.5	6.5
Lateral incisors (LI)	8	7
Canines (C)	16–20	16–20
First molars (M1)	12–16	12–16
Second molars (M2)	20–30	20–30
Permanent teeth	*Maxillary* (years)	*Mandibular* (years)
Central incisors (CI)	7–8	9
Lateral incisors (LI)	8–9	10
Canines (C)	11–12	12–14
First premolars (P1)	10–11	12–13
Second premolars (P2)	10–12	13–14
First molars (M1)	6–7	9–10
Second molars (M2)	12–13	14–15
Third molars (M3)	18+	18–25

proximately 3% of the population. In Angle's Class III occlusion, the mesiobuccal cusp of the maxillary first molar is distal to the buccal groove of the mandibular first molar. Any alteration in normal maxillary overbite is considered a crossbite. It can be further defined as a crossbite occurring in the lateral posterior or the anterior teeth. Apertognathia or open bite occurs when some teeth fall into occlusion while others remain apart. Open bite can further be described by its site, such as anterior or posterior open bite.

II. DISTURBANCES OF DENTAL DEVELOPMENT DURING THE GERMINAL PHASE

A. Ectodermal Dysplasia

This autosomal recessive disease involves all ectodermal structures including the teeth. The patient may have no teeth (anodontia) or a decreased number of teeth (hypodontia). Teeth that do form are often rudimentary and conical in shape. They may be of little functional value and may require coverage with full crowns or removal and replacement with full dentures.

B. Anodontia

This term refers to the complete absence of dentition. The disorder must be distinguished from false anodontia, a disease of tooth eruption in which the teeth form but do not erupt. Anodontia usually affects both the deciduous and the permanent teeth. Occasionally, anodontia affects only the permanent teeth, and the deciduous teeth are present. The reverse does not happen, however. Patients with true anodontia require full dentures.

C. Accessory and Supernumerary Teeth

Accessory or supernumerary teeth are teeth in excess of the normal complement. They are usually abnormal in form. Such teeth are generally described by their position relative to the normal arch. For example, a periodens occurs buccal to the arch, whereas a mesiodens occurs between the maxillary central incisors. In general, supernumerary teeth are extracted once it has been determined that they are not part of the normal complement of teeth.

D. Predeciduous Dentition

Predeciduous teeth are present at or soon after birth. These teeth are usually aborted in structure and are a form of supernumerary teeth. Like supernumerary teeth, they should be extracted once it is clear that they are not part of the normal complement of teeth.

E. Postpermanent Dentition

Such teeth erupt well after the normal eruption of the permanent dentition. In general, these teeth are accessory teeth impacted by delayed eruption. Under most circumstances, they should be extracted when they appear.

III. DISTURBANCES OF DENTAL DEVELOPMENT DURING THE STAGE OF MORPHODIFFERENTIATION

A. Hutchinson's Teeth

Hutchinson's teeth occur in 10 to 30% of patients with congenital syphilis. The teeth are generally screwdriver shaped or show notching of the incisal edges. The maxillary central incisors demonstrate this abnormality much more commonly than the mandibular central incisors. The enamel abnormalities that may occur in these teeth predispose them to dental caries. Therefore, careful dental follow-up is indicated.

B. Mulberry Molars

This disorder, which is present in approximately 30% of patients with congenital syphilis, is primarily an abnormality in the amount and configuration of enamel of the first molars. Varying elements of enamel hypoplasia may occur. In the most severe form of this disease, enamel may occur as small, spherical globules on the surface of the dentin. These teeth may require restoration, with new crowns.

C. Macrodontia

Macrodontia is the presence of abnormally large teeth throughout the dentition. This disorder may require treatment if the jaw is not correspondingly enlarged. Tooth crowding caused by macrodontia can be treated by extraction and orthodontic procedures.

D. Microdontia

Microdontia is the presence of abnormally small teeth throughout the dental arch. No specific treatment is necessary for this condition.

E. Dens in Dente

This term literally means a tooth growing within a tooth. The disorder is present in 2% of the population and may occur within the pulp chamber or within the root canal. It is generally asymptomatic and is diagnosed by incidental radiography. Some of these teeth possess pits connecting the fusiform internal tooth to the outside. These pits may predispose the affected teeth to caries. These teeth must be watched closely because carious lesions progress rapidly in the poorly formed enamel of the invaginated tooth. Another condition related to dens in dente is the so-called dilated odontoma, in which the deeply invaginated tooth within a tooth expands and causes a physical ballooning of the outer tooth. These teeth must be extracted.

F. Gemination and Fusion

Gemination refers to a single root with two completely or partially separated crowns. Fusion refers to two separate tooth germs that fuse into a large crown with a grooved or separated root and separate root canals. It is difficult to distinguish between gemination and fusion. Problems arise in that the fused teeth may be aesthetically unacceptable or the increased bulk of the fused crowns may lead to crowding problems, maleruption, or impaction. Moreover, the line of cleavage between adjoining crowns may be deep and vulnerable to caries. The disorder usually occurs in the incisors and often necessitates extraction.

IV. DISTURBANCES OF DENTAL DEVELOPMENT DURING ODONTOGENESIS AND AMELOGENESIS

A. Enamel Hypoplasia

Also known as hereditary brown teeth, enamel hypoplasia is caused by a reduction in the thickness of enamel. This reduction may be local, occurring in one or several teeth secondary to such local causes as trauma or local infection. A general form of the condition secondary to systemic infection during the formation of enamel may be caused by rickets, smallpox, or rubella. A hereditary form of this disorder has also been described. The disturbance in the thickness of the enamel may leave these teeth both aesthetically unappealing and subject to rampant dental caries. Depending on timing, the condition may affect the primary or secondary dentition or both. Enamel hypoplasia may also be accompanied by enamel hypocalcification. Like hypoplasia, hypocalcification may affect single teeth, multiple teeth, or all teeth. The process involves the deeper layers of enamel and so may not predispose teeth to dental caries. Once the teeth become carious, however, the erosive process is of greater magnitude in the presence of hypocalcification. Both hypoplastic and hypocalcified teeth may show thermal sensitivity. Treatment of this disorder is generally full coverage of the crown. A hereditary subgroup of enamel hypoplasia and hypocalcification is amelogenesis imperfecta. Some forms of the disease seem to follow a sex-linked dominant pattern, whereas others seem to follow an autosomal dominant pattern. The teeth may range from normal in shape, with an opaque, chalky white appearance in some areas and a burnt-sugar brown in others, to grossly malformed dentition. Enamel replacement with full-crown coverage remains the treatment of choice.

B. Dentinogenesis Imperfecta

This disorder, also known as hereditary opalescent dentin, may occur as an isolated disorder or as part of a more widespread systemic disturbance, such as osteogenesis imperfecta and generalized albinism. The mode of inheritance appears to be autosomal dominant. The disorder is characterized by a generalized grayish discoloration of all teeth. In addition, the teeth have bulbous crowns and brittle enamel that often flakes off and separates at the dentinoenamel junction. A predisposition to caries formation exists, and once caries are established, they spread in an accelerated manner. The treatment for the disorder is the coverage of all teeth with full, protective crowns. Because the roots of these teeth are more brittle than normal, these teeth should not be used as abutments for bridges or attachments for arch bars. Hereditary shell teeth and dentinal dysplasia are two variations of dentinogenesis imperfecta. In each of these variants, the teeth have essentially normal enamel with an abnormal quantity and quality of dentin. In both cases, root formation is incomplete or nearly absent, with resultant early atresia.

C. Enamel and Dentin Pigmentation

A number of neonatal factors produce abnormal pigmentation in developing teeth, such as erythroblastosis fetalis, congenital hematoporphyrinuria, ochronosis, lead poisoning, and tetracycline ingestion. Of these factors, the most notable is the administration of tetracyclines, both in pregnancy and in children up to the age of 6 years. Tetracycline crosses the placenta and has an affinity for all developing calcified tissue. When given during pregnancy, the drug affects the deciduous dentition. Because tooth formation continues until the age of 6 years, when all permanent teeth are developed, except the third molars, tetracycline should be avoided until after that age. The discoloration caused by tetracycline is initially bright yellow or yellow green but gradually becomes darker with the eruption of the tooth. Both the enamel and the dentin are affected, and some associated hypoplasia and hypocalcification of the enamel may be present. For the most part, these teeth have no functional problems, and treatment is directed toward the cosmetic effect, by means of bleaching, bonding, or full-crown coverage. Fluoride, occurring naturally or added to the drinking water at concentrations above 1.8 parts per million, can cause small areas of hypocalcification of enamel that appear as flecks of chalky white discoloration in the crowns of teeth.

D. Cemental Hypoplasia

Patients with cemental hypoplasia have a decreased amount of and rate of production of cementum, the specialized avascular bone covering the roots of teeth. This disorder results in premature atresia of the teeth. It is rare and can be associated with hereditary hypophosphatasia, an autosomal recessive condition that causes bone and metabolic lesions similar to those of rickets. The anterior deciduous teeth are most frequently affected; however, the permanent teeth may also be involved. Such teeth are usually lost and must be replaced with fixed or removable prosthetic appliances.

V. DISTURBANCES IN DENTAL ERUPTION

A. Retarded or Delayed Eruption

This disorder most often follows a familial pattern without association with any specific malady. Both systemic and local factors can play a role. For example, systemic disorders such as hypopituitarism, hypothyroidism, and vitamin D deficiency can delay tooth eruption; delayed eruption is also associated with cleidocranial dysostosis. Local factors, such as tooth crowding, dentigerous cysts, and eruption cysts, can interfere with the eruption of a single tooth or group of teeth. Ankylosis, the obliteration of the periodontal ligament with the fusing of the tooth root and surrounding bone, can interfere with tooth eruption in two ways. First, ankylosis of a deciduous tooth, most often seen in deciduous molars, prevents the loss of a deciduous tooth and thereby the normal eruption of the permanent tooth; this fusion is most often caused by chronic apical inflammation. Second, ankylosis can occur in the developing permanent tooth, thus directly inhibiting its eruption. These teeth often come to lie in an abnormal position, with the crown lying apical to the surrounding occlusal plane. Such teeth are referred to as submerged. The treatment for retarded tooth eruption is directed toward the specific cause whenever possible. Treatment of the systemic disorder often allows the teeth to emerge. Removal of crowded conditions or associated cysts can allow for eruption of individual teeth. Teeth may also be aided in their eruption orthodontically.

B. Supraeruption

This term refers to the eruption of a tooth apical to the surrounding occlusal plane. This disorder is associated with the loss of opposing dentition. Surrounding teeth act as guides and stops for eruption, and the loss of these guides and stops allows for the supraeruption of teeth. For this reason, lost teeth should be replaced whenever possible, to provide continuity and stability of the dental arches.

C. Premature Eruption

This condition almost always has a familial pattern. It rarely accompanies any major systemic disease and requires no specific treatment.

D. Pseudoanodontia

This term refers to the condition in which the teeth develop normally but do not erupt. This disorder gives the appearance of anodontia. In patients with anodontia, it is important to ascertain radiographically the presence or absence of tooth formation. One may thus determine whether the problem is one of tooth formation or of tooth eruption. In evaluating a patient with an unerupted tooth, one should first consult a table of normal tooth-eruption ages (see Table 18–2), to consider whether the situation is truly pathologic. Only when eruption age falls outside these normal values is a further workup necessary.

VI. ACQUIRED DENTAL DISEASE

A. Dental Caries

Dental caries, considered to be the most common disease of man, results in decalcification and disintegration of the dental hard tissue.

1. **Clinical manifestations** Caries begins in the grooves and pits of teeth and in the interproximal areas, where food debris becomes lodged. Less commonly, caries can occur on the smooth surfaces of teeth. The teeth most commonly affected by dental caries are the first molars. The occlusal surfaces are involved most frequently, followed by the interproximal areas. In the earliest form, caries appears as a chalky area on the enamel that progresses to gross, identifiable erosion of tooth structures. Acute caries occurs most frequently in the primary teeth of children and shows rapid development and progression. Chronic caries is found mostly in the permanent teeth of older individuals and develops slowly. Caries may arrest during formation, to leave a permanent lesion in the enamel of the tooth. Previously treated caries may reoccur at the margin of a previously placed restoration. Although gross caries is readily identifiable even by the untrained eye, incipient caries requires careful examination. The dental practitioner generally uses the tip of a dental explorer to look for "sticky areas." Careful examination of the spaces between the enamel and existing dental restorations is important. Radiographic examination is also important, especially in the interproximal areas.
2. **Prevention** Caries is a bacterially related disease. Bacteria present on areas of dental plaque react with sugars from the

diet to produce acids that decalcify the dental enamel. The best treatment is prevention. The most important prescription is a balanced diet and good oral hygiene, including a fluoride dentifrice and dental flossing to remove food particles from the interproximal areas. The administration of systemic fluoride, either in the drinking water or by oral supplement, as well as professionally applied topical treatment with 10% stannous fluoride, can increase the enamel's resistance to decalcification. In young children, the teeth can be sealed with a plastic-like material that bonds to the surface of the enamel and produces a coating impervious to the caries-producing acids. Vaccines against cariogenic bacteria are now being developed.

3. **Treatment** Once caries forms, it must be removed in its entirety and replaced with a substance that will restore the function of the tooth. The type of restoration depends on the location of the dental caries and on the amount of tooth structure destroyed. The involved tooth structure is removed with a combination of rotary instruments and other special hand instruments. The pattern in which the structure is removed depends on the type of restorative material to be used. The most common material is amalgam, a mixture of silver, tin, and mercury, that can be placed immediately into the prepared area. The average life span of an amalgam restoration is 20 years. Other restorative materials include gold foil, composite resin (tooth-colored plastic materials), and cast gold or nonprecious metal restorations. Cast restorations are indirect. Impressions of the dental arch are needed to form the restoration in the laboratory. The formed restoration is then cemented into place in the patient's mouth.

4. **Caries associated with radiation therapy** A form of dental caries of particular concern to head and neck surgeons is secondary to radiation therapy. These lesions generally occur 2 to 3 weeks to 2 to 3 months from the start of radiotherapy. They are most often located at the cervix of the tooth and progress rapidly. The loss of saliva secondary to radiation therapy is believed to play an important role in the development of radiation-related caries. Careful dental restoration prior to and during radiotherapy is the most important means of prevention of radiation-related caries. Dental consultation prior to radiotherapy is recommended. See Chapter 19.

B. Erosion and Abrasion

The term erosion refers to the loss of dental hard tissue at the gingival margin of the tooth. This lesion usually appears as a groove running parallel to the margin of the gingiva. Its cause is obscure, but it may be related to tooth-brushing technique, neurologic disorders, hyperthyroidism, mucosal gland secretions, or gingival pocket discharge. Abrasion is indistinguishable from erosion; however, it is definitely traceable to tooth-brushing technique or to the use of an excessively abrasive dentifrice. The primary treatment is the use of a soft-bristled brush and a mild dentifrice; patients must be instructed to brush perpendicular to rather than parallel to the gingival margin. Occasionally, erosion and abrasion are so severe that the exposed dentin becomes sensitive to various stimuli. This problem can sometimes be helped by the use of a special dentifrice for sensitive teeth. When this treatment is not successful, the best alternative is full-crown coverage of the tooth.

C. Attrition

This term refers to the loss of tooth structure related to mastication. This disorder occurs primarily on the occlusal surface of teeth and appears as flattened areas known as wear facets. The presence of these wear facets points to parafunctional occlusal habits such as bruxism, or the grinding of teeth at night, and clenching, or the the grinding of teeth during the day. These habits can lead to secondary disorders of the temporomandibular joint.

D. Hypercementosis

Hypercementosis, the excessive deposition of cementum on the root surface, may cause the tooth root to become bulbous and malformed. The process can be idiopathic, or it may be associated with local or systemic disorders such as periapical granulomas, Paget's disease, acromegaly, gigantism, or local trauma. Hypercementosis is generally of little clinical significance, except during the extraction of teeth, when the malformed and enlarged roots may complicate the extraction process.

E. Trauma

Patients with individually traumatized teeth are frequently seen by the otolaryngologist. Such patients should be referred as soon as clinically feasible to a trained dental practitioner. The dental arch should be thoroughly examined, to determine the presence and absence of individual teeth and their condition. Fractured tooth fragments often find their way into associated perioral and intraoral lacerations. Radiographic examination is helpful in ascertaining the presence of retained tooth structures and tooth-material foreign bodies. Table 18–3 summarizes the classes of dental trauma and their treatment.

F. Pulpitis

1. **Acute pulpitis** occurs secondary to physical agents such as heat or cold, chemical agents such as irritants applied to exposed dentin, and bacterial invasion secondary to deep caries. The major symptom is pain, either continuous or throbbing, which is usually increased when lying down. Pain also increases with changes in temperature. The teeth are often sensitive to extremes of temperature, especially cold. The diagnosis is made

TABLE 18–3

Classification and Treatment of Dental Trauma

Class		
Class I		
	Definition:	Simple fracture of the crown involving enamel only
	Treatment:	Occlusal grinding or simple restoration
Class II		
	Definition:	Fracture of the crown involving enamel and dentin, but not dental pulp
	Treatment:	Standard dental restoration
Class III		
	Definition:	Extensive fracture of the crown, involving enamel and dentin and exposing dental pulp
	Treatment:	Root-canal therapy and restoration
Class IV		
	Definition:	Traumatized tooth becoming nonvital, with or without loss of tooth structure
	Treatment:	Root-canal therapy
Class V		
	Definition:	Teeth lost as a result of trauma
	Treatment:	The tooth in question should be transported with the patient by gently pushing the tooth back into the socket (if not completely avulsed) or in a sterile saline-soaked gauze (if completely avulsed); permanent teeth can be reimplanted and splinted into place; deciduous dentition should not be replanted; if replantation is unsuccessful or if the condition of the tooth or patient does not allow replantation, the tooth should be replaced with a bridge as soon as feasible; the sooner the tooth is replanted, the better the prognosis
Class VI		
	Definition:	Fracture of the root of a tooth, with or without loss of crown structure
	Treatment:	The closer the fracture is to the crown of the tooth, the poorer the prognosis for retention of that tooth; when possible, endodontic therapy followed by crown restoration is recommended
Class VII		
	Definition:	Displacement of a tooth without fracture of the crown or root
	Treatment:	Gentle repositioning in the socket and splinting to adjacent stable teeth
Class VIII		
	Definition:	Fracture of the crown en masse
	Treatment:	Usually extraction of the remaining root with replacement of the tooth by a dental bridge
Class IX		
	Definition:	Traumatic injuries to deciduous teeth
	Treatment:	Similar to that for permanent teeth; the exception is that primary dentition should not be replanted; careful follow-up, to ensure that no injury has occurred to the developing permanent dentition is mandatory

by vitality testing of the tooth. Treatment may include root-canal therapy.

2. **Chronic pulpitis** is a more protracted form of acute pulpitis in which the symptoms are intermittent, dull aching with hot and cold sensitivity. The teeth generally test as vital, but at a higher level than normal. The treatment is root-canal therapy.

3. **Hyperplastic pulpitis** or pulp polyp is most common in deciduous molars. The lesion appears as a fleshy red mass in a grossly carious tooth. Treatment is by removal of the pulp with pulp capping.

4. **Periapical abscess** When infection of the pulp spreads to the area around the tip of the root, a periapical abscess can occur. It is acute in onset and causes severe pain in the area of the alveolus of the involved tooth. One often sees swelling and fluctuance over the alveolus. Occasionally, the tooth is elevated in the socket. Percussion tenderness of the involved tooth is present. Treatment is by incision and drainage, either through the pulp chamber of the tooth or through the periapical tissues.

VII. PERIODONTAL DISEASE

A. Gingivitis

1. **Chronic gingivitis** The most common inflammation of the gingiva is chronic gingivitis. It is caused by local irritation from plaque, calculi, or dental restorations. The edematous type of the disorder is characterized by swelling of the gingival tissues that gives them a shiny, glossy appearance. Normal gingival stippling is lost. The gingivae are friable, and the gingival papillae are blunt. Chronic edematous gingivitis is reversible on removal of the locally irritating factors. Another form of chronic gingivitis is the fibrous type. This later and more developed stage of the edematous type has symptoms similar to those of edematous gingivitis. The treatment of chronic fibrous gingivitis is by gingivectomy.

2. **Infective gingivitis** is generally caused by streptococci and is characterized by a red, swollen, and painful gingiva. The inflammation extends to the oral mucosa. It is treated with penicillin.

3. **Hyperplastic gingivitis** results in exuberant fibrous overgrowth of the gingiva. It is frequently associated with phenytoin (Dilantin) intake; the disorder is present in 78% of patients taking phenytoin and is generalized in 10 to 30% of patients taking the drug. It is also associated with hereditary fibromatosis gingivae and with long-term mouth breathing. The treatment is by gingivectomy and withdrawal of the phenytoin, if possible, in patients with phenytoin-associated hyperplasia.

4. **Hormonal gingivitis** is similar to chronic edematous gingivitis in appearance and is associated with adolescence, menstruation, and oral contraceptive use. It is present in about 50% of pregnant women to one degree or another. The disorder is generally associated with poor hygiene and resolves spontaneously after pregnancy. The lesions begin in the interproximal spaces and may be either local or generalized. Treatment consists of periodontal hygiene.
5. **Desquamative gingivitis** starts as vesicles that rupture and leave raw patches on the gingiva. It is associated with menopause and with systemic diseases such as erosive lichen planus, pemphigus, and erythema multiforme. The patient may have a positive Nikolsky sign, with separation of gingival epithelium from underlying tissue under a moderate amount of finger pressure. The treatment consists of good oral hygiene, topical pain medication, and corticosteroid administration.
6. **Acute necrotizing ulcerative gingivitis** or Vincent's gingivitis is associated with Fusobacterium plautivincenti. The disease causes fever, cervical lymphadenopathy, malaise, necrosis of the interdental papillae, pseudomembranous formations, fetid breath, and swollen, red, painful, and bleeding gingiva. The treatment consists of rest, fluids, aspirin, debridement and scaling, penicillin, and the placement of a periodontal dressing.
7. **Allergic gingivitis,** also known as plasma cell or idiopathic gingivitis, involves the marginal and attached gingiva ending at the mucogingival junction. The disorder produces a red, swollen gingiva with a burning sensation or pain that is less severe than the clinical appearance would indicate. It can be local or generalized. The condition is usually secondary to a contact allergy; chewing gum is the most common allergen. Treatment involves removal of the offending agent and good oral hygiene.

B. Periodontitis

This inflammatory process, which involves the periodontal membrane and associated alveolar bone, results in the destruction of the bone and the formation of pockets between the tooth and alveolar bone. Periodontitis causes changes in the color of the gingiva, loss of stippling, edema, hypoplasia or recession of the gingiva, gingival cleft formation, pocket formation, increased tooth mobility, and radiographic evidence of bone destruction. The treatment consists of scaling, to remove plaque, calculus, and irritants. In addition, the surgical removal of any bony pockets, with recontouring of the underlying bone, is indicated. If the condition is allowed to progress, an abscess may form in the bony pockets. These lesions, referred to as periodontal abscesses, are uncomfortable and sometimes painful small, circumscribed swellings of the gingiva lateral to the associated teeth. Occasionally, the patient has a purulent discharge from the gingival sulcus. Treatment consists of incision and drainage, as well as elimination of the periodontal pocket.

C. Periodontosis

This disease of indefinite origin may be associated with gram-negative anaerobic infection. It is characterized by migration of teeth, formation of diastemas, extrusion of teeth, progressive malocclusion, pocket formation with inflammation, and secondary periodontitis. Unlike periodontitis, the disorder is most common in the first two decades of life. Treatment consists of scaling, pocket removal and recontouring of bone, splinting of loose teeth, elimination of occlusal prematurities, and antibiotics administration. A hereditary syndrome consisting of hyperkeratosis of the palms and soles and juvenile periodontosis is called the Papillon-Lefèvre syndrome.

D. Occlusal Traumatism

Occlusal traumatism results from pathologic occlusal forces secondary to malocclusions or parafunctional habits such as bruxism or clenching. The trauma of abnormal occlusal force damages the periodontium and leads to bony destruction, secondary inflammation, and periodontitis. Prolonged exposure can lead to loosening of teeth and their eventual attrition. The treatment includes scaling and pocket removal, as well as the removal of all occlusal interferences.

VIII. ODONTOGENIC CYSTS

These lesions are outlined in Table 18–4.

A. Periodontal Cysts

Periapical and lateral periodontal cysts are derived from epithelial rests referred to as the rests of Malassez. Lateral periodontal cysts are rare and develop within the periodontal tissues adjacent to the

TABLE 18–4

Odontogenic Cysts
Periodontal cysts
periapical
lateral
residual
Dentigerous (follicular) cysts
primordial
true follicular
eruption
Odontogenic keratocysts
Calcifying odontogenic cysts (Gorlin cysts)

lateral surface of a tooth. On roentgenograms, these cysts appear as radiolucent defects in bone. These cysts generally occur in the mandibular bicuspid areas. Periodontal cysts are usually asymptomatic and are detected incidentally on routine radiologic examination. Cysts arising from the epithelial rests of Malassez at the apex of the root of a tooth are known as periapical or radicular cysts. These lesions are asymptomatic unless they become secondarily infected. They may either enlarge or remain static. Enlargement may cause movement of the associated teeth and resultant local malocclusion. As cysts continue to enlarge, they may cause the cortical plates of the alveolus to expand, with accompanying external deformities of the jaw bones. Treatment of these cysts is by curettage, when possible, or marsupialization. When a tooth involved with a periapical cyst is extracted and the cyst is inadvertently left behind, it becomes known as a residual cyst.

B. Dentigerous (Follicular) Cysts

Cystic odontomas can be subdivided into simple follicular or primordial cysts, true follicular or dentigerous cysts, and eruption cysts.

1. **Primordial cysts** arise from the epithelium of the dental organ at an early stage in development and are the simplest and most undeveloped of the odontogenic cysts. They usually arise from the most distal part of the dental lamina in the mandibular molar region. Primordial cysts are most prevalent between the ages of 10 and 30 years and are most common in the region of the mandibular third molars. They appear as an asymptomatic, circumscribed radiolucency within bone, sometimes with a coarse, soap-bubble type of multiloculation. The treatment, in most cases, consists of enucleation or, when large size does not permit adequate enucleation, marsupialization.

2. **True follicular or dentigerous cysts** are similar to primordial cysts, except they are associated with the crown of an unerupted tooth. These cysts seem to arise from the reduced enamel epithelium that normally covers the crown of an unerupted tooth. Because dentigerous cysts are most common in teeth whose normal eruption has in some way been impeded, these cysts most frequently occur in impacted mandibular third molars. They may expand rapidly and may cause enlargement of the jaw. These cysts may be associated with migration of a neighboring tooth toward the inferior border of the mandible. The treatment of the dentigerous cyst is by enucleation when possible, in association with removal of the impacted tooth. Occasionally, the impacted tooth is left in place when its function is helpful to the dental arch. Dentigerous cysts are of further significance because of their association with ameloblastomas; these tumors may develop from the walls of dentigerous cysts. In addition, multiple dentigerous cysts are part

of the basal cell nevus syndrome that includes multiple basal cell nevi, bifid ribs, and multiple odontogenic cysts.

3. **Eruption cysts** are a superficial, extraosseous type of dentigerous cyst that occur in association with the crown of a nearly erupted tooth. These cysts cause fluctuant swelling in the soft tissues overlying the crown of such a tooth. The cyst is usually blue. Treatment, which consists of simple excision of the superficial cyst wall, usually allows for eruption of the associated tooth to proceed normally.

C. Odontogenic Keratocysts

These lesions are similar in origin and appearance to primordial cysts; however keratocysts are filled with keratin material. The significance of this cyst is that its expansion is thought to be secondary to the benign neoplastic proliferation of its epithelium rather than merely to the expansion of its keratin count. These cysts should be removed by enucleation. Removal must be complete, to prevent recurrence.

D. Calcifying Odontogenic Cysts (Gorlin Cysts)

Calcifying odontogenic cysts may be true cysts, but they have also been described as solid tumors. These lesions are generally intraosseous in location and occur primarily in the second decade of life. They show equal sex distribution and occur in equal numbers in the maxilla and the mandible. These cysts appear radiographically as a well-circumscribed radiolucency. Their significance is their association with ameloblastomas, ameloblastic odontomas, ameloblastic fibro-odontomas, and complex odontomas. Total excision is the treatment of choice; these cysts do not usually recur. Because of their association with odontogenic tumors, the excised specimen should be examined carefully by the pathologist, to ensure that treatment has been adequate.

IX. ODONTOGENIC TUMORS

These tumors are outlined in Table 18–5.

A. Ameloblastoma

Although no absolute agreement exists, ameloblastomas probably arise from cells of the dental lamina. This rare lesion affects both sexes and shows a peak incidence around 30 years of age. Eighty percent of ameloblastomas occur in the mandible, and 75% of these occur in the region of the angle. These tumors are seen as slow, painless, expansile lesions. The average delay from the time when swelling is first noted to the time medical care is sought is 6 years. Usually, the tumor breaks through bone and begins to invade overlying soft tissue. Unlike simple dental cysts, ameloblastomas expand toward both buccal and lingual plates simultaneously. Adjacent teeth are often loosened secondary to loss of bony support. Occasionally, these teeth are extracted, and the tumor is thereby able

TABLE 18–5

Odontogenic Tumors
Ameloblastoma
Adenomatoid odontogenic tumor (adenoameloblastoma)
Calcifying epithelial odontogenic tumor
Ameloblastic fibroma
Ameloblastic fibrosarcoma
Odontoma
compound
complex
ameloblastic
Dentinoma
mature
immature
Odontogenic fibroma
Odontogenic myxoma and fibromyxoma
Cementoma
Gigantiform
Fibrocementoma
Benign cementoblastoma
Periapical osteofibroma

to grow out of the socket of the tooth. Initially, multiple, punched-out locular lesions of bone are present, with little absorption of root structure. Some reactive sclerosis may be evident. One-third of ameloblastomas are associated with dentigerous cysts and appear to grow from the walls of these cysts. These lesions are said to have a high recurrence rate, although most recurrences are probably secondary to inadequate original treatment. The malignant spread of an ameloblastoma has been reported; however, documentation remains questionable. Treatment is by wide local surgical excision.

B. Adenomatoid Odontogenic Tumor (Adenoameloblastoma)

These tumors appear primarily as localized mural proliferations in dentigerous cysts. In fact, these tumors bear no relation to ameloblastomas. They are rare lesions; most occur before the age of 20 years, and a slight female predominance has been reported. These tumors, which are most often associated with an unerupted or impacted maxillary canine tooth, grow in a well-circumscribed manner and are entirely benign. Treatment consists of removal by curettage. The incidence of recurrence of these tumors is low.

C. Calcifying Epithelial Odontogenic Tumor (Pindborg Tumor)

These rare tumors, which seem to be most often associated with the crown of an impacted tooth, share many features with ameloblastoma. The lesion is not considered to be as aggressive as an ameloblastoma. Histologically, these tumors show focuses of calcification. Treatment is by wide local excision.

D. Ameloblastic Fibroma

This term refers to a rare odontogenic tumor associated with proliferation of both odontogenic epithelium and fibrous connective tissue. The tumor most commonly involves the bicuspid and molar regions. This lesion usually occurs in the second decade of life and causes slow expansion of the jaw, with progressive separation of the roots of adjacent teeth. The patient is usually asymptomatic, but mild pain may be associated. The tumor is well encapsulated, and simple curettage is curative. Recurrence is rare.

E. Ameloblastic Fibrosarcoma

This tumor is similar to ameloblastic fibroma, except malignant fibroblasts are revealed by careful analysis of the connective tissue component. This aggressive tumor has considerable local destructive capacity. Wide local excision is the treatment of choice.

F. Odontoma

Odontomas are benign tumors composed of adult tooth material. They may contain mixtures of enamel, enamel matrix, dentin, predentin, cementum, pulp, or periodontal tissues.

1. **Compound odontoma** contains multiple tiny teeth, either bizarre or rudimentary in shape. The arrangement of the individual tooth tissues is generally normal, with enamel overlying dentin and some sort of central pulp tissue.
2. **Complex odontoma** also contains a mixture of various adult tooth tissues, but the relationship among these tissues is abnormal.
3. **Ameloblastic odontoma** is rare. It is basically a compound or complex odontoma with proliferation of the odontogenic epithelium. This benign and noninvasive lesion has no behavioral association with ameloblastoma.
4. **Prevalence and treatment** Compound odontomas occur most frequently in the incisal region, whereas complex odontomas occur most frequently in the molar region. They are most common in the second or third decades of life and are usually asymptomatic. These lesions are often discovered serendipitously on routine radiologic examination. Occasionally, they become large enough that their bulk causes expansion of the jaw bone or movement of adjacent teeth. Conservative enucleation is the treatment of choice.

G. Dentinoma

This rare tumor is made up of dentin and supporting connective tissue. Mature dentinomas consist primarily of hard tissue with characteristics of mature dentin; immature dentinomas contain only focal deposits of immature dentin. These tumors occur most frequently in the mandibular molar area and increase in size gradually. The presenting features often include enlargement of the jaw, spreading of adjacent tooth roots, and impaction of adjacent teeth. These lesions usually occur in the second and third decades of life. Local conservative removal is the treatment of choice.

H. Odontogenic Fibroma

This lesion is similar to fibromas elsewhere, but it arises from fibrous tissue of the forming tooth. These benign tumors have no local invasive potential. They are rare, and the treatment is by local enucleation.

I. Odontogenic Myxoma and Fibromyxoma

These tumors, which arise from the connective tissue of the dental papillae, cause painless swelling of the jaws. They are benign, but can be locally invasive. Radiographically, these lesions appear as unilocular or multilocular cysts. The treatment of choice is by wide local excision.

J. Cementoma

1. **Gigantiform cementoma** (familial multiple cementoma) consists of large sheets of calcified tissue resembling cementum. This familial lesion is often multiple and may grow to considerable size within the jaw bones. Treatment is by conservative removal.
2. **Fibrocementoma** (cementifying fibroma) is found in older individuals, usually in the posterior region of the mandible. Radiographically, it appears as a predominantly radiolucent lesion with varying degrees of radiopacity, depending on the degree of calcification. The lesion may or may not be associated with individual teeth. Local conservative excision is the treatment of choice.
3. **Benign cementoblastoma** is a true benign lesion of cementoblasts. The tumor grows slowly and has a dense fibrous encapsulation. The patient is usually asymptomatic; however, some percussion tenderness of the associated tooth may be present. Palpable expansion of bone may also be evident. Treatment consists of extraction of the tooth and conservative enucleation of the associated cementoblastoma.
4. **Periapical osteofibrosis** is also known as a cementoma, cementoblastoma, cementifying fibroma, and periapical fibrous dysplasia. It is the most common lesion of the cementoma group and often appears as an asymptomatic periapical radiolucency on a roentgenogram. The manner of its presentation has led to the unnecessary extraction of many involved teeth. Lesions may affect single or multiple teeth, and the mandible is involved approximately 10 times more frequently than the maxilla. The incisors are the most frequently affected

teeth. The patient is invariably asymptomatic. Vitality testing of the associated tooth generally shows a normal response. The presence of a periapical radiolucency associated with a normal and vital tooth is the hallmark of periapical osteofibrosis. Therapeutic intervention is only rarely necessary, if the lesion becomes large enough to expand the jaw bone.

19

ORAL CARE AND REHABILITATION OF THE PATIENT WITH HEAD AND NECK CANCER

MATTHEW J. JACKSON

Nowhere in the health sciences are dentistry and medicine so closely integrated as in the management of the patient with head and neck cancer. The status of the oral cavity is of paramount importance in today's multidimensional approach to cancer of the head and neck. Proper oral form and function are the objectives of the dentist in managing patients who are undergoing cancer therapy. Only close collaboration among the members of the "head and neck team" can accomplish these goals.

I. ORAL CARE OF THE IRRADIATED PATIENT

The complications of irradiation to the oral cavity and adjacent structures are manifested in numerous ways. The severity of these sequelae are directly related to the dosage, fractionation, type, and duration of radiation. The institution of proper dental care may minimize or eliminate these problems. The side effects of tumoricidal irradiation to the oral tissue are xerostomia, radiation decay, infection, necrosis of soft and hard tissue, trismus, mucositis, severe mucositis, and loss of taste.

A. Pretreatment Assessment and Therapy

1. **Objective** Prior to the initiation of radiation therapy in the patient with head and neck cancer, a thorough dental examination must be performed. Such an examination is essential if therapy will involve the oral cavity or contiguous structures such as the major salivary glands, no matter which combination

of therapeutic techniques is employed. The goal is to ensure that the patient's dentition is in optimal condition, to obviate the need for high-risk procedures in the post-treatment period.

2. **Evaluation and treatment** The initial oral examination must use all necessary diagnostic aids to assess the hard and soft structures of the mouth. The objective of this pretreatment evaluation is to render the patient asymptomatic and free of any infection that might hamper the therapeutic regimen. After completion of the initial evaluation and the presentation of the findings to the head and neck team, the dentist must perform all necessary preirradiation dental procedures. Any unsalvageable teeth should be removed before radiation therapy starts. If the patient is to undergo an operation before radiation therapy, any teeth to be extracted should be removed during that surgical procedure. This method usually provides adequate healing time and eliminates the need for additional anesthesia. If radiation therapy is to be the primary therapeutic technique or if it is to be given preoperatively, however, these teeth should be extracted beforehand, and treatment should be delayed until adequate healing has occurred. Wound breakdown at the extraction sites is thus prevented. Generally, sufficient healing cannot occur in under 10 days. Difficult tooth extractions are associated with greater surgical trauma and require a longer healing period. Impacted or ankylosed teeth may take 4 or more weeks to heal. Inadequate healing invariably leads to necrosis of soft or hard tissues. In addition, if the teeth and their supporting bone are within the field of irradiation or adjacent to it, all necessary alveoloplasties and ridge contouring must be performed at the time of the oral surgical procedure. The removal of all loose spicules and sharp projections of bone, to provide an ideal edentulous ridge, ensures the primary approximation of the tissue. This precaution may enhance healing by preventing puncture or erosion of the bone through the gingival tissues, as well as by preventing the accumulation of debris in the tooth sockets. Patients with sound teeth are instructed in proper oral hygiene, dental care, and daily fluoride treatments. If a radiation stent or maxillofacial prosthetic device is indicated, construction should be initiated at this time. The preservation of as many sound teeth as possible is critical to maximal oral form and function, especially in patients who need maxillofacial prosthetic devices because of surgical resection.

B. Complications of Irradiation

1. **Xerostomia** Irradiation of the major salivary glands produces a permanent quantitative and qualitative reduction of saliva. Radiation-induced xerostomia is related to the dose and duration of the ionizing radiation. Histologically, one sees a progressive, radiation-induced inflammatory and degenerative

change in the acinar and ductal elements. It is rapid in onset, usually noted by the end of the second week of therapy, is pronounced, and is irreversible.

a. ***Alteration of oral environment*** The watery or serous secretions are lost initially. The residual salivary secretions are of the mucin type and are thick, ropy, and tenacious. Complaints of difficulty in swallowing food, of the presence of phlegm, and of extreme dryness are common. The intraoral soft tissues are altered by the loss of the lubricating effect of saliva; cracking and bleeding are common clinical signs. The fragile and damaged tissue is painful and distressing to the patient, especially when eating. Moistening or liquifying the food facilitates eating and swallowing and helps the patient to maintain adequate nutritional intake. Liquid high-calorie nutritional supplements are recommended.

b. ***Management*** Treatment for radiation-induced xerostomia is palliative. Frequent rinsing with nonirritating substances is recommended. Saliva-substitute rinses should be prescribed. Numerous rinses have been developed, with varying success, and are commercially available; examples are Xero-Lube and Oralube. The advantage of these elixirs is that their viscosity and electrolyte composition are similar to those of normal saliva. In addition, fluoride is added for enhancing the mineralization capacity of the solution, which is high in calcium and phosphate. Other preparations can also be used to coat and lubricate the dehydrated soft tissues and to relieve symptoms.

2. **Radiation decay and its prevention** With the onset of xerostomia, the oral environment changes. The inherent mechanical and chemical defenses of saliva against tooth decay are impaired. The residual saliva is no longer able to debride the teeth mechanically. Serous secretions are lost; the remaining saliva is stringy, thick, and tenacious and allows plaque and micro-organisms to accumulate on the teeth.

a. ***Chemical and microbial changes*** Chemically, the saliva becomes more acidic, with a drastic diminution in its protective salivary electrolytes and immunoproteins. With these changes, cariogenic microflora and plaque appear, regardless of the use of topically applied fluorides, artificial saliva, or meticulous oral hygiene. Significant changes in the aerobic and anaerobic microflora parallel the alterations of the salivary secretions. Populations of yeast-like fungi such as candida, of lactobacilli, and of Streptococcus mutans are increased. Moreover, the patient's diet changes from a detergent to a nondetergent type, as a consequence of mucosal dryness and discomfort. The additive effect of all these factors is a potentially enormous risk of caries. The magnitude of the potential cariogenic insult is imposing also because most patients who develop carcinoma of the head and neck are in the fifth, sixth, and seventh decades of life. Most patients who still have an intact or partially intact dentition exhibit varying amounts of gingival recession and incisal or occlusal wear. The net result is exposure of cementum or dentin, which is less resistant to decay than enamel. Because radiation decay characteristically occurs along the cervical regions of the teeth, the potential sensitivity, wear, and cariogenic devastation can be realized. This type of decay can be prevented by the daily use of fluoride and by meticulous oral hygiene. Areas of demineralization can be remineralized and hardened by the long-term use of fluoride. Associated tooth sensitivity and incisal or occlusal wear diminish with fluoride treatments.

b. ***Management of the dentition*** Various fluoride protocols have been devised for the irradiated patient. They may include fluoride rinses, fluoride gel in flexible trays, fluoride tablets, fluoride gum, or any combination. A 1% neutral sodium fluoride gel containing a disclosing agent is used. The gel is placed into flexible carriers made on dental casts of the individual patient's dental arches. A neutral fluoride gel and smooth flexible carriers are used to minimize trauma to the fragile and sensitive oral mucosa. The common commercially available acidulated fluoride preparations used routinely in dental practice are contraindicated because of the potentially irritative effect of the acid on the compromised irradiated soft tissues. The patient must brush and floss the teeth following proper technique. The carriers are then coated with the fluoride gel, are positioned over their respective arches, and are left in place for a minimum of 5 minutes. Intimate fluoride contact of all tooth surfaces is accomplished by the use of customized trays and by the pumping effect of clenching teeth. After the prescribed period of contact, the carriers are removed, and the gel is rinsed. The mouth is reinspected. Areas that have not been properly brushed or flossed appear red from the disclosing agent incorporated into the gel. The patient then must rebrush and refloss those deficient areas. The fluoride is used every day indefinitely. Discontinuing the fluoride initiates the decay process, no matter how long the interval after radiation therapy. Fluoride applications can be increased as needed if demineralization is evident. The use of the previously mentioned protocol or of similar regimens in conjunction with routine dental checkups and prophylaxis can virtually eliminate radiation decay. Both patient and dentist must know the problems, risks, and available therapeutic methods. Soft and hard dental tissues in or immediately adjacent to the field of treatment cannot receive any type of surgical trauma without possible serious consequences.

3. **Infection** During this period of change in the oral environment, the possibility of fungal overgrowth and infection also exists. The objective is to prevent secondary infection and the interruption of therapy. The overgrowth of yeast-like fungi such as Candida albicans in the mouth is common especially during therapy. Oral rinses of nystatin are effective.

4. **Soft and hard tissue necrosis** Osteoradionecrosis is a major complication and potentially the most debilitating sequela of cancerocidal doses of ionizing radiation to the oral cavity. This disorder has been reported to occur in 5 to 37% of patients receiving therapeutic radiation to the oral cavity and the naso- and oropharyngeal regions. It may occur within a few months of therapy, or it may occur up to 20 years later.
   a. ***Histologic changes*** Therapeutic doses of radiation to the bone and soft tissues cause basic pathophysiologic alterations. These include the following: impaired blood supply resulting in a decreased ability of the tissue to respond to injury; extracapillary fibrosis and decreased diffusion through the capillary wall; thickening of the basement membrane of the capillaries; arteriolocapillary intimal hyalinosis; inhibited capillary sprouting and vascular remodeling; vascular occlusion and a decrease in the number of small vessels per area, with a compensatory dilatation of the remaining capillaries (telangiectasia); separation of periosteum or endosteum from the underlying bone that denudes the bone, which frequently dies from the lack of blood supply; and disturbance of the well-balanced process of destruction and reconstruction of bone because of direct damage to the osteoclasts or osteoblasts. The effects of cancerocidal radiation on bone are due to injury to both cellular and vascular osseous components. The additional insult of reduced metabolic activity inevitably leads to bone death. The result is osteoporosis leading to osteonecrosis. This radiation-induced bone death is not of great significance, however, as long as the bone does not become infected or subjected to great stress or trauma.
   b. ***Predisposing factors*** Dental surgical procedures, operations on the jaw, pulp exposure from radiation decay, denture irritation, and traumatic occlusion may all cause osteoradionecrosis. Necrosis can also be spontaneous and of unknown origin; such a condition perhaps reflects the inability of the mucosa to maintain its normal integrity. Characteristics typical of these patients include the following: history of a previous surgical procedure, performed shortly before the initiation of radiation therapy with an inadequate period of healing; irradiation of lesions in close

proximity to the bone relative to medially located lesions; treatment with high doses of ionizing radiation with or without proper fractionation; therapeutic regimens of external radiation and interstitial implants; poor oral hygiene and the continued use of irritants such as alcohol and tobacco; lack of cooperation in managing radiation-induced tissue changes; elective or necessary surgical procedures in irradiated tissues including oral, periodontal, and endodontic surgical manipulation; indiscriminate use of prostheses after radiation therapy without resolving all treatment sequelae; the lack of preventive measures to avoid trauma to the irradiated area; the selection of poor candidates with numerous physical and nutritional problems for radiation therapy; the use of large treatment portals with greater radiation volume; and the presence of advanced tumors

c. ***Conservative management*** Necrosis, generally the result of trauma and infection to the irradiated tissue, may arise from a chemical, mechanical, or microbial insult. The primary treatment of soft or hard tissue necrosis is conservative management. Treatment objectives are to keep the area of necrosis free of infection and to promote healing. No radical surgical intervention should be attempted unless all conservative procedures prove fruitless and the patient's symptoms remain. The onset of soft tissue necrosis usually leads to an ulceration that is painful and enlarges unless treatment is instituted. This ulceration is slow to heal, and immediate conservative therapeutic intervention is indicated. The patient is advised to avoid irritants such as hot or cold liquids, spices, alcohol, and smoke. Irrigations with mild solutions of salt and soda and gentle debridement promote healing. In more severe cases, additional medicaments are recommended. Topical applications of zinc peroxide, carboxymethyl cellulose, and hydrogen peroxide pastes or of 1% neomycin solutions are effective. If soft tissue necrosis continues, the underlying hard tissues become exposed to the oral environment and develop osteoradionecrosis. Intense conservative procedures are indicated and include the removal of all irritants, the application of topical medicaments of zinc peroxide paste or 1% neomycin solution, meticulous oral hygiene, irrigations, and the gentle debridement of loose necrotic bone spicules. In patients with gross infection and severe pain, systemic antibiotics and analgesics are indicated.

d. ***Surgical management*** Only if conservative methods are unproductive and if the patient continues to have intractable pain, severe infection, trismus, and impaired function should more radical surgical procedures be employed; such operations often have severely debilitating results.

Surgical treatment can vary from simple sequestrectomy to mandibulectomy. Extraoral resections have been abandoned because of the high incidence of complications. An intraoral approach is recommended to reduce the danger of an orocutaneous fistula. This approach does not violate the irradiated skin, and the cosmetic deformity is minimized because no external scar is produced. The morbidity rate is lower, and no need exists for multiple reconstructive procedures.

5. **Trismus** When the muscles of mastication or of the temporomandibular joint are irradiated, a strong risk of trismus exists. The radiation causes tonic spasms and fibrosis of the muscles or fibrotic changes in the capsular elements of the joint. Trismus may become evident during the radiation therapy, but this condition is usually related to the degree of mucositis rather than to fibrosis or muscle spasms. Generally, radiation-induced trismus develops 3 to 6 months after termination of therapy.
   a. ***Treatment regimens*** If the foregoing anatomic sites are within the field of treatment, the patient should perform prophylactic mouth-opening exercises. In general, opening one's mouth as widely as possible 20 times, 3 to 4 times per day, usually minimizes fibrotic changes in the muscle and capsular components and loss of interarch space. If frank trismus does develop, more intensive measures will be indicated to minimize the loss of opening and to permit proper oral function. The amount of mouth opening is measured and is recorded. Intensive exercises and prosthetic aids are employed to regain the lost interarch space. Conservative approaches, including exercises and appliances, should be attempted before any radical surgical procedure is considered.
   b. ***Treatment devices*** Numerous devices can be constructed to counteract trismus. The objective of these appliances is to stretch the muscles and the fibrotic contractures. Varying designs such as wedges, screws, springs, or elastics are incorporated into these devices to achieve the necessary stretching. The dynamic bite opener is commonly employed for severe trismus. The advantage of this appliance is its ability to function in any position, whether during opening, closing, or lateral movement of the mouth. The dynamic bite opener permits a more gradual and more comfortable resolution of the problem than forced-opening corrective procedures. It allows a constant but firm pressure over a protracted period, and the amount and magnitude of force can be readily controlled.

6. **Mucositis** This complication of radiation therapy can become serious enough to interrupt treatment if it is not dealt with properly.

a. ***Signs and symptoms*** Oral mucosa within the field of radiation undergoes a series of transient and permanent changes. The mucositis is related to the overall dose, the number of doses given, the type of radiation, and the length of each dose. Mucositis generally develops by the end of the second week of treatment. The patient complains of pain, burning, and soreness and experiences discomfort during therapy and for several weeks afterwards. Clinically, the tissue becomes edematous and red. This tissue later becomes white, denuded, and finally ulcerates, covered by a fibrinous exudate.

b. ***Oral care*** Treatment is palliative. The objective is to provide both analgesic and antiseptic effects. Preparations such as viscous lidocaine, colloidal silver solutions, salt and soda rinses, Orabase, and peroxide rinses have all been used in controlling this problem. If treatment is successful, the patient will be comfortable, free of secondary infection, and able to maintain proper nutrition. Uncontrolled mucositis can lead to nutritional problems. The patient finds eating a difficult task, both psychologically and physically. It actually becomes easier not to eat. The patient must maintain a positive nitrogen balance to maximize the therapeutic effect of irradiation. Coarse and seasoned foods should be avoided. Topical viscous lidocaine, swished in the mouth several minutes before eating, anesthetizes the sensitive oral tissues and permits more comfort while masticating and swallowing. Other topical medicaments may also help; colloidal silver solutions have the twofold effect of being demulcents and mild antiseptics.

7. **Severe mucositis** In severe cases of mucositis, the use of systemic analgesics is indicated. If discomfort becomes overwhelming and if the nutritional status of the patient becomes compromised, a nasogastric tube must be placed, to allow proper nutrition and a positive nitrogen balance. Despite all efforts, it is impossible to eliminate the discomfort totally. Mucositis is a reversible situation, and the patient should be aware that the pain and discomfort are temporary and subside in several weeks. Then, although free of pain and apparently healed, the patient must realize that this tissue has been compromised permanently.

8. **Loss of taste sensation** Hypogeusia occurs early in therapy and is noted at approximately 3000 rads. Histologically, one sees radiation-induced injury to the microvilli or the surfaces of the taste buds. Generally, it is a transient sequela, but doses greater than 6000 rads may lead to some permanent taste loss. Partial taste sensation is re-established within 20 to 60 days of the last dose of radiation. In 2 to 4 months, the patient's sense of taste should be fully restored. The combination of mucositis, xerostomia, and hypogeusia leads to a loss of appetite and the

desire to eat. It is easier and more comfortable for the patient to abstain from food. Careful daily monitoring of the patient's nutritional intake and body weight is imperative, to prevent debilitation during treatment. See Chapter 17.

II. RADIATION THERAPY PROSTHESES

The radiotherapist may need to use prosthetic devices to facilitate the treatment program. In addition to optimizing the effects of head and neck irradiation, these devices can also prevent some of the sequelae.

A. Design

A team approach requiring close collaboration between the prosthodontist and the radiotherapist is necessary to accomplish treatment goals. The radiotherapist must outline the area to be treated, and the prosthodontist must analyze and explain to the therapist the limitations in the construction of the device. The size and shape of the prosthesis depend on the fields of radiation planned for any given primary site. The consequences of the prosthodontist's design can be assessed at the completion of therapy and thereafter. A sharply defined exudative mucositis is the best evidence that the appropriate geometric configuration has been reproduced at every period of irradiation.

B. Objectives

Some of the sequelae of radiation therapy can be severe and debilitating, even when the patient is free of disease. The objective is to eliminate or to minimize the side effects of therapy. The use of prostheses can be of great benefit in meeting these objectives. The reasons for using treatment prostheses are as follows: to outline and define fields of treatment; to assist with the proper direction of the radiation beams; to provide protection for contiguous normal tissues; to displace the tongue, lips, or cheeks; to serve as carriers for radium sources; to make it easier for the patient; to ensure accuracy of beam directions; and to simplify dosimetry in the tumor and in normal tissue.

C. Types of Prostheses

1. **Tissue displacers** This type of device ensures that the tissues to be irradiated (such as the tongue) are positioned within the radiation fields and that the tissues to be spared are correctly displaced.
2. **Tissue shields** With the use of various types of radiation sources, such as electron beam or orthovoltage, shielding devices may be used to protect contiguous intraoral structures that need not be irradiated. Lead, or alloys of lead, of varying thickness may be embedded into the prosthesis to shield such structures as the tongue and gingiva. In addition to the shield-

ing effect, the tissue is usually thereby displaced away from the radiation beam. This type of device minimizes the sequelae of radiation in normal structures.

3. **Carriers** A carrier appliance is indicated when a radioactive source is administered by means of beads, capsules, or needles; usually, radium or cesium-137 is the radiation source. The device is designed and constructed to place and to hold the radiation source accurately and securely in the same position during each period of treatment.
4. **Cone-locating devices** This prosthesis positions the radiation beam precisely to the tumor. An acrylic stent is custom-fabricated to the intraoral cone, and a custom baseplate or occlusal index is attached to the acrylic cone. The cone-locating device is inserted by the patient. The prosthesis positions the radiation beam accurately throughout treatment and simplifies and improves intraoral radiotherapeutic technique.

III. DENTURE USE FOLLOWING RADIOTHERAPY

The placement of dental prostheses over irradiated tissue is a controversial subject. In one series, 5% of patients irradiated to the oral cavity developed osteoradionecrosis related to denture irritation. With no prosthetic device, the mucosa would not be subjected to the trauma of denture bases caused by normal masticatory forces. Our aesthetically oriented society often dictates the replacement of lost teeth with some type of prosthetic device, however. Before prescribing prosthetic treatment, the dentist must accumulate as much information as possible from the patient, the radiotherapist, and the surgeon, to determine the general health of the patient, prognosis, treatment portals, and doses received. Oral evaluation provides information concerning friability and fragility of the mucosa. Signs and symptoms such as telangiectasia and scarring indicate tissue friability and areas of potential breakdown. Xerostomia results in the loss of the lubricating and retentive character provided to the dentures by saliva. Exostosis and bony undercuts are areas of high risk for developing osteoradionecrosis. Generally, a year is the waiting period before construction of dentures. This rule is not hard and fast, but an adequate period of time must be provided to allow the tissues to heal and to manifest radiation-related changes. Some patients are able to wear dentures before the end of the first year, and some have such drastic tissue changes that they are denied any prostheses at all. Patients who do wear dentures over an irradiated foundation necessitate careful construction and follow-up. Any irritation must be taken seriously. The prostheses should be removed and adjusted and not reinserted until healing has occurred.

IV. MAXILLOFACIAL PROSTHETIC DEVICES

Surgical resection of large oral and paraoral structures produces severe alterations of form and function. Prosthetic intervention is often the only method for rehabilitating the patient back into society. Maxillofacial prosthetic restoration may involve the palate, mandible, face, or any combination of these structures.

A. Maxillectomy

The prosthetic replacement following the resection of the hard or soft palate is termed the obturator. It restores oral form, communication, mastication, and deglutition. The three types of obturators used at different intervals during the healing process are the surgical, transitional, and definitive appliances.

1. **Types of defects** Prosthetically, two distinct defects can be created following maxillectomy. Unlike removal of the soft palate, resection of the hard palate leaves a static defect. The prosthesis (obturator) needs only to restore palatal form. The obturator is modified to improve speech and to prevent leakage of food and liquids around its borders. Removal of the soft palate produces a functional defect, however. Velopharyngeal competence is lost and must be re-established with a static prosthetic restoration that is physiologically acceptable to the residual velopharyngeal mechanism.
2. **Planning treatment** When a palatal resection is anticipated, the patient must be evaluated preoperatively. All diagnostic aids should be employed to render the oral cavity asymptomatic and optimally healthy. As many teeth as possible should be saved to provide support, stability, and retention of the obturator. Pretreatment dental casts are made of the maxillary and mandibular arches. The surgeon must then outline the extent of the resection and any possible modifications. The prosthodontist can then provide information to the surgeon that might improve the tissue foundation needed for rehabilitation. Such recommendations may include making a surgical cut through the middle of the tooth socket most proximal to the defect, repositioning of a palatal mucosal flap into the nasal cavity, removal of the inferior turbinate on the side of the defect, and maintenance and creation of subtle undercuts and scar bands.
3. **Surgical obturator** For hard palate resection, an immediate surgical appliance is recommended because it permits immediate oral feeding and eliminates the need for a nasogastric tube, it allows verbal communication, it aids in maintaining packing and dressing, it improves oral hygiene, it reduces postoperative morbidity and hospitalization time, and it improves the patient's psychologic outlook. Soft palate prosthetic restoration is not initiated until after operation because of the dynamic nature of the defect. For the dentulous arch, denture retention is obtained by the use of wrought-wire clasps attached to the residual teeth. These clasps are incorporated into the base of the prosthesis. The base is constructed from a clear acrylic, which permits visualization of the underlying tissue.

On the other hand, obturators for an edentulous arch must be retained by placement of suspension wires. The base is designed and constructed from clear acrylic. Generally, the prosthesis can be suspended posteriorly by circumzygomatic wires and anteriorly by a nasal-spine wire. On completion of the resection, the obturator is fitted and adjusted. The surgical obturator is removed at the initial pack removal and, if necessary, is modified with resilient liners to compensate for any changes in the defect.

4. **Transitional obturator** During subsequent healing or radiation therapy the surgical appliance is modified as needed to improve speech and prevent the reflux of food and liquid through the nose. A new prosthesis can be constructed, or the original surgical appliance can be modified and used during this period.
5. **Definitive obturator** Following healing, a new prosthesis is constructed of more substantial materials. At this stage, the occlusion is re-established on the side of the defect for the dentulous arch, or the entire occlusion is re-established for the edentulous patient. The defect is obturated with a hollow bulb, which reduces the weight of the prosthesis. Acrylics or siloxanes are used most often for bulb construction.
6. **Soft palate resection** Obturation is initiated approximately 10 to 14 days postoperatively, when healing has started and the patient is more comfortable and is alert. The obturator must accommodate to the dynamics of the musculature of the lateral and posterior pharyngeal walls. The pharyngeal extension of the appliance is usually in the same plane and is functionally constructed to Passavant's cushion. The sequence following initial obturation is similar to that used for the hard palate appliance.

B. Mandibular Resections

The three categories of mandibular resections are marginal, segmental, and total. Marginal resection is the least severe of the three procedures. The continuity of the mandible is maintained, to preserve the proper maxillomandibular relationship. Constructing a prosthesis to restore form and function is not difficult. A partially resected mandible results in a muscle imbalance; the proper maxillomandibular relationship, imperative for proper mastication, swallowing, speech, and facial form, is disturbed. The greater the amount of mandible removed, the greater the debilitation. Total removal ultimately leaves the patient a helpless oral cripple, eliminates oral competence, and produces a severe cosmetic deformity ("Andy Gump" appearance). Rehabilitation of such patients can be achieved prosthetically with a mandibular implant, a resection appliance, or a palatal augmentation device.

1. **Implant prostheses** Re-establishment of the continuity of

the mandible restores form, function, and aesthetic effect. Often, this type of appliance is contraindicated following large cancer resections of the mandible because of the lack of adequate tissue to close the wound, residual disease, or the postoperative use of cancerocidal doses of ionizing radiation. If indicated, the prosthetic implant can be fabricated to fit the residual tissue bed and may be altered as needed.

a. ***Design*** Prosthetic mandibular implants are made from biologically acceptable inert materials such as tantalum, acrylic, siloxane, stainless steel, titanium, or chrome-cobalt alloys. They are usually fenestrated to allow for tissue ingrowth and to provide greater adaptability.
b. ***Segmental implants*** are shaped and fastened to the residual bone by screws or wire. Intermaxillary fixation should be used if possible.
c. ***Total mandibular implants*** present a different problem. Structures normally suspended from the mandible must be resuspended from the implant and allowed to heal and fibrose. The hyoid bone must be supported, to prevent the attached structures from falling back onto the larynx and choking the patient. The use of a Barton type of bandage or an extraoral head frame helps to stabilize these structures and the implant. Intermaxillary fixation is not usually employed for total mandibular replacement because of possible pressure necrosis of the intraoral mucosa and exposure of the implant.
d. ***Telescopic implants*** For cancer operations, the most adaptable implant is the telescopic type fashioned from a chrome-cobalt alloy. It is circular, small in diameter, of an open wire mesh design, and can be adjusted to any size during a segmental or total resection.

2. **Resection appliances** Often, following composite resections, the amount of tissue is inadequate to reconstruct the mandible with an implant. The remaining mandible deviates toward the side of the defect. After healing, the deviation can become severe, with scar formation and contracture.
   a. ***Surgical appliance*** To alleviate this deviation and to maintain flexibility of the residual mandible, the patient should be placed into intermaxillary fixation at the time of the operation. This fixation is maintained intermittently during the healing period with training elastics, to minimize scar contracture. In addition, the patient is instructed in jaw exercises. Most patients have some deviation toward the side of the defect.
   b. ***Lingual guide*** When the training elastics have been removed, a prosthesis can be made to guide the jaw into the proper occlusion and maxillomandibular relationship. The lingual-guide ramp appliance directs closure as the mandible closes from the deviated position into occlusion.

Without this device, the patient often has difficulty in guiding the mandible into proper closure. Initial contact is made at an open position on the ramp, and closure is terminated in maximal occlusal contact.

c. ***Buccal-guide plane*** Scar contracture may be too severe for the mandible to be guided into proper closure. In such cases, a buccal-guide prosthesis is indicated. When this appliance is engaged, the mandible can make only a vertical movement. The objectives are to provide occlusion and to stretch the scar tissue. Generally, use of the prosthesis can be discontinued within 6 months, or it can be exchanged for a lingual-guide ramp appliance.

3. **Palatal augmentation** Often, the tongue is partially resected and is used to close the surgical wound in composite resections. This situation limits tongue movement and alters the patient's ability to swallow and to speak. The palatal augmentation device can be incorporated into one of the previously mentioned prostheses, or it may function as a separate appliance. A functional impression is made of the new dynamics of the tongue and is then incorporated in acrylic into the palatal appliance.

C. Facial Prosthetic Restoration

The face is the center of attention during social interaction. Loss of part of the face can destroy a patient's self-image and may leave him psychologically and functionally a cripple.

1. **Advantages of prosthetic restoration** Rehabilitation can be accomplished rapidly by the use of a prosthesis. Often, plastic surgical correction is contraindicated because of the nature of the disease, the size of the defect, or the type of cancer treatment. In addition, a facial prosthesis permits the surgical site to be easily checked for recurrence, it is usually cosmetically superior to surgical correction, it can be remade as needed, and it eliminates the need for hospitalization.

2. **Requirements for facial prosthetics** The patient is evaluated preoperatively. Records are made of the face by means of a facial moulage and photographs. Recommendations can be made to the surgeon to produce a defect better able to receive a facial restoration for fit and cosmetic effect. Such suggestions are to minimize the size of the defect if possible, to terminate surgical margins near or at a natural anatomic landmark, and to remove rudimentary or bulky tissue. Specific recommendations are as follows:

   a. ***Ear resection*** One should remove residual ear lobe, maintain as much of the cartilage as is feasible for cosmetic effect, retention, and orientation, and preserve the tragus and external auditory canal.

   b. ***Nasal resection*** One should maintain the continuity of the upper lip to the margin of the nasal cavity, retain the bridge of the nose for retention and orientation, and remove residual tissue in the area of the alar process.

c. ***Orbital exenteration*** One should maintain the eyebrow and inferior and superior orbital ridges, and one should remove residual eyelids.

3. **Characteristics of facial prostheses** Facial prostheses are fabricated from flexible, biologically acceptable materials such as polyvinyl chloride, acrylic, polyurethanes, or siloxanes. They are held in place by skin adhesives. The restoration can be colored, shaded, and characterized specifically for the patient. These appliances do need to be replaced periodically, however, and they are static, unable to adjust and blend completely to the dynamics of the face.

20

SALIVARY GLAND DISEASE

DAVID E. SCHULLER

Salivary gland disorders encompass inflammatory, congenital, and neoplastic abnormalities. The development of antibiotics has lowered the incidence of inflammatory salivary gland disorders. A critical factor in the differential diagnosis of salivary gland problems is the patient's age. Physical abnormalities of the salivary glands in children have a significance different from those in adults and, therefore, are discussed separately. This chapter provides a sequential means of evaluating the patient with salivary gland disease. Rather than discussing all possible abnormalities representing or mimicking salivary gland disorders, the chapter focuses only on those entities that are commonly encountered.

I. ADULT SALIVARY GLAND DISEASE

A. Medical History and General Considerations

An accurate medical history is critically important in reducing the number of possibilities in the differential diagnosis. As a result of information gained from the patient's medical history, one can narrow the range of possible diagnoses and therefore the number of diagnostic studies needed for the evaluation. Information about glandular tenderness, the size of the salivary gland and its relation to eating, the chronologic order of symptoms, and concomitant medical problems facilitates and expedites the definitive diagnosis.

1. **Gland tenderness** Tenderness over one of the salivary glands suggests some type of inflammatory disorder. The tenderness caused by inflammation is usually persistent because it is a function of tissue pressure resulting from edema. This constant tenderness is in contrast to a salivary gland abnor-

mality that causes tenderness only on palpation and suggests a possible neoplasm involving the facial nerve.

2. **Gland size** One should determine whether the change consists of a multiglandular, symmetric increase in size or whether it is an asymmetric localized involvement in just one particular gland. Systemic disorders, such as Sjögren's syndrome, often cause an enlargement not only of the parotid gland bilaterally, but also of the submandibular and sublingual glands. This finding is in contrast to inflammatory or neoplastic conditions, which usually involve just one gland, and are thus described as asymmetric enlargements.

3. **Effect of eating** Often, an obstructive component is seen, not only in inflammatory conditions, but also in neoplastic disorders. It is important to seek this information in the patient's medical history. Salivary flow results from gustatory stimuli during eating or even from olfactory stimulation. Therefore, a patient should be asked whether any change has occurred in the size of the involved gland and whether the symptoms are potentiated while eating. Such findings suggest an obstructive disorder, such as sialolithiasis.

4. **Order of gland involvement** Acute inflammatory disorders usually result in an increase in size of infected glands within a couple of days. Chronic inflammatory problems cause glandular enlargement over a long period of time; the size of the gland increases even more during an acute exacerbation of the condition. This type of glandular enlargement is in contrast to discrete masses within a gland that are considered to be neoplastic in origin. A rapidly enlarging discrete mass is, of course, more worrisome than a mass that grows slowly over an extended period.

5. **Concomitant medical conditions** Certain systemic disorders involve the salivary glands. These disorders are primarily of endocrine or metabolic origin. Therefore, it is important to document whether the patient has a diagnosis of or any systemic symptoms suggesting diabetes mellitus, changing estrogen levels such as in the menopausal female, or chronic alcohol abuse. Patients with these conditions often develop bilateral symmetric enlargement of the parotid glands. Such a finding is usually asymptomatic. Chronic alcohol abuse can also result in parotid and submandibular gland enlargement.

B. Inflammation

The information obtained on these five general categories may permit one to subgroup the diagnostic possibilities. If the patient states that an asymmetric enlargement of the gland has occurred over a period of a few days, that the gland is persistently tender, and that it seems not to be associated with a change in size or symptoms while the patient is eating, then the following list of diseases must be considered:

1. **Acute sialadenitis** predominantly involves the parotid gland and is usually asymmetric in adults. The incidence of this problem has dramatically decreased with the introduction of antibiotics. Acute sialadenitis most commonly has a bacterial origin, usually involving multiple organisms. The incidence of staphylococcal infection is high enough to warrant appropriate antibiotic treatment, however. The infection is often the result of an ascending ductal inflammatory process. This ductal inflammation, coupled with some level of dehydration, may be a precipitating factor in acute sialadenitis. The disorder used to be common in postoperative patients because of dehydration, but it currently is most frequent in severely debilitated patients, such as those with an underlying malignant disease who are receiving immunosuppressive treatment either as radiation therapy or as chemotherapy. These patients require aggressive treatment because their tolerance for additional medical stress is minimal. Acute sialadenitis usually produces pain and tenderness of the involved gland. Fever is not always present, perhaps because of the immunosuppressed or debilitated status of the patient. One should massage the involved gland, in an effort to elicit any purulent exudate from the corresponding ductal orifice. Such a finding is no longer consistent, however. It is still important to culture the involved ductal orifice during gland massage. Initial management of such patients consists primarily of judicious hydration, high doses of antibiotics, and possibly, application of local heat overlying the involved gland. Abscess formation may be a feature of acute sialadenitis and requires prompt surgical drainage. The multiple septa coursing through the parotid gland prevent the formation of a single, easily diagnosable, large abscess. A diagnosis of a parotid abscess is made on the basis of the patient's clinical response to aggressive medical therapy, rather than on the usual physical finding of localized erythema in an area of a fluctuant mass. Once again, because the patients most commonly affected by acute sialadenitis are unable to tolerate excessive medical stress, it is advisable to consider the possibility of abscess formation early on, if one does not see obvious clinical improvement with antibiotics and hydration. The septa within the parotid gland usually allow the formation of multiple small abscesses. Therefore, surgical drainage must be performed by elevating a standard parotidectomy skin flap, by making multiple perforations with a blunt instrument, such as a hemostat, through the parenchyma of the gland, by spreading it parallel to the presumed course of the facial nerve fibers, and by draining the abscesses so as to minimize the possibility of injury to the facial nerve.

2. **Chronic sialadenitis** This disease has also decreased in incidence since the advent of effective antimicrobial agents. The

factor that distinguishes chronic from acute sialadenitis is a history of persistent symptoms over an extended period of time. Usually, just one of the salivary glands is involved, with recurrent episodes of pain and swelling and, less frequently, symptoms and signs of an acute inflammatory event such as fever or systemic toxicity. Duct stones are sometimes implicated in the development and persistence of the problem. The medical history includes the administration of multiple courses of antibiotics taken over the years in an effort to control the problem. The pathophysiologic features involve progressive fibrosis and destruction of the parenchyma and ductal portions of the involved gland. Sialography may well show a spectrum of abnormalities ranging from a normal ductal system to cavity formation within the gland parenchyma. Because no sialographic findings unequivocally confirm the diagnosis of chronic sialadenitis, treatment usually depends on the severity of the symptoms and their impact on the patient's daily activities. When the condition is severe enough, a total parotidectomy with attempted preservation of the facial nerve is recommended. That the tissue about the facial nerve has been inflamed and has become progressively more fibrotic over the years complicates the operation, and the patient must clearly understand the risk of temporary or permanent paresis or paralysis of one or more branches of the facial nerve. Resection of the submandibular gland for chronic sialadenitis is not as great a surgical challenge as parotidectomy in these patients.

3. **Other considerations** Two other disorders may cause the previously described symptoms. They are not as common as acute or chronic sialadenitis, but they are encountered frequently enough to warrant awareness.
   a. ***Mycobacterial infection*** Although the incidence of tuberculous sialadenitis has dramatically decreased with the introduction of antituberculous agents, atypical mycobacteria can still involve not only cervical lymph nodes, but also the parotid or submandibular glands. Such a condition usually becomes manifest as a tender gland enlargement that is less painful than acute bacterial sialadenitis. The diagnosis should be suspected if one does not observe the expected response to appropriate antibiotics. The tenderness usually subsides, but the mass in the involved gland persists, with eventual sinus tract formation to the overlying skin. Diagnosis can be made microscopically. Recommended treatment involves complete excision of the mass and of its sinus tract. Of course, if this mass involves the parotid gland, facial nerve dissection is required.
   b. ***Actinomycosis*** has clinical features almost identical to those of atypical mycobacterial infection; both disorders cause an almost painless swelling of one salivary gland that

eventually forms a sinus tract. The existence of "sulfur granules," noted microscopically, confirms the diagnosis. Proper medical management entails an extended course of antibiotics, usually penicillin for the patient who is not allergic to the drug. If a sinus tract has developed, however, then surgical intervention is required, to excise the tract and the involved tissue. Once again, facial nerve dissection is mandatory if the parotid gland is involved.

C. Obstruction (Sialolithiasis)

If a patient has unilateral painful swelling of one salivary gland, and if the swelling or pain seems to dramatically increase either during or shortly after eating, sialolithiasis must be considered. A change either in the patient's symptoms or in the gland's size directly associated chronologically with eating is almost pathognomonic of some type of ductal obstruction, usually involving a stone. In patients with obstruction caused by a stone, the salivary gland most commonly involved is the submandibular gland. The secretions of the submandibular gland are primarily mucous in character. Furthermore, the submandibular duct drains in a nondependent fashion, exiting the parenchyma of the gland at a point inferior to the orifice of the duct at the midline of the floor of the mouth. Therefore, the submandibular duct drains tenacious, high-viscosity fluid in a superiorly directed, tubular system. Any dehydration increases the viscosity of this fluid and potentiates the possibility of stone development from stasis of inspissated secretions. While massaging the gland, one cannot rule out the possibility of a stone if one notes saliva draining from the orifice of the duct. The duct is rarely totally obstructed.

1. **Diagnosis** This diagnosis can be confirmed by dilating the submandibular ductal orifice with lacrimal probes and then probing the duct system until a stone is encountered. A moderate-sized stone can often be palpated on bimanual examination of the floor of the mouth, but even when bimanual examination and lacrimal probing do not confirm the suspected diagnosis, the possibility of a stone cannot be completely excluded. A stone in the hilum of the gland may periodically move into position, to obstruct the submandibular duct. When the diagnosis is still unconfirmed after the foregoing maneuvers, then radiographs are advisable. The diagnostic evaluation of most salivary gland problems does not require many adjunctive tests; however, in cases of obstruction, certain radiographic procedures are helpful. The initial radiograph should be a dental occlusal view, which uses a dental plate and subsequently exposes the floor of the mouth. Salivary calculi are dissimilar to renal calculi in that approximately 85% are radiopaque. If no stones are identified with the dental occlusal view, then sialographic study is advisable. Multiple stones are common.

2. **Treatment** A stone occurring in the portion of the duct that is in the submucosal area of the floor of the mouth is often easily removed under local anesthesia, by placing a suture medial to the stone and incising the duct in a retrograde fashion from the orifice until the stone is released. It is not usually necessary to marsupialize the new duct opening intentionally at that point because the flow of saliva effectively maintains its patency. If the stone is located in the hilum of the gland, gland excision is usually necessary when symptoms are incapacitating enough to indicate such surgical intervention. No medical means exist by which to dissolve such stones at present.

D. Systemic Diseases

1. **Benign lymphoepithelial disease** is more common in women than in men. The glandular enlargement is usually nontender and most commonly involves both of the same glands. This disease may affect all the major and even the minor salivary glands. The patient often has evidence of systemic involvement manifested by symptoms in other organ systems, such as the lacrimal system. When this diagnosis is suspected, sialography does not provide pathognomonic information. The early stages of the disease are marked by a normal radiographic appearance of the ductal system. Later, a sialogram may reveal punctate sialectasis. In the serious stages of the disease, the patient may even have cavitary sialectasis. If the disease is suspected and if sialography does not provide supplemental evidence, then a biopsy of minor salivary glands, such as from the buccal or labial mucosa, will provide the histologic diagnosis. No specific medical treatment is available for this problem. Surgical intervention is usually reserved for patients in whom extreme gland enlargement is a cosmetic problem or for those with sialographic evidence of significant sialectasis that precludes the proper function of the gland.

2. **Endocrine abnormalities** The most common endocrine abnormality manifesting itself in this fashion is diabetes mellitus. Such an enlargement is usually asymptomatic, however. It is therefore mandatory to modify treatment, based on the impact of the problem on the patient's health and on normal daily activities. Sialography usually offers minimal diagnostic information. The pathophysiologic process is one of either fatty degeneration of the involved gland(s) or progressive fibrous displacement of normal gland parenchyma. Because the condition does not usually involve all the salivary glands, problems such as xerostomia are not encountered. Therefore, surgical intervention is rarely indicated, and treatment is expectant. The menopausal female sometimes has such asymmetric glandular enlargement. Once again, the indication for treatment is based on cosmetic criteria.

3. **Alcohol-related abnormalities** Chronic ethanol abuse can

result in asymptomatic glandular enlargement that is usually symmetric. This disorder commonly involves not only the parotid glands, but also the submandibular and sublingual salivary glands. The affected glands are smooth in contour on palpation, and histologic diagnosis is probably unnecessary unless focal areas of irregularity are noted in the physical examination. Sialography, once again, provides no unique diagnostic information. Surgical treatment is not recommended unless one suspects something besides alcohol-induced glandular enlargement.

E. Neoplasms

If a patient has a discrete, unilateral mass involving one salivary gland, certain items in the medical history will be critically important. The duration of the presence of the mass provides information on the speed of growth. Tenderness on palpation indicates some sensory nerve involvement. An assessment of facial nerve function is mandatory during the initial evaluation of such a patient. One must then consider the following:

1. Benign tumors

a. ***Differential diagnosis*** Many entities may produce discrete salivary gland abnormalities. One must be aware of all these possibilities before automatically assuming that such a discrete abnormality represents a salivary neoplasm. Probably, the most common finding that can be confused with a salivary gland tumor is an enlarged lymph node. The submandibular gland has lymph nodes intimately involved with it; if these become enlarged, it is difficult to distinguish the lymph node from the submandibular gland. It is even more difficult with the parotid lymph nodes because extraglandular and intraglandular nodes are located right within the gland substance. Often, the distinction cannot be made without the aid of a histologic study. With the exception of a submandibular lymph node and possibly the existence of a floor-of-mouth cyst, few other entities mimic a submandibular gland tumor. The situation is different with the parotid gland, however, because a variety of abnormalities can be confused with a parotid neoplasm. Mandibular or temporomandibular joint tumors or cysts, such as dentigerous cysts, aneurysm of the temporal artery, localized hypertrophic segment of the masseter muscle, a winged mandible, or facial venous thrombosis may all suggest parotid disease to the uninformed physician. It is beyond the scope of this chapter to discuss in detail the distinction of all these entities. Rather, it is hoped that the reader will keep these possibilities in mind when making the differential diagnosis and will take necessary action when suspicion arises. The reason for aggressiveness in evaluation of these lesions is that approximately 25% of all parotid gland and 50% of all submandibular gland tumors are malignant. No currently available noninvasive procedures give enough specific information to be relied on for such a critical determination. Sialograms and gallium scans are not accurate enough to rely solely on their results. Therefore, tissue diagnosis is mandatory.

b. ***Pleomorphic adenoma*** is the most common of all salivary gland tumors, including benign and malignant varieties. This lesion usually displays all the usual clinical criteria of a benign lesion; it is painless, slow growing, not fixed to any overlying or underlying structures, and does not cause facial nerve paralysis. The tumor is usually described as a discrete mass within the parenchyma of the gland, usually the parotid gland. Once again, in view of the lack of noninvasive studies for tissue diagnosis, surgical intervention is mandatory, both for diagnosis and for treatment. These lesions were formerly treated by simple enucleation. The disturbingly high recurrence rate following such a technique was used as the basis of documentation of "satellitosis" of benign mixed tumors. Serial histologic sectioning of such tumors subsequently demonstrated, however, that true satellitosis was unusual in benign mixed tumors, which more commonly had pseudopod-like extensions from the main tumor mass. Simple enucleation most likely transected some of these finger-like extensions, with the subsequent return of new palpable tumors because of persistent disease in retained tumor tissue, rather than because of satellite tumors. Lateral parotid lobectomy has become the mainstay of proper diagnostic technique for benign mixed tumors of the parotid gland. This procedure ensures adequate tissue for diagnosis, as well as generous removal of salivary parenchyma, to decrease the chance of retained tumor. Benign mixed tumors in submandibular glands are treated by total gland excision. The incidence of recurrent benign mixed tumors has decreased since the popularity of lateral lobectomy in the parotid gland. It still exists, however, and is often a troublesome problem (Conley, J. (ed.): Salivary Glands and the Facial Nerve. New York, Grune & Stratton, 1975). Some deaths have even been reported to have resulted from benign mixed tumors that possessed the histologic criteria of benign tumors, but became lethal because of persistence of the disorder.

c. ***Other lesions*** with a similar clinical presentation are hemangiomas, lymphangiomas, and congenital cysts, such as first branchial cysts. It is unusual for such lesions to go undetected until adulthood. Their presentation and management are discussed in more detail in the section of this chapter on pediatric salivary gland disorders.

2. **Malignant tumors**

a. ***General considerations*** Certain general features in the presentation of a discrete salivary mass should cause concern. The rapid growth of a discrete mass is a worrisome feature in a patient's medical history. It was formerly believed that certain symptoms were almost uniformly present in patients with malignant salivary gland tumors; such symptoms included pain and tenderness, paresis or paralysis of a branch of the facial nerve, and fixation of the lesion to the overlying skin. Now, however, sufficient evidence shows that a malignant salivary tumor may appear as an asymptomatic mass with no sign of facial nerve involvement or of skin fixation. Because sialograms are not pathognomonic, and no other noninvasive technique can confirm this diagnosis, histologic study, requiring either a total submandibular gland excision or a lateral parotid lobectomy, is mandatory. The usual routine is to perform a frozen section, to determine the histopathologic features at the time of operation, and then to proceed with an additional surgical procedure, depending on the pathologist's interpretation of the neoplasm. Malignant salivary tumors are not always easy to identify by the frozen-section technique. It is therefore imperative for the surgeon and pathologist to have a clear understanding of the importance of their collaborative efforts. It certainly would do a disservice to the patient to resect part of or the entire facial nerve intentionally, based on a frozen-section diagnosis that is later changed after review of the permanent histologic sections. If a pathologist is confident about the interpretation of the frozen section and is aware of the consequences of the ensuing decision, however, one should proceed with whatever supplemental operation is advisable, provided the patient has been duly informed preoperatively. The psychologic impact of facial paralysis cannot be minimized. Although several reconstructive techniques are now available for reinnervating the paralysed face, none can approximate the quality of normally innervated mimetic musculature. The surgeon and pathologist cannot underplay their responsibility to the patient in this respect.

b. ***Mucoepidermoid carcinoma*** Although this lesion involves any of the salivary glands, it is most common in the parotid gland. These malignant tumors are classified as either low grade (well differentiated) or high grade (undifferentiated). The low-grade mucoepidermoid carcinoma is clinically similar to a benign mixed tumor because it is a slow-growing, asymptomatic mass. Lateral parotid lobectomy is the recommended diagnostic procedure. If the pathologist is secure in the frozen-section diagnosis of mucoepidermoid carcinoma, then resection of branches of the facial nerve adjacent to this mass is recommended, with completion of the resection to a total parotidectomy. Nerve grafting is undertaken using microsurgical technique. The 5-year survival rates for patients with low-grade mucoepidermoid carcinomas are favorable, in sharp contrast to survival rates for the so-called high-grade mucoepidermoid carcinoma, whose biologic behavior is aggressive. The treatment of these high-grade cancers reflects an awareness of the behavior of this particular tumor and usually involves aggressive resection, including excision of the total parotid gland in continuity with the facial nerve and, often, associated neck contents, with additional resection of the parotid compartment, including musculature, occasionally a portion of the mandible, skin, auricle, and a portion of the temporal bone. Some advocate a combined treatment regimen, with postoperative radiation therapy, for these ominous neoplasms.

c. ***Adenoid cystic carcinoma (cylindroma)*** has a behavior pattern distinctly different from that of other malignant tumors. This lesion, which can involve any of the major or minor salivary glands, distinguishes itself by its persistent nature and its propensity for developing clinically silent distant metastases. The lesion often mimics a benign tumor; however, total eradication of this disease is difficult and mandates an aggressive treatment program. It is beyond the scope of this chapter to discuss this particular neoplasm in detail. The reader is referred to other excellent sources (Conley, J. (ed.): Salivary Glands and The Facial Nerve. New York, Grune & Stratton, 1975). Certain generalizations help to provide the rationale for treatment programs. Adenoid cystic carcinoma arising in minor salivary glands has a worse prognosis than that arising in other salivary glands. This tumor is generally considered to be radiosensitive, but not radiocurable. These lesions have a propensity for extension along the nerves in the area of involvement. For this reason, one must suspect an adenoid cystic carcinoma in the patient with a salivary tumor who shows signs of neural involvement manifested as hyperesthesia, paresthesia, or hypesthesia. This lesion does not usually metastasize to regional lymphatic vessels. Five-year survival rates are meaningless because of the persistent nature of the tumor. One needs to speak in terms of 15- or 20-year survival rates to be more accurate. Therefore, this factor must be considered when planning a treatment program for the elderly patient. Treatment usually involves resection of the primary disease, including a cuff larger than for squamous cell carcinoma. Radical neck dissection is usually not indicated, unless it is performed in an effort to excise a large cuff of tissue around the primary tumor, such as with submandibular gland cylindromas. The histologic pattern of cylindromas, whether tubular, cribriform, or solid, has recently been found to offer some prognostic information. The tubular pattern carries the most favorable prognosis, and the solid pattern the least favorable. (Cancer, *42*:265, 1978.)

d. ***Adenocarcinoma*** also has an unfavorable prognosis. The symptoms of this tumor reflect more aggressive behavior; many of these tumors have already caused infiltration of surrounding tissue, fixation of the overlying skin, and facial nerve paresis at the time of diagnosis. They are able to metastasize to regional lymphatic vessels as well as systemically. Treatment, once again, is governed by the aggressive nature of this lesion. Wide resection, in the form of radical parotidectomy, often including adjacent tissues, is coupled with postoperative radiation therapy.

e. ***Malignant mixed tumor*** usually seems to arise as a result of transformation or malignant degeneration of a previously benign mixed tumor. Most patients with this histologic diagnosis have a previous history of benign mixed tumor. Suspicion of malignant degeneration often arises from the development of rapid growth and pain in the area of a salivary tumor present for many years. Treatment is aggressive, and total parotidectomy with excision of the facial nerve is recommended, with immediate nerve grafting.

f. ***Squamous cell carcinoma*** is similar to adenocarcinoma; the clinical symptoms suggest a malignant tumor because the lesion grows rapidly, becomes fixed to the skin and ulcerates, causes pain, and frequently produces facial paresis or paralysis. Total parotidectomy with facial nerve resection is the cornerstone of aggressive treatment; however, it is common to include portions of surrounding tissue, such as the temporal bone, the mandible, and overlying skin in the resection. Combined therapy using postoperative irradiation seems to be a reasonable approach for such an aggressive lesion with a grave prognosis.

g. ***Acinic cell carcinoma*** causes symptoms similar to those of a benign tumor. They have no special propensity for neural involvement. Therefore, total parotidectomy, with either total facial nerve preservation or resection of a branch of the facial nerve, represents adequate treatment.

h. ***Other considerations*** The parotid gland, as well as the submandibular gland, can act as a focus for metastatic disease, as a result of the intimate relationship with the lymph nodes surrounding the capsule of the gland and even within it. Because these glands drain areas of the head and neck that are frequently involved by primary neoplasms, they become secondarily involved by metastatic disease. The treatment of such metastatic disease must be included in the overall program for the primary neoplasm.

Parotid lymph nodes are frequently a metastatic site for scalp melanomas. Lymphomas involving parotid and submandibular lymph nodes may also occur. When this diagnosis is made, the patient must undergo staging to define the level of malignant involvement.

II. PEDIATRIC SALIVARY GLAND DISEASE

A. General Considerations

Although inflammatory disorders are usually the most common salivary gland problem in the pediatric population and are certainly more common than neoplasms, actual neoplasms are the cause of salivary masses more frequently than either inflammatory or congenital diseases. The approach to children with salivary gland abnormalities is dictated by an awareness of this unusually high incidence of neoplasms (*In* Symposium on salivary gland diseases. Otolaryngol. Clin. North Am., *10*:399, 1977).

B. Inflammatory Diseases

1. **Mumps** is the most common inflammatory cause of salivary gland enlargement. The parotid gland is most frequently affected and can be involved either unilaterally or bilaterally. The submandibular gland can also be infected and therefore involved by the mumps virus. The disease usually causes swelling and tenderness associated with systemic toxicity, rather than a discrete tumor mass. Treatment is expectant.
2. **Chronic sialadenitis with or without sialolithiasis** seems to involve the parotid more frequently than the submandibular or sublingual glands. One usually sees diffuse enlargement of the gland, but it can also be localized. The disorder is associated with local pain and tenderness on palpation. The treatment in children is essentially the same as in the adult population. The other inflammatory disorders discussed with reference to adults are rare in children.

C. Congenital Diseases

1. **Cysts** Congenital salivary abnormalities are not common. They primarily represent abnormalities of the first branchial pouch (Conley, J. (ed.): Salivary Glands and the Facial Nerve. New York, Grune & Stratton, 1975). If the first pouch is just a cyst, it will gradually enlarge because the inner respiratory epithelium will secrete mucus into an enclosed space; the secretion rate usually exceeds the absorption rate, with subsequent enlargement of the mass. If a fistula is associated with this cyst, however, the orifice of the fistula will be in the ear canal at the bone-cartilage junction. Such a structure is susceptible to recurrent infections. Treatment for these first branchial cleft cysts is excision, usually involving facial nerve dissection for complete resection.

2. **Ranula,** another consideration, is an asymptomatic, fluctuant mass usually associated in the midline or at one side of the floor of the mouth. This lesion appears to be a retention cyst; it also has an epithelial lining. It does not represent a difficult diagnostic problem, however, and is readily amenable to surgical resection.

D. Neoplasms

Because neoplasms of a child's salivary gland are a more common cause of glandular masses than inflammatory or congenital disorders, it is mandatory to approach such a child in an orderly fashion during evaluation and treatment. It is first mandatory to determine whether the salivary mass is fluctuant or firm.

1. **Fluctuant mass** If this mass is determined by physical examination to be fluctuant, then two major possibilities exist:
   a. ***Hemangioma*** of a capillary variety causes purplish discoloration and involvement of overlying skin; cavernous hemangioma does not directly involve the overlying skin, but usually the vascularity transmits through the skin as a bluish discoloration. When the clinical diagnosis of hemangioma is confirmed, observation is recommended. Excision of the lesion is indicated only if it causes, because of its size, recurrent infections, bleeding, or coagulation disorders such as platelet trapping.
   b. ***Lymphangioma*** If the clinical diagnosis is a lymphangioma (cystic hygroma), then it is prudent to observe the infant until he is large enough to tolerate the general anesthesia necessary for surgical excision. Lymphangiomas are characterized as a fluctuant mass with no discoloration and with a multilobular nature. Excision is recommended because these lesions may become spontaneously infected, with rapid enlargement of the mass. This problem is especially crucial if the lymphangioma involves anatomic structures that might restrict the airway, such as the submandibular gland, with extension into the floor of the mouth. If one cannot distinguish between hemangioma and lymphangioma on the basis of the clinical findings, it will be advisable to proceed with a small open biopsy, to make a tissue diagnosis, so appropriate therapy can be instituted.

2. **Firm mass** If the mass in a child's salivary gland is firm, then subsequent diagnostic procedures and treatment must be governed by the knowledge that approximately 60% of all firm, unilateral salivary gland masses in children are malignant. Although these tumors are malignant, the overwhelming histologic type is a low-grade mucoepidermoid carcinoma, which has a favorable prognosis. Therefore, in the child with a firm, unilateral salivary lesion, wide local excision, such as subman-

dibular gland excision or lateral parotid lobectomy, is recommended.

a. ***Benign lesion*** If the lesion is histologically benign, no further treatment is recommended.
b. ***Low-grade malignant tumor*** If the tumor is of low-grade malignancy, such as a low-grade mucoepidermoid carcinoma, lateral parotid lobectomy or submandibular gland excision should be adequate, and no further treatment is recommended.
c. ***High-grade malignant tumor*** When a high-grade malignant tumor is diagnosed, additional treatment depends on the particular histologic type of tumor. The prognosis in patients with high-grade mucoepidermoid carcinoma is considerably worse than in those with a low-grade tumor and justifies more aggressive excision, such as total parotidectomy with resection of adjacent branches of the facial nerve. Undifferentiated carcinoma precludes any attempt at cure with a radical surgical procedure. Rhabdomyosarcoma now seems to be sufficiently managed with a reasonable surgical resection, coupled with radiation therapy and chemotherapy.

21

SORE THROAT

COLLIN S. KARMODY

I. GENERAL PRINCIPLES

A. Presentation

Pain or soreness of the throat is a frequent complaint with many causes. Sore throats afflict all age groups, but are most common in children and young adults. Most sore throats are part of the spectrum of viral upper respiratory infections, but they may be caused by bacterial infection in younger patients. Prolonged pain in the throat in the middle-aged or elderly adult is cause for concern, particularly in the heavy consumer of alcohol and tobacco. One must consider the presence of a neoplasm. A complaint of soreness of the throat demands a thorough physical examination of the oral cavity, oropharynx, hypopharynx, larynx, thyroid gland, and neck. Pain is sometimes referred to the throat from the esophagus, stomach, and heart.

B. Evaluation

When diagnosis is not immediately obvious on physical examination, adjunctive studies may be necessary. Routine cultures for bacteria and viruses, routine hematologic studies, lateral roentgenograms of the neck, barium studies of the pharynx, esophagus, and stomach, and computed tomographic (CT) scanning may be of value. Scans of the thyroid gland (iodine 131^{+}) and evaluation of thyroid function are sometimes helpful. If pain in the throat is initiated or accentuated by exertion, then assessment for cardiopathy will be needed. Rare causes of throat pain include glossopharyngeal neuralgia and an elongated styloid process. The styloid process is clearly seen on a Towne view of the skull. Soreness and dryness of the throat are common problems in mouth breathers and in smokers, as well as in the winter, owing to the dry atmosphere of a heated house. Allergic reactions may also cause soreness of the throat, sometimes with obvious angioedema, but mostly with minimal, positive physical findings. Frequent recurrent, particularly bacterial, infections of the pharynx may be an expression of immunodeficiency, such as seen in the DiGeorge syndrome or acquired immune deficiency syndrome (AIDS). When evaluating patients with sore throat, one should swab white patches with a cotton-tipped applicator; candida patches bleed easily. One should not examine the throat with an ungloved finger, particularly when the patient has ulcerations, because venereal diseases are still prevalent. Cultures for routine study of aerobic and anaerobic bacteria and fungi, should be taken when deemed clinically necessary. In the young child in whom epiglottitis (supraglottitis) is suspected, examination may precipitate respiratory obstruction and should therefore be deferred. In heavy smokers and heavy drinkers, who are at risk for carcinoma of the aerodigestive tract, palpation of the oral cavity and of the oropharynx is sometimes valuable. Patients with a hyperactive gag reflex should be examined with a transnasal fiberoptic endoscope.

II. BACTERIAL PHARYNGITIS

A. Clinical Features of Common Infections

Bacterial pharyngitis is usually an acute infection causing pain in the throat, fever, and midjugular lymphadenopathy. Leucocytosis is present, with elevated numbers of polymorphonuclear leukocytes. At first, the patient has hyperemia of the pharyngeal mucosa, particularly of the tonsillar pillars. Later, an exudate appears as yellow patches on the crypts of the tonsils and other pharyngeal lymphoid aggregates. Odynophagia prevents adequate intake of solid food, and even liquids may be difficult to swallow. The commonest infecting organisms are Streptococcus pyogenes, Haemophilus influenzae, and neisseria.

B. Treatment of Common Infections

Whenever possible, the pharynx should be swabbed for culture before treatment is begun. Penicillin controls streptococci and neisseria species. Haemophilus influenzae responds to ampicillin and amoxicillin. Oral antibiotics are useful in the early stages of the disorder, when swallowing is still possible. Later, however, intramuscular or intravenous routes may be necessary. Antibiotics are traditionally given for 10 days, but evidence suggests that, if response to the drug is immediate in the earliest stages of the disease, a 5-day regimen is adequate. Local treatment is important for relief of symptoms. Irrigations with a warm, dilute salt solution are soothing, and so is gargling with a suspension of aspirin made by disintegrating two 300-mg tablets of aspirin in a glass of warm water. This suspension is first gargled, then swallowed. Aspirin is a mild topical anesthetic. Most of the lozenges available for treatment of sore throat contain the topical anesthetic benzocaine and are useful for short-term symptomatic relief around mealtime. Viscous topical anesthetics, such as viscous lidocaine, are sometimes prescribed for acute bacterial pharyngitis. In advanced cases when the respiratory passage is compromised, these drugs may even be dangerous. Systemic analgesics are usually necessary. Aspirin is effective, provided the patient has no history of aspirin sensitivity. Typical adult dosage is 10 grains (600 mg) q.i.d. In children, dosage depends on body weight; up to the age of 3 years, 1.25 grains (75 mg) q.i.d., and from 3 to 6 years, 2.5 grains (150 mg) q.i.d. Codeine, 30 mg, is useful, but it is addictive. For stronger analgesia, one should prescribe meperidine (Demerol), 50 to 100 mg orally or 50 mg by intramuscular injection. The patient should be encouraged to drink as much liquid as possible. When oral intake is inadequate, intravenous fluids may be necessary to prevent dehydration.

C. Treponemal Infections

Two forms of spirochetes cause soreness of the throat and pharyngitis, Treponema pallidum, the organism of syphilis, and Treponema microdentium, which, together with a fusobacterium, cause Vincent's angina (necrotizing gingivitis).

1. **Syphilis** may cause painful lesions in the mouth and throat in all three stages.
   a. ***Primary*** A chancre may be found on the tongue, buccal mucosa, or tonsil, but rarely on the pharyngeal wall.
   b. ***Secondary*** Serpiginous mucosal patches are the classic signs of secondary syphilis. These painful superficial ulcerations occur on the buccal mucosa, palate, and pharynx. The patient has associated fever, lymphadenopathy, and a papular rash.
   c. ***Tertiary*** The classic lesion is a gumma with a painful, localized zone of necrosis. Gummas may occur in the tongue, palate, pharynx, epiglottis, or larynx. Diagnosis is confirmed by serologic tests. One should not examine a patient suspected of having syphilis with an ungloved hand. Treatment of syphilis, regardless of its stage, requires massive doses of penicillin, 2 million U daily, to a total of 12 to 15 million Units intramuscularly or intravenously. Some centers use smaller doses.
2. **Vincent's angina (necrotizing gingivitis, trench mouth)** is a contagious infection of the oral cavity and pharynx more frequent in young adults and caused by Treponema microdentium and a fusiform bacterium acting synergistically. These extensive, malodorous, painful, bleeding ulcerations are covered by a dirty, gray necrotic membrane along the margins of the gums. The patient may have an underlying debilitating

disease such as diabetes or leukemia. Treatment is with penicillin, 4 million U daily systemically for 5 days, followed by 1 g phenoxymethyl penicillin per day, in divided oral doses. Meticulous oral hygiene is mandatory. A warm, dilute salt solution is recommended as an irrigation and gargle at least 4 times per day. A liquid diet is advisable until the gums heal. Acetaminophen, 600 mg q6h, is helpful to reduce pain. Aspirin should be avoided because of the tendency of the gums to bleed. All feeding utensils should be sterilized after use by boiling, or they should be discarded. Close personal contact should be avoided. See Chapter 18.

III. INDICATIONS FOR TONSILLECTOMY AND ADENOIDECTOMY

Tonsillectomy and adenoidectomy are frequently performed together. Although the indications for each procedure are different, they do sometimes overlap. Former indications for tonsillectomy have included recurrent sore throat, recurrent or persistent streptococcal pharyngitis, peritonsillar abscess, respiratory obstruction, dysphagia, recurrent bronchitis, rheumatic fever, and neoplasms of the tonsil. Former indications for adenoidectomy have been respiratory obstruction, whether consisting of nasal obstruction only, stuffy nose, or mouth breathing or combined with tonsillar hypertrophy causing cor pulmonale; recurrent otitis media; benign cysts and neoplasm; and recurrent nasopharyngitis, a rare, usually streptococcal, infection. The indications for adenoidectomy are not firm. Criteria are loose and are still controversial.

A. Recurrent Sore Throat

Recurrent sore throat is an arbitrary indication. No consensus exists as to a meaningful frequency of recurrence. A rate of six episodes per year is commonly used, but no logical reasons exist for selecting six over four or eight. The complaint of sore throat should be carefully considered. When observed over a one-year period, patients with previous episodes of frequent sore throat had many fewer attacks and so did not meet the criteria for tonsillectomy. Recurrent, culture-proved streptococcal pharyngitis and other types of bacterial pharyngitis are reasonable indications for tonsillectomy, but the frequency and severity of such episodes must be considered, and every child must be assessed individually.

B. Nasal Obstruction

Whether posterior nasal obstruction is harmful to the developing child is still unknown. The high arching of the hard palate and the narrowing of the maxillary arch supposedly caused by nasal obstruction are probably not significant. Furthermore, nasal obstruction is usually diagnosed by the patient's medical history, as given by the parents. Therefore, findings on clinical examination of the nasopharynx and adjacent structures should be correlated with the general health of the child before adenoidectomy is considered. A soft tissue lateral film of the nasopharynx is useful for assessing adenoid size.

C. Recurrent Otitis Media

The role of adenoidectomy in the treatment of recurrent otitis media is under re-evaluation. The lack of well-controlled prospective studies on this topic is appalling. Recurrent infection confined to the adenoid is rare. It has been common practice to perform a tonsillectomy and an adenoidectomy, or an adenoidectomy only, as routine therapy for serous otitis media and recurrent suppurative otitis media, but this approach is no longer considered acceptable. Tonsillectomy and adenoidectomy should be considered on their own merits in the treatment of chronic serous otitis media.

D. Peritonsillar Abscess

Recently, the concept of peritonsillar abscess as an indication for tonsillectomy has been challenged because peritonsillar abscess in adults rarely recurs. The presence of such an abscess, however, remains a valid indication for tonsillectomy. These abscesses, which develop lateral to the tonsil and secondary to acute bacterial tonsillitis, are more common in teenagers and young adults, but they can occur in any age group. The most frequent site is at the superolateral aspect of the tonsil, and the predisposing factor is probably the presence of a small salivary gland (Weber's gland) lateral to the capsule of the tonsil. The incidence of peritonsillar abscess is also higher in the black population. (See also Chap. 28).

1. **Clinical features** This seriously ill patient is febrile, with signs of toxicity, has severe pain in the throat, considerable odynophagia, and has marked trismus. One usually sees unilateral, tense swelling of the junctional area between the soft palate and tonsil, and the tonsil is displaced inferomedially. The uvula is edematous, and the patient speaks with a "hot potato" voice.
2. **Treatment** consists of the administration of antibiotics, preferably intravenously and in high doses, such as penicillin G, 1 million U q6h. Irrigating the mouth and pharynx with warm saline solution is soothing. Analgesics are given liberally, except aspirin; acetaminophen with codeine, 30 mg q6h, is helpful. Narcotics should not be prescribed, to prevent suppression of the respiratory center. Peritonsillar abscesses may be treated either by immediate incision and drainage, with tonsillectomy several weeks later, or by tonsillectomy after 12 to 24 hours of intravenous antibiotics (tonsillectomy au chaud). Either way, symptoms usually disappear immediately after drainage of the abscess.

E. Parapharyngeal Abscess

Infection of the parapharyngeal space frequently occurs secondary to acute pharyngitis and probably represents severe lymphadenopathy. Parapharyngeal space infections are potentially dangerous because the parapharyngeal space communicates with the mediastinum along the major vessels and without natural barriers.

1. **Clinical features** The patient complains of a sore throat of long duration, followed by painful swelling of the side of the upper neck, fever, toxicity, and mild trismus. The lateral pharyngeal wall is displaced medially, with consequent displacement of the tonsil. The patient may have some generalized swelling of the soft palate and the pharyngeal mucosa. It is clinically important to differentiate between a parapharyngeal space infection and a peritonsillar abscess because treatment of these two disorders is radically different. See Chapter 28.
2. **Treatment** of a parapharyngeal space infection is with high doses of intravenous antibiotics, such as penicillin G, 1 million U q6h, or dicloxacillin, 1 million U q6h. Analgesics and warm compresses to the side of the neck are important for symptomatic relief. The patient's airway must be monitored carefully. Drainage may be necessary, by means of an external incision, displacement of the sternocleidomastoid muscle, and gentle blunt dissection until the abscess cavity is entered. A drain should be placed, and intravenous antibiotics should be continued until drainage ceases and the inflammatory response subsides completely. Parapharyngeal abscess is not an indication for tonsillectomy unless there is a coexisting peritonsillar abscess.

F. Other Indications

Recurrent bronchitis is a tenuous indication for tonsillectomy. Because the incidence of rheumatic fever is declining rapidly, the disorder is no longer a common indication for tonsillectomy.

IV. FUNGAL INFECTIONS

Fungal infections of the mouth and pharynx are common in otherwise normal infants, but in adults, they usually are associated with intercurrent diseases such as diabetes or immunosuppression, as in patients receiving chemotherapy. Fungal infections may also occur secondary to antibiotic therapy. Candida is the most common offending organism; phycomycetes occurs only occasionally, and blastomyces is confined to selected geographic areas.

A. Clinical Features

Candidiasis usually causes white patches to appear on the buccal mucosa and on the tongue and palate. These painful lesions bleed when the white deposit is rubbed with a cotton-tipped probe. Phycomycetes is a dangerous organism that occurs more frequently in middle-aged and elderly diabetics than in other populations. Phycomycetes invades the blood vessels and rapidly causes intraluminal thrombosis with devascularization of large segments of tissue. The patient therefore has a rapidly progressive necrosis of the palate and adjacent maxilla and ethmoid sinuses. Blastomyces, which causes painful ulcerations with a typical, punched-out appearance, may involve any part of the oral cavity, oropharynx, or larynx. Blastomycosis is confined to the southern United States and to Central America and parts of South America. See Chapter 23.

B. Treatment

For all fungal infections, the only effective systemic therapeutic agent currently in use is amphotericin B, given intravenously by slow infusion. Therapy is initiated with a daily dose of 0.25 mg/kg, and daily doses are gradually increased as tolerated, to a maximum of 1.5 mg/kg. Long-term treatment is usually necessary; one may need at least 2 weeks, and sometimes even 6 weeks, to eliminate the fungus and to effect simultaneous clinical improvement. Amphotericin B may produce angina pectoris in susceptible patients. If this complication occurs, the daily dose may have to be reduced or temporarily suspended. Nystatin suspension, used as a mouthwash, is frequently effective against superficial candida. This agent is the drug of choice for infants, as a suspension painted onto the buccal mucosa with a cotton-tipped applicator. Painting the pharynx with a solution of gentian violet is sometimes effective against candida. Lozenges containing a topical anesthetic, such as benzocaine, are useful to relieve pain. Antibiotics should be avoided in patients with a fungal infection of the buccal mucosa.

V. VIRAL INFECTIONS

Viral infection is probably the most frequent cause of pharyngitis. The sore throat is usually part of an upper respiratory infection. A number of different viruses are implicated, such as influenza virus, herpes simplex virus, adenoviruses, rhinoviruses, Coxsackie virus, and Epstein-Barr virus.

A. General Clinical Features

The usual picture is of severe pain with comparatively mild clinical findings. One may see mild hyperemia and edema of the pharynx, particularly along the faucial pillars and the posterior pharyngeal wall. The lymphoid aggregates of the pharyngeal mucosa are pink and edematous, and one may see mild-to-moderate enlargement of the jugulodigastric nodes. In general, the findings on physical examination are not nearly as severe as in patients with bacterial pharyngitis, although viral infection can cause severe ulcerative stomatopharyngitis. Routine blood studies usually allow one to differentiate between viral and bacterial infections. In viral infections, the white blood cell count is not elevated, nor is the number of polymorphonuclear leukocytes increased. On the contrary, some patients have mild leukopenia. Viral pharyngitis and upper respiratory infections may be accompanied by fever, ranging from slight to high.

B. Herpes Stomatitis

Herpes stomatitis can be classified as primary, recurrent nonvenereal (herpes simplex virus type I), or venereal (herpes simplex virus type II). Primary and nonvenereal recurrent herpes are discussed in Chapter 16.

1. **Features of venereal herpes (stomatopharyngitis)** Among the viral infections that afflict mankind, infection with the herpes virus is unique. Antibodies are formed against herpes virus, and peak titers may remain high for many months. Any immunity that develops limits, but does not prevent, episodic recurrences. Venereal herpes is acquired by kissing or by sexual contact and is caused by herpes simplex virus type II. It is primarily a disease of young to middle-aged adults, but recent reports have noted infection in the newborn children of infected mothers. The disease causes multiple, painful, initially punctate then confluent, superficial ulcerations of the mucosa of the cheek, tongue, and oropharynx. Each episode consists of a prodrome of discomfort in the mouth, followed by eruption lasting from 7 to 10 days; the eruption subsides, only to recur 2 to 4 weeks later. Episodes may continue to be a problem for many years. Mild cervical lymphadenopathy may accompany the episode. Some evidence suggests that the eruptions are excited by emotional factors and by local trauma.
2. **Treatment of venereal herpes** is difficult; at present, the only successful agent is intravenous Acyclovir. Acyclovir is most effective if used promptly to treat the first episode of herpes stomatitis. Thereafter, its efficacy is less obvious, although evidence suggests a reduction in the duration of subsequent episodes if Acyclovir is used immediately following the onset of symptoms. Acyclovir applied topically may shorten the duration and may lessen the severity of symptoms. Other immune system-bolstering agents such as levamisole are not of much value. Symptomatic treatment is helpful, particularly with diazepam (Valium), 5 mg t.i.d., at the first suspicion of symptoms. The exact role of diazepam is still not clear. Lozenges containing benzocaine or lidocaine viscous 2% solution, 2 teaspoonfuls held in the mouth for as long as possible, also provide some relief. Symptomatic relief may be obtained by using a standard antacid preparation, such as aluminum hydroxide or magnesium hydroxide, as a mouthwash q.i.d. Patients who have herpes stomatitis need counseling because of the prospect of a recurrent, incurable, painful disease for the rest of their lives.

C. Treatment of Viral Pharyngitis

No specific treatment exists for common viral pharyngitis. Treatment is primarily symptomatic and is directed particularly to relieve pain. Aspirin, 600 mg, or acetaminophen, 650 mg, at 6-hour intervals is useful. Irrigation or gargling with warm dilute salt water is comforting. Salt water is made by adding a teaspoonful of household salt to 8 oz warm water. Lozenges that contain a topical anesthetic such as benzocaine are also useful, and so is lidocaine viscous 2% solution. Soreness of the throat usually subsides in 5 to 10 days, but it may persist long after all signs of infection have disappeared.

VI. ALLERGIC REACTIONS

Allergic reactions that affect the upper aerodigestive tract cause soreness of the throat either directly, by an allergic pharyngitis, or indirectly, secondary to nasal obstruction. Allergic pharyngitis causes a sore, scratchy throat. The patient has neither fever nor leukocytosis. Antihistamines, such as diphenhydramine hydrochloride, chlorpheniramine, or brompheniramine, are all useful at their appropriate dosages. True delayed-sensitivity reactions are usually not life-threatening, as is the acute angioedematous type of reaction. Iodine compounds, usually ingested in shellfish, cause soreness and sometimes acute swelling of the throat. Less acute reactions are controlled by oral antihistamines, but more urgent problems require subcutaneous injections of epinephrine or intravenous corticosteroids. Hydrocortisone, 100 mg intravenously, is particularly effective. Chronic pharyngeal irritation with tobacco is a common cause of sore throat. The only solution is to stop smoking. See Chapter 23.

VII. IDIOPATHIC DISORDERS

A. Aphthous Ulcers

Aphthous lesions are painful, superficial ulcers, 0.5 to 10 mm in diameter, that occur mostly on the lips, buccal mucosa, tongue, and pharynx. They occur episodically and may be recurrent for most of the patient's life. No specific treatment exists for aphthous ulcers, but one may prescribe any of the following symptomatic treatments: cautery of the ulcers with silver nitrate; administration of topical corticosteroids, such as triamcinolone acetonide in a carboxymethyl-cellulose base (Kenalog in Orabase); nystatin mouthwash; topical administration of tannic acid; topical application of gentian violet; and lidocaine viscous solution used as a mouthwash and gargle, 2 teaspoonfuls 4 times per day. Although aphthous ulcerations are self-limiting, they are painful and unpleasant. See Chapter 18.

B. Pemphigus

Pemphigus is a debilitating, potentially fatal epithelial disease characterized by large, painful, vesicular lesions on the skin and mucosal surfaces accompanied by lethargy and eventually extreme debility. Pemphigus requires prompt treatment with corticosteroids, such as prednisone, 10 mg q.i.d., until the disease is controlled. The dosage should then be reduced to a maintenance level, usually about 10 mg per day. Consultation and management by a dermatologist are recommended. See Chapter 16.

C. Erythema Multiforme

This disease is similar to pemphigus and requires the same treatment. Differentiation between the two entities is made by biopsy.

D. Stylalgia (Eagle's Syndrome)

This controversial entity causes pain in the tonsilar fossa that is usually unilateral, presumably because of an elongated styloid process. The pain is usually sharp and confined to the region of the tonsil. It is difficult to distinguish between stylalgia and glossopharyngeal neuralgia. Occasionally, the tip of the styloid process is palpable in the tonsillar fossa. Treatment is by surgical excision of the lower 1.5 cm of the styloid process, usually as an intraoral procedure after tonsillectomy. See Chapter 25.

E. Glossopharyngeal Neuralgia

Glossopharyngeal neuralgia is characterized by episodes of severe, sharp, stabbing, usually unilateral pain in the throat and is described as open "tic douloureux of the throat." Patients are usually highly motivated, compulsive personalities. If no obvious etiologic factors are found, glossopharyngeal neuralgia can usually be treated conservatively with analgesics and antidepressants, such as amitriptyline (Elavil), beginning with 25 mg daily and increasing the doses. If conservative measures fail, resection of the roots of the glossopharyngeal nerves will be necessary, by means of an occipital craniectomy. See Chapter 25.

F. Carotidynia

This ill-defined condition usually afflicts middle-aged women. The patient complains of pain in the neck and throat that frequently radiates to the ear. No history of trauma or infection is elicited. The only positive finding is tenderness along the line of the common carotid artery and its major branches, sometimes even along the peripheral facial vessels. No specific pathologic descriptions of carotidynia exist, and, therefore, treatment is empiric. Analgesics may not help. Anesthetizing a segment of the vessel by local infiltration with a 1% lidocaine solution is sometimes useful and may break the cycle of constant discomfort. Corticosteroids taken orally are not generally helpful. See Chapter 25.

VIII. MUSCULAR PAIN

Pain in the throat caused by muscle disease is rare. Muscle spasm occurs secondary to local-irritation phenomena such as infection or trauma. Pain is not a symptom of dysfunction of the constrictor muscles.

IX. PAIN OF SKELETAL ORIGIN

Soreness of the throat can be caused by pathologic processes in the cervical spine, particularly inflammatory or neoplastic disorders. Osteomyelitis of the cervical spine is rare today, but it can occur directly from penetrating wounds or from bacteremic seeding. Complaints are of pain in the deep throat, stiffness of the neck, and odynophagia. The patient has fever, obvious swelling and tenderness of the posterior neck, and edema of the posterior pharyngeal wall, which feels boggy. Whenever possible, cultures should be obtained, and a specific organism should be identified. Treatment is with antibiotics, given intravenously in large doses. For infections of the bone, the antibiotic of choice is clindamycin, 150 mg q6h, or in higher doses as indicated. Clindamycin must be used carefully because it may cause severe colitis. For soft tissue infection, dicloxacillin or penicillin G, 1,000,000 Units q6h intravenously, is helpful. Alternatively, cefazolin sodium, 500 mg q6h intravenously, has a broader spectrum of coverage. High doses of antibiotics are necessary because infections in this area are potentially dangerous and must be controlled promptly. Collections of pus should be drained. These collections can now be identified by CT scanning. See Chapter 28.

X. BLEEDING DISORDERS

All bleeding disorders may cause spontaneous submucosal bleeding into the oral cavity and pharynx. Some of these disorders may cause soreness of the throat; others may produce ill-defined sensations in the throat. The patient has no fever, and the white blood cell count is not elevated, but the platelet count may be diminished. One sees patches of ecchymosis on the tonsils, posterior pharyngeal wall, buccal mucosa, and even on the tongue. Treatment of these conditions must be biphasic. First, one must deal with the immediate sequela of coagulopathy, and then, one must institute long-term therapy of the basic problem. Transfusions of platelets, of cryoprecipitate, of whole, fresh blood, or other factors may be necessary to control the tendency to bleeding. Corticosteroids, intravenously or orally, may be helpful. Immediate consultation with a hematologist is essential.

XI. THYROIDITIS

Acute or subacute thyroiditis causes pain in the neck or throat. In the acute phase of the disorder, the patient has no difficulty in localizing the problem to the neck. Patients with subacute thyroiditis, however, frequently complain of a persistent soreness of the throat. The discomfort is constant, is aggravated by swallowing, and is associated with a sensation of a lump in the throat. Patients are intolerant of constriction of the neck, for example with shirt collars and necklaces. The patient has no fever, and the pharyngeal mucosa is normal. Diagnosis is made by careful, systematic palpation of the thyroid gland, all or part of which may be tender. Treatment of acute or subacute viral thyroiditis is with suppression of glandular function with levothyroxine sodium (Synthroid) or thyroid extract. If symptoms are sufficiently severe, corticosteroids may be used initially and concomitantly. The corticosteroids should be slowly withdrawn when symptoms subside, but the thyroid medication should be continued for an extended period. One should prescribe thyroid extract, 1 grain daily for 14 days; the dose should be increased by 0.5 grain every 14 days as response dictates, to a maximum of 3 grains per day. One must monitor the patient's pulse rate, body weight, and symptoms of nervousness. Alternatively, one may administer levothyroxine sodium, beginning with 0.025 to 0.04 mg daily and increasing by 0.025 to 0.05 mg weekly, to a maximum of 0.1 to 0.2 mg per day, with careful monitoring of pulse rate, nervousness, and tremor. One should maintain the dose at the patient's maximum level of tolerance. For corticosteroids, one should prescribe prednisone, 30 mg daily in divided doses for a week; then one should gradually reduce the dosage over a 2-week period, to complete withdrawal. See Chapter 30.

XII. REFLUX ESOPHAGITIS

Reflux esophagitis usually causes vague symptoms of soreness in the throat or a sensation of a lump in the throat. The patient may have chronic hoarseness. Pain may be aggravated after meals or at night, when the patient is recumbent. Frequently, heartburn is associated with the disorder. Patients are often overweight, but no anthropomorphic type is spared. Diagnosis of reflux esophagitis must be suspected from the history, and may be confirmed by radiologic contrast studies, although these studies can be falsely negative. Esophagoscopy and pH probe studies may also be helpful. Reflux esophagitis is treated by elevating the head of the bed at night; just elevating the back on pillows is not usually sufficient. Meals should be small and light, as for patients with peptic ulcerations, and antacids should be given at least 4 times per day, particularly after the evening meal. Finally, surgical treatment is indicated only if absolutely necessary. The current surgical procedure of choice is fundoplication. See Chapter 22.

22

DYSPHAGIA

R. KIM DAVIS AND STANLEY M. SHAPSHAY

I. GENERAL PRINCIPLES

Dysphagia, or difficulty with swallowing, results from interference with the passage of food. The three phases of food passage are transfer from the mouth to the esophagus, transport along the esophagus, and entrance into the stomach. The otolaryngologist is mainly concerned with the first two phases, and the discussion is focused on these areas.

A. Physiologic Features

The first phase of swallowing involves the voluntary movement of food through the oral cavity and the involuntary movement of food from the pharynx to the cervical esophagus. This passageway is shared by the respiratory system to the level of the larynx and is governed by a specific set of muscle balances that propel the food while protecting the airway. Food is moved from the oral cavity by the posterior sweeping of the tongue, the medial movement of the fauces, and the superior movement of the soft palate to seal off the nasopharynx. As food passes into the pharynx, the airway is protected by the superior movement of the larynx posterior to the base of the tongue and by the closure of the larynx by the epiglottis, ventricular bands, and true vocal cords. Food moves through the hypopharynx and gains entrance into the cervical esophagus by relaxation of the cricopharyngeus muscle. Any imbalance in this system results in either dysphagia or aspiration.

B. Pathophysiologic Features

Dysfunction of the first phase of swallowing is either anatomic or neuromuscular. Anatomic changes most often occur secondary to infection, neoplasia, or trauma, especially postsurgical tissue loss. Neuromuscular disorders are either diffuse or localized. Table 22–1 lists the most common problems. Symptoms frequently described by patients with these disorders are difficulty in swallowing (dysphagia), painful swallowing (odynophagia), alteration in voice, especially a muffled or "full" voice, aspiration and choking, regurgitation through the nose, and a sensation of a lump or mass. When a patient has difficulty in swallowing, one must determine whether this problem exists with solids, liquids, or both. Difficulty in swallowing solids suggests obstruction at some level in the digestive tract. When a patient has difficulty in swallowing liquids and solids, a greater degree of obstruction is probably present. Difficulty with liquids only is usually due to aspiration and suggests a disorder of the larynx. Odynophagia, a serious symptom, is almost always due to an organic lesion. The cause may be readily apparent, as in the

TABLE 22–1

- Phase I Disorders
  - Infections
    - Faucial tonsillitis (viral or bacterial)
    - Stomatitis (viral or fungal)
    - Peritonsillar and parapharyngeal abscess
    - Lingual tonsillitis and abscess
    - Ludwig's angina
    - Supraglottitis
  - Neoplasms
    - Oral and oropharyngeal carcinoma, especially of the base of the tongue
    - Hypopharyngeal carcinoma, especially of the pyriform sinus
    - Laryngeal carcinoma, especially supraglottic
  - Trauma
    - Facial fractures, especially mandibular
    - Surgical tissue loss
      - After glossectomy
      - After composite resection
      - After palatectomy
      - After laryngectomy (total or partial)
    - Thyrohyoid dysfunction secondary to tracheotomy
  - Neuromuscular disorders
    - Myasthenia gravis
    - Bulbar lesions
    - Peripheral cranial nerve lesions, especially of cranial nerve X
  - Cricopharyngeal dysphagia
    - Secondary to reflux esophagitis
    - Related to recurrent paralysis
    - Poliomyelitic
    - Thyrotoxic
    - Postsurgical
    - Secondary to foreign body impaction
    - Inflammatory
  - Zenker's diverticulum

case of an obvious oral cavity infection, or it may be obscure and require extensive use of available diagnostic methods.

C. Diagnostic Evaluation

A great advantage in the diagnosis of phase I swallowing disorders is that most of the area is accessible to direct examination. The oral cavity can be readily inspected, and the pharynx and larynx can be examined in almost all cases by the indirect mirror technique. Each anatomic area must be visualized and considered. In addition, palpation must be done because it may reveal a disorder that is not apparent by visualization alone.

The postcricoid area is difficult to examine clinically. To gain information about the cricopharyngeus muscle and the esophagus, additional tests are necessary. The barium swallow, the usual next step in diagnosis, is an excellent screening examination. When greater detail is needed, cinefluoroscopic studies may provide further physiologic information. If the barium swallow does not furnish sufficient information, direct pharyngoesophagoscopy may then be considered. Differential-diagnostic lists of phase I and II disorders are given in Tables 22–1 and 22–2.

II. PHASE I DISORDERS

A. Infections

The infectious disorders listed in Table 22–1 are usually readily diagnosed. Candida stomatitis appears as white, plaque-like lesions that are easily removed by gentle scraping, to reveal an underlying erythematous base. When the white lesions are absent, however, patients have only a diffusely erythematous oral cavity and pharynx and complain of severe oral pain or odynophagia. These lesions do not respond to antibacterial agents, but rapidly respond to nystatin (Mycostatin). The possibility of lingual tonsillitis or abscess should be considered in patients with severe oral pain or odynophagia. The diagnosis is made by indirect mirror examination. Supraglottitis is well recognized because of obstructive airway symptoms, but the significance of dysphagia in the symptom complex must be stressed. Dysphagia almost always predates the respiratory symptoms. See Chapter 23.

B. Neoplasms

Neoplastic processes produce dysphagia by several mechanisms. Ulcerative lesions cause pain and lead to voluntary limitation of swallowing, to avoid discomfort. Trismus develops when the muscles of mastication are invaded by tumor. Dysphagia results from bulky oral cavity or oropharyngeal lesions purely because of a mass effect. Invasive tumors interfere with the normal rhythm of swallowing. Pyriform sinus lesions produce mechanical obstruction or additionally interfere with laryngeal function leading to aspiration.

TABLE 22–2

Phase II Disorders (transport)
- Presence of foreign bodies
- Structural disorders
  - Extrinsic compression
    - Thyroid, parathyroid, thymus disorders
    - Osteoarthritic spurs
    - Mediastinal tumors, cysts, and inflammation
    - Vascular disorders
      - Congenital anomalies
      - Dilated tortuous common carotid artery
      - Aneurysm of descending thoracic aorta
  - Diverticula
  - Webs
- Neoplasms
  - Benign
  - Malignant
- Inflammatory disorders
  - Benign esophageal strictures or stenosis
  - Postsurgical or postradiational stenosis
  - Caustic ingestion
  - Plummer-Vinson syndrome
- Motor disorders
  - Diffuse spasm
  - Localized spasm (achalasia)
- Congenital or developmental anomalies
  - Tracheoesophageal fistula and esophageal atresia
  - Compression by anomalous blood vessels
  - Chalasia
- Other
  - Dermatomyositis and scleroderma
  - Infectious diseases (rare)
    - Candida esophagitis in immunosuppressed patients
    - Viral esophagitis
    - Syphilitic esophagitis

C. Dysphagia Related to Cancer Therapy

Treatment of malignant head and neck tumors that have caused dysphagia may eliminate the tumor, but it may fail to solve or may accentuate the difficulty in swallowing. Many chemotherapeutic agents cause mucositis and subsequent dysphagia or odynophagia. Radiation therapy produces xerostomia and mucositis in varying degrees resulting in subsequent dysphagia. When considering surgical treatment one should bear in mind the following "rule of thumb": when more than 50% of any region is resected, or when resection incorporates several regions or organs, interference with the function of swallowing will be severe. Rehabilitation of the oral and laryngopharyngeal cavities is not within the scope of this text, and the reader is referred to an excellent discussion by Conley (Complications of Head and Neck Surgery. Philadelphia, W.B. Saunders, 1979, p. 124).

D. Dysphagia Related to Tracheotomy

Dysphagia related to tracheotomy is a common problem and has been associated with an anterior tracheal flap technique (Lancet, *1*:954, 1966). Dysphagia following tracheotomy is due to restriction in the elevation of the thyroid cartilage during the act of swallowing secondary to immobilization caused by the tracheal tube.

E. Myasthenia Gravis

Neuromuscular disorders that lead to dysphagia are not usually exclusively phase I disorders. An exception, however, is myasthenia gravis, a condition characterized by weakness or paralysis of voluntary muscles after activity, followed by recovery of strength after a rest period of several minutes to several hours. Although clinical symptoms vary, approximately 20% of patients have difficulty in chewing and swallowing (Medical Neurology. New York, Macmillan, 1975, p. 724). When the bulbar muscles are involved, patients commonly develop a nasal quality to the voice, with dysphagia and nasal regurgitation of food when eating. Diagnosis of this disorder, which is seldom difficult in severe or moderately severe cases, is normally made by a neurologist. The otolaryngologist should consider this diagnosis in patients with otherwise unexplained dysphagia. The diagnosis is confirmed by observing the patient's response to the rapid intravenous injection of edrophonium chloride (Tensilon). See Chapter 23.

F. Bulbar Palsy

Bulbar palsy rarely produces dysphagia alone; it is usually associated with aspiration and respiratory insufficiency. The most common causes are vertebrobasilar insufficiency, poliomyelitis, and ascending paralyses, such as Guillain-Barré syndrome; or amyotrophic lateral sclerosis. The treatment is by airway establishment, protection from aspiration, enteral alimentation with a nasogastric feeding tube, and cervical esophagostomy or gastrostomy. Release of cricopharyngeal spasm by myotomy or sympathectomy is occasionally necessary. See Chapter 23.

G. Cranial Nerve Paralysis (Peripheral)

Peripheral paralysis of cranial nerves is often seen by the otolaryngologist. The most important nerve producing dysphagia is the vagus nerve. If this nerve is interrupted near or at the base of the skull, the patient will experience severe dysphagia and hoarseness associated with aspiration. The role of the vagus nerve and of the cricopharyngeal muscle is discussed in the section of this chapter on cricopharyngeal dysphagia. Seventh nerve paralysis leads to drooling and to a loss of buccal tone that may interfere with posterior pulsion. Isolated lesions of the ninth (glossopharyngeal) nerve are rare. Loss or diminution of the gag reflex usually occurs in patients with lesions of this nerve, rather than the vagus. Peripheral twelfth nerve paralysis is seldom a severe problem as long as the loss is unilateral. When this nerve was voluntarily sectioned for the purpose of anastomosing nerves VII to XII, approximately 22% of patients had minimal tongue atrophy, 53% had moderate atrophy, and 25% had severe atrophy (Trans. Am. Acad. Ophthalmol. Otolaryngol., *84*:763, 1977). Of the entire group, only 3% had speech or swallowing difficulties. Bilateral twelfth nerve paralysis leads to a severe swallowing handicap with aspiration and difficulty in moving a bolus of food.

H. Cricopharyngeal Dysphagia

One of the most common disorders of swallowing is cricopharyngeal dysphagia. This condition bridges a gap between phase I and phase II disorders and is a poorly defined entity in which the cricopharyngeus muscle fails to relax in the presence of a bolus of food.

1. **Physiologic features** Cricopharyngeal dysphagia is analagous to achalasia in that the sphincter fails to relax. In 1958, Kirchner studied the relation of the cricopharyngeus muscle to the vagus nerve and sympathetic nerve trunks in dogs (Laryngoscope, *68*:1119, 1958). He found that the cricopharyngeus muscle maintains a normal state of tonus. It relaxes to receive the passage of the bolus and then contracts to a pressure level equal to or higher than its resting state, to assist in the movement of the bolus. Unilateral section of the vagus nerve at the base of the skull reduced the relaxation phase. When both vagus nerves were sectioned at the base of the skull, the relaxation phase was abolished, with ensuing severe dysphagia. Stimulation of the superior cervical ganglion caused a sharp rise in pressure, whereas stimulation to the vagal branch of the nerve to the cricopharyngeus muscle caused marked relaxation of pressure. In summary, relaxation was found to be mediated by parasympathetic fibers, and contraction mediated by sympathetic fibers. Dysphagia would then result from sympathetic overactivity or vagal loss. Surgical treatment would require division of the muscle itself or of its sympathetic nerve supply. Lund isolated the nerve to the cricopharyngeus muscle and demonstrated that the reflex arc involving the nerve to that muscle was essential for normal peristalsis from the pharynx to the esophagus. Isolating the pharynx from the sphincter immediately superior to the superior border of the muscle, that is, afferent limb, prevented relaxation of the cricopharyngeus muscle. Conversely, section of the motor efferent limb by severing the nerve prevented the normal increase in pressure seen after the bolus passed the muscle (Acta Otolaryngol. (Stockh.), *59*:497, 1964). Cricopharyngeal function is also influenced by the distal esophagus. Henderson studied 50 patients with gastroesophageal reflux and 10 control subjects by high-speed esophageal manometric techniques (Laryngoscope, *86*:1531, 1976). Twenty of the 50 patients with gastroesophageal reflux had muscle incoordination during swallowing,

manifested by premature cricopharyngeal contraction. This disorder was not present in the control subjects.

2. **Causes** Cricopharyngeal dysphagia has been associated with reflux esophagitis, recurrent laryngeal nerve paralysis, poliomyelitis or other bulbar palsies, thyrotoxic myopathy, and pharyngectomy. By far the most common association is with reflux esophagitis. Distal esophagitis can lead to gastroesophageal motor dysphagia, peptic stricture, or cricopharyngeal spasm. Obstruction at the gastroesophageal level gives rise to discomfort that radiates to the neck and is relieved either by passage of the bolus into the stomach or by regurgitation. Obstruction at the level of the cricopharyngeus muscle presents similar discomfort, but it commonly leads to simultaneous aspiration, in contrast to aspiration at night seen with distal motor dysphagia or stricture. The space posterior to the larynx has only a 5-ml volume, whereas an average swallowed food bolus has a volume of 15 ml. Therefore, food spills into the larynx and causes aspiration. If the degree of aspiration is mild, patients develop hoarseness and chronic coughing. When aspiration is more severe, recurrent respiratory infections occur. Henderson studied 200 patients who were to undergo surgical repair of severe reflux esophagitis (Laryngoscope, *86*:1531, 1976). The total incidence of dysphagia was 79.5%; 100 patients (50%) had cricopharyngeal dysphagia. After surgical correction of reflux, only 10 of the 100 patients had residual symptoms; 8 of these had mild symptoms, without coughing or choking. Cricopharyngeal dysphagia is associated with recurrent laryngeal nerve paralysis. Eighteen patients who developed recurrent laryngeal nerve paralysis were studied by Henderson (J. Thorac. Cardiovasc. Surg., *68*:507, 1974). Fifteen patients had bronchogenic carcinoma, 2 patients had thyroid resections, and 1 patient had viral neuritis. Eleven of the 15 patients with bronchogenic carcinoma had cricopharyngeal dysphagia and vocal cord paralysis of simultaneous onset. Aspiration, the dominant clinical symptom associated with dysphagia, was relieved in 3 patients by cricopharyngeal myotomy. Recurrent nerve paralysis should be considered in patients with unexplained dysphagia, especially if aspiration is present. On the other hand, in patients with known recurrent nerve paralysis and aspiration, the aspiration may not be solely due to incompetence of the larynx. See Chapter 23.

3. **Diagnosis**
   a. ***Medical history*** Predisposing factors, as noted in the previous section, should be sought when obtaining the patient's medical history. Patients with cricopharyngeal dysphagia are said to be "nervous individuals" and commonly complain of a "lump" in the throat. They may complain of the inability to force food from the mouth into the esophagus and the need to make several attempts at

swallowing. When patients describe a persistent lump in the throat that is present even when they do not try to swallow, the cause may be neurotic, that is, globus hystericus. This disorder commonly occurs in association with emotional disturbance. The emotional disturbance may be masked, and the only manifestation may be the persistent lump sensation. Globus hystericus differs from organic disease in that the symptoms are not worse during swallowing and may, in fact, be improved. This diagnosis is one of exclusion, and such patients must be thoroughly evaluated. Although patients with cricopharyngeal dysphagia are commonly 40 to 60 years old, this is not exclusively a disorder of adults. Reichert and associates reviewed the histories of 15 infants with cricopharyngeal achalasia (dysphagia) (Ann. Otol. Rhinol. Laryngol., *86*:603, 1977). The symptoms were poor eating, congestion in the throat, choking and coughing while eating, regurgitation, and nasal reflux. Most patients had symptoms at birth; the latest diagnosis was made at 6 months of age. Eleven of 15 infants had associated disorders such as meningomyeloceles and Arnold-Chiari malformations (4 patients) and congenital anomalies associated with the central nervous system (7 patients).

b. ***Specific tests*** Radiologic and manometric studies have been disappointing in delineating cricopharyngeal problems. When cricopharyngeal hypertrophy is present, a shelf-like or semicircular filling defect can be seen in the area under question. The barium may pool and may overflow into the valleculae. Spillage of radiopaque material into the tracheobronchial tree can also be seen. The role of manometric studies was discussed earlier. These studies may show incoordination at the cricopharyngeal area, especially abnormally high cricopharyngeal pressure. Endoscopic study performed with the patient under general anesthesia is seldom helpful because of the relaxation obtained. Spasm may be seen if endoscopic examination is done under local anesthesia. If distal esophagitis is present, secondary cricopharyngeal spasm may be inferred, but not proved.

4. **Treatment** should be first directed to any predisposing factors. Esophagitis may be treated medically and, when indicated, referral may be made for the evaluation of possible antireflux procedures. Cricopharyngeal myotomy has been reported to relieve cricopharyngeal dysphagia successfully, and the technique and indications have been reviewed by Chodosh (Laryngoscope, *85*:1862, 1975). The procedure should be routinely done in association with supraglottic laryngectomy and should be considered with other ablative head and neck procedures. It also should be considered when dysphagia accom-

panies vagal lesions, cerebrovascular accidents, dermatomyositis, poliomyelitis, or other bulbar palsies. The operation may be helpful when dysphagia persists in patients with reflux esophagitis who are not helped by antireflux procedures. When dysphagia is due to section of the vagus nerve at or near the skull base, resection of the denervated pharyngeal muscle on the paralyzed side in the manner of a partial pharyngectomy may be indicated (Trans. Am. Acad. Ophthalmol. Otolaryngol., *84*:57, 1977). The rationale is that the newly constructed food passage has a balanced sphincteric function.

I. Zenker's (Pharyngoesophageal) Diverticulum

Closely related to cricopharyngeal disorders is Zenker's diverticulum. This rare disorder, which most often occurs after the age of 60 years, originates in the posterior pharyngeal wall at or superior to the level of the cricopharyngeus muscle. Although the exact cause is unknown, the disorder is commonly seen in association with other diseases of the esophagus, especially cricopharyngeal dysphagia. It is most clearly related to a developmental weakness of the muscular coat of the posterior pharynx between the oblique fibers of the inferior constrictor muscle and the horizontal fibers of the cricopharyngeus muscle. During the first stage of swallowing, the pharynx is converted into a closed space. When the cricopharyngeus muscle relaxes, the pressure wave forces the bolus of food into the cervical esophagus. If the cricopharyngeus muscle fails to open, the pressure is directed throughout the pharynx. If a developmental weakness exists posteriorly, this area will herniate and will eventually form a true diverticulum.

1. **Symptoms** of Zenker's diverticulum are characteristic. Commonly, the patient has only mild dysphagia initially and notices a gurgling sensation when drinking. Regurgitation of undigested food hours after eating is a classic symptom. These symptoms can exist for years. If regurgitation occurs at night, aspiration may take place and may lead to episodes of severe coughing and, eventually, to chronic pulmonary disease. Patients may be aware of food lodged in the diverticulum and may be able to dislodge it by twisting the neck or by massaging the angle of the mandible. Significant dysphagia occurs when the diverticulum enlarges and blocks the cervical esophagus. Spontaneous bleeding or perforation is rare. Weight loss is common.

2. **Diagnosis** is usually made by the patient's medical history and is normally confirmed by barium study. The barium-filled pouch first projects posteriorly and then to the left of the midline in the space between the prevertebral fascia and the pretracheal fascia. Esophagoscopic examination may be necessary to exclude another lesion, but the procedure may be hazardous. Perforation can occur because such a diverticulum is often confused with the esophageal lumen, and undue force

applied in directing the esophagoscope distally results in perforation. Small filiform dilators ("lumen finders") or a swallowed string can be used to define the esophageal lumen, which is always anterior to the diverticulum.

3. **Treatment** depends on the size of the diverticulum and on the patient's symptoms. Small diverticula in mildly symptomatic patients are not surgically treated. When operation is necessary, the approach can be by external incision, as described by Montgomery (Surgery of the Upper Respiratory Tract. Vol. 2. Philadelphia, Lea & Febiger, 1973, p. 283) or endoscopic, as described by Dohlman (Arch. Otolaryngol., *71*:744, 1960). External diverticulectomy is the operation of choice in all healthy, younger individuals. The main risk is of damage to the recurrent laryngeal nerve. In high-risk patients and in patients aged 60 years and over, the Dohlman procedure should be considered. Contraindications to endoscopic division are the lack of proper instrumentation or experience, the presence of a pouch too small for instrumentation, or the inability to gain medical clearance for anesthesia (South. Med. J., *68*:1260, 1975).

III. PHASE II DISORDERS

Phase II or transport disorders of the body of the esophagus are listed in Table 22–2. Otolaryngologists are most commonly involved with the anatomic disorders, whereas gastroenterologists generally treat the motor disorders. Of course, these fields overlap.

A. Presence of Foreign Bodies

One of the most common problems is the presence of a foreign body. Patients are usually small children or edentulous adults. Symptoms are generally dysphagia, odynophagia, and pooling of secretions. When large foreign bodies lodge in the postcricoid area, respiratory distress may be present. Symptoms are usually precipitous, with a history of sudden choking or gagging on something hard. This finding is associated with pain, which is generally localized to the cervical esophagus. The presence of a foreign body should also be considered, however, in patients with dysphagia of longer duration and in children who develop poor feeding habits, regurgitation, weight loss, or unexplained pulmonary symptoms. When the presence of a foreign body is suspected on the basis of the patient's medical history, the first diagnostic step is the physical examination. Indirect mirror examination may reveal the foreign body. Chest films are necessary and may reveal radiopaque objects. The role of the barium study is controversial. A negative test result in a patient with a suggestive history should not preclude esophagoscopy. The quantity of barium used should be as small as possible. When the normal procedure is followed in a patient with complete or near complete obstruction, the barium pools superior to the obstruction and becomes a potential source of aspiration. The presence of residual barium in the esophagus may make the identification of foreign bodies at esophagoscopy more difficult. To obviate these problems, one should place a small quantity of barium on a piece of cotton or use water-soluble contrast agents. When chest roentgenograms or barium studies reveal objects that normally would be expected to pass uneventfully through the esophagus, one should consider a pre-existing esophageal disorder. Removal of foreign bodies has clearly been presented (Pediatric Otolaryngology. Vol. II. Philadelphia, W.B. Saunders, 1972, p. 1242).

B. Structural Disorders

Anatomic structural disorders can be divided into those secondary to external compression and those due to diverticula or webs. The most common source of external (extraluminal) compression is osteoarthritic spurs (ORL, *38*:45, 1976). These spurs are usually easily demonstrated on routine lateral neck films or by xeroradiography. Extrinsic compression by tumors is most commonly seen in adults, with tumor masses, especially benign goiters, the most frequent cause. In children, extrinsic compression is usually due to vascular anomalies, especially of the innominate artery. Mid-esophageal and epiphrenic diverticula are rare and have no specific symptoms. They may obstruct and perforate, however, like any other diverticulum. Inferior esophageal webs are seen in 6 to 14% of routine barium studies, but these lesions are symptomatic only in one-third of these patients. Symptomatic patients are usually over age 40. Episodic, short-lived dysphagia is the main symptom. Treatment, which is rarely necessary, is by dilatation. See Chapter 38.

C. Esophageal Cancer

Neoplasms of the esophagus are almost always malignant; 95% or greater are squamous cell carcinoma. The association of alcoholism with esophageal carcinoma has long been documented, and the association of other head and neck squamous cell carcinoma to synchronous or metachronous esophageal carcinoma has also received attention. A review of 150 consecutive head and neck cancer patients over a 22-month period revealed a multiple primary cancer rate of 19%, with 9 patients (6%) having simultaneous esophageal primary tumors (Otolaryngol. Head Neck Surg., *88*:373, 1980). Dysphagia is the presenting symptom in 75 to 85% of these patients. Weight loss may be profound; the average patient in one series lost 25 pounds over a 5-month period (Surg. Gynecol. Obstet., *105*:465, 1957). Chest pain may be persistent and usually signals local extensions of the tumor. Rarely, massive upper gastrointestinal bleeding or metastasis to thyroid or bone are the presenting symptoms. Physical examination is rarely helpful. The role of barium and endoscopic studies has already been mentioned. Treatment is often by irradiation because many lesions are inoperable when diagnosed. Encouraging results have been noted in early lesions treated with induction chemotherapy, with *cis*-platinum and bleomycin, followed by irradiation (Otolaryngol. Head Neck Surg. *88*:373, 1980).

D. Inflammatory Disorders

1. Benign esophageal strictures

a. ***Postsurgical or postradiational stricture*** The most common inflammatory disorders seen by the otolaryngologist are postsurgical and postradiational strictures of the cervical esophagus. Stenosis of the cervical esophagus is commonly seen after laryngectomy, with or without pre- or postoperative radiation therapy. Because radiation therapy incites an inflammatory response in squamous epithelium, the incidence of stricture or stenosis is probably higher in patients receiving combined therapy than in those receiving surgical or radiation therapy alone, but such a finding has not yet been documented. The most common site of stenosis is at the inferior margin of the closure. Stenosis may occur anywhere along the suture line. It rarely occurs as a web at the base of the tongue, where redundant folds of soft tissue (pseudoepiglottis) block the esophageal introitus. Stenosis is most common where too much mucosa is resected, and a tight primary closure is attempted. The onset of symptoms is most common in the first postoperative year. Stenosis in the early postoperative period should alert the clinician to the possibility of residual carcinoma. When pharyngocutaneous fistula complicates the patient's postoperative course, stenosis may develop at the fistula site. Residual carcinoma must again be ruled out by careful biopsy. The incidence of stenosis or stricture related to the presence of fistula is probably higher than the incidence of cancer-associated stenosis. Diagnosis is made by barium study, in which the area of stenosis appears as a constriction of the esophageal lumen, usually 2 to 3 cm in length. Stenosis longer than 3 cm, in the absence of any postoperative trauma, such as the untimely removal of the nasogastric tube or early oral feeding, should alert the clinician to the possibility of residual tumor. Barium studies may be done 10 to 14 days after the surgical procedure. Definitive diagnosis is made by esophagoscopy, which should not be attempted until 6 weeks postoperatively. The use of a small, filiform dilator, which serves as a "lumen finder" in advance of the esophagoscope, is recommended at endoscopy. Biopsy specimens of suspicious areas should be obtained. Treatment may be started at the time of endoscopic study. The mainstay of therapy is repeated dilatation. This procedure can be preceded by laser excision in areas of firm stenosis. No attempt should be made to remove the entire area of stenosis. Sections of stenosis can be removed in each quadrant to facilitate dilatation. Dilatation is most safely performed in a retrograde manner using Jackson dilators. A small dilator that may readily pass the obstruction is first placed. With the first dilator in place, a second small dilator is passed. If necessary, this procedure can be repeated. The dilators are then pulled together through the area of stenosis. Care must be taken that the additive size is not too great, to prevent linear lacerations on withdrawal of the instruments. When the area of stenosis is long, or when the stricture is almost complete, an open procedure may be necessary, including reconstruction with regional flaps.

b. ***Caustic ingestions*** Most ingestions of caustic substances are either accidental ingestions in children or suicide attempts in adults. By far the most common agents are strong alkalis, which produce severe liquefaction necrosis. If the ingestants are dry pellets or flakes, the insult will be a segmental esophageal injury that may progress to later stricture. Individuals who swallow these agents accidentally expectorate most of the material in a reflex action because of the intense, burning pain. When liquid lyes are ingested, and particularly during a suicide attempt, the liquid rapidly descends the esophagus, enters the stomach, and possibly is discharged into the duodenum. In transit, the liquid caustic contacts all esophageal mucosa and leads to widespread necrosis. In contrast to alkalis, acid ingestants cause a coagulative necrosis. Because squamous epithelium is resistant to the acid's effect, the injuries are usually more superficial and less severe. The possibility of caustic ingestion is usually clear from the patient's medical history. The precise identity or volume of the ingestant is often much less apparent. In the presence of buccal or pharyngeal burns, esophageal damage must be suspected; such damage is discovered during endoscopic study in approximately one-third of these patients. No correlation exists between the degree of buccal and of esophageal burns, however. Patients may have esophageal damage in the absence of pharyngeal or mouth burns. All patients with a medical history suggestive of ingestion of caustic substances or with evidence of oral or pharyngeal burns should be hospitalized and should be given corticosteroids and broad-spectrum antibiotics. Diagnostic esophagoscopy is recommended under the following circumstances: suicide attempts, ingestion by children or alcoholics with an unknown chemical, or known chemical with documented tissue injury potential, corrosive injuries in the mouth or pharynx, hematemesis, and epigastric pain. This procedure should be performed as soon as possible, but not later than 48 hours after the ingestion of caustic substances (Laryngoscope, *88*:1300, 1978). Examination of the hypopharynx and superior esophagus can be done with an open esophagoscope to the point of any mucosal burn. No attempt should be made to pass the scope beyond the burn. In such a case, a soft feeding tube may be passed directly without force, or a string may be placed for the patient to swallow. If no burns are found, the remainder of the esophagoscopic study is best done with a flexible gastroscope. This instrument also allows examination of the stomach and duodenum. When significant injury is present, corticosteroids should be continued for 4 to 6 weeks. At that time, dilatation may be attempted, most safely in a retrograde manner (Ann. Otol. Rhinol. Laryngol., *83*:1, 1974).

2. **Plummer-Vinson syndrome** comprises iron-deficiency anemia and dysphagia. Ninety percent of cases are in women, predominantly of the northern hemisphere. Iron deficiency, the essential element in the diagnosis, is the causal factor. Dysphagia is due to web formation just inferior to the cricopharyngeus muscle. The web may be eccentric and is usually less than 2 mm in width. At esophagoscopy, it appears as a smooth, gray, diaphragmatic opening with an eccentric lumen. Myxedema occurs in 50%, achlorhydria in 30 to 40%, pernicious anemia in 30%, and atrophic gastritis in 40% of these patients. Over 50% of patients with this syndrome develop carcinomas of the aerodigestive tract. Treatment of anemia is essential and may alleviate the dysphagia. Dilatation may be necessary. Careful follow-up of patients is critical because this condition is precancerous.

E. Motor Disorders

Diffuse spasm of the esophagus is defined by Spiro as simultaneous, repetitive, nonperistaltic, and often abnormally powerful contractions of the esophagus (Clinical Gastroenterology. New York, Macmillan, 1977, p. 42). This entity is often associated with other organic disorders of the esophagus, but it may exist in the absence of any demonstrable lesion. It is often produced by emotional stress and is manifested by dysphagia and substernal chest pain. Symptoms are intermittent. If a barium study is done when the patient is symptomatic, one may see a change in the normal sequential flow of barium. Peristalsis is often diminished in the inferior esophagus, and the esophagus is thereby passively dilated. Treatment consists first of reassuring the patient the pain is not of cardiac origin. When this approach is not helpful, passage of an esophageal dilator often reduces the frequency of attacks. This condition should be differentiated from achalasia, which is a disorder of esophageal motility characterized by failure of the inferior esophageal sphincter to relax normally. Achalasia is thought to be caused by vagal denervation. Patients with achalasia rarely have pain, often vomit or regurgitate food, and exhibit decreased esophageal emptying. Patients with diffuse spasm have pain, rarely regurgitate food, and have prompt esophageal emptying.

F. Congenital Anomalies

1. **Tracheoesophageal fistula** is a congenital abnormality in which normal canalization of the foregut does not occur. Ninety percent of children with tracheoesophageal fistula have a large, thick-walled superior esophagus that ends as a blind pouch in the mediastinum, with the inferior esophagus connected to the trachea as a fistula. Several other variations of atresia and fistula include esophageal atresia alone, fistula with the superior esophageal segment, fistula with both superior and inferior esophageal segments, and H-type tracheoesophageal fistula. Approximately 50% of infants with tracheoesophageal fistula have other abnormalities, 35% of these children are premature, and 16% had hydramnios present during their mother's pregnancy. Presenting symptoms are copius salivation, choking, dyspneic attacks, coughing, and cyanotic spells. When esophageal atresia is considered, one should initiate diagnostic studies immediately. Chest films may show pneumonia. Abdominal films show marked abdominal distension, with gas throughout the gastrointestinal tract. Small French catheters can be passed through the nose, and small quantities of water-soluble contrast material may be instilled in the superior esophagus, to document the atresia or fistula. Treatment is surgical.

2. **Dysphagia lusoria** is the term applied to esophageal obstruction by an anomalous right subclavian artery. This rare entity occurs in under 1% of the population and has no specific age of onset. "Dysphagia lusoria" has been loosely applied to any number of vascular malformations involving the embryologic structures of the aortic arches, most commonly the third and fourth arches. A complete vascular ring can be present or only an anomalous vessel. In children, a double arch is the most common abnormality, whereas in adults, the aberrant right subclavian artery is most frequent. In children, dysphagia is rarely present at birth, but is usually first seen when the child starts to eat solid food. Urgent respiratory distress precipitated by swallowing is a rare presenting symptom. Diagnosis is suggested on the barium study by an indentation in the posterior wall of the esophagus near the level of the aortic arch. Treatment is rarely necessary in adults. Surgical intervention may be necessary in children who aspirate regurgitated food.

3. **Chalasia** is the persistent reflux of food from the stomach into the lower esophagus in infants. Vomiting, developing 3 to 10 days after birth, is characteristic. This condition is probably an accentuation of a normal phenomenon and is treated by sitting or propping the infant upright.

G. Dermatomyositis and Scleroderma

Patients with these diseases, which affect esophageal motility, are rarely seen by the otolaryngologist. Scleroderma is characterized by induration of skin and fibrous replacement of the smooth muscle of internal organs. It affects the smooth muscle of the esophagus and leads to loss of tone in the distal esophageal high-pressure zone and loss of normal peristalsis. The resultant gastroesophageal reflux, coupled with impairment of the inferior esophagus to clear refluxed gastric contents, causes reflux esophagitis. Dermatomyositis is a collagen-vascular disorder that causes degeneration of striated muscle and weakening of smooth muscle. For this reason, it is a disease of the superior esophagus that often produces dysphagia or hoarseness. Because laryngoesophageal muscle tone is low, the lumen of the diseased portions of the esophagus is gaping and contains air. Active propulsion of a bolus of food is defective; progress is due only to gravity. In lateral plain roentgenograms of the neck, air may be seen in the superior, flaccid segment of the esophagus with a distended hypopharynx. Approximately one-third of all patients with dermatomyositis have stomatitis. In adults over age 40, the incidence of co-existing malignant disease is 17%. Treatment is with corticosteroids (Laryngoscope, *88*:147, 1978).

23

LARYNGEAL DISORDERS

J. KEVIN FORTSON AND M. STUART STRONG

The role of the larynx in protecting the airway is well understood. This organ is important as a sphincter during deglutition, parturition, cough, and defecation. As the sounding source of speech, the larynx performs its most fascinating role. In treating disorders of the larynx, one attempts to restore the ability to perform all these functions whenever possible.

I. CONGENITAL ANOMALIES

A. Laryngomalacia

This disorder comprises about 75% of all congenital anomalies of the larynx. In this condition, excessive flaccidity of the cartilaginous superglottic larynx causes inspiratory stridor. Symptoms may start shortly after birth and are diminished by rest and sleep. Symptoms are worse when the patient is crying, and the disorder may be associated with respiratory distress. The diagnosis is made by direct laryngoscopy, during which stridor stops as the laryngoscope passes under the epiglottis. The epiglottis is frequently omega shaped, and the arytenoid cartilages move anteriorly into the glottic opening during inspiration. One should perform an esophagogram to rule out the presence of vascular compression of the trachea. Treatment of this condition is generally conservative. One may observe the patient in the hospital, although this procedure is usually unnecessary. Dyspneic episodes are usually terminated when the child is placed in a prone position, and tracheostomy is rarely needed. Parents should be instructed to interrupt feeding after each 2 to 3 swallows, to allow the infant to breathe. Most children recover by 18 months of age.

B. Congenital Subglottic Stenosis

This condition is the third most common congenital abnormality of the larynx, after laryngomalacia and neurologic lesions. The patient usually has inspiratory and expiratory stridor, and a soft tissue roentgenogram of the neck may reveal subglottic swelling. Approximately 50% of these patients have recurrent episodes of tracheobronchitis, and 40% require tracheostomy. Endoscopic dilatation at regular intervals may be helpful, but major reconstructive surgical procedures should be delayed until adolescence.

C. Congenital Laryngeal Webs

Seventy-five percent of laryngeal webs are at the glottic level and cause an abnormal cry or squeak. Respiratory distress, asthma-like breathing, dyspnea, cyanosis, or croupy cough may be present in patients with laryngeal web. Treatment involves division of the web and dilatation to prevent reformation. Placement of a McNaught Keel may be necessary to prevent reformation of extensive webs.

D. Congenital Laryngeal Atresia

Complete atresia of the larynx is present in 5% of patients who have laryngeal webs as their sole abnormality of the airway. This condition is incompatible with life unless it is immediately recognized at birth or unless it is associated with a tracheoesophageal fistula. Immediate treatment includes passage of a bronchoscope through the most posterior part of the atresia, followed by an emergency tracheotomy. This disease must be suspected in infants making a vigorous, unsuccessful attempt to breathe, with increasing cyanosis. Untreated, this condition leads to cardiopulmonary arrest.

E. Congenital Laryngeal Cysts (Laryngoceles)

Congenital cysts of the larynx are rare. Eighty percent of congenital laryngoceles are diagnosed in adults. These cysts may be internal, external, or both, depending whether the lesion herniates through the thyrohyoid membrane. Symptoms include respiratory obstruction, dysphagia, feeble or absent cry, and a soft neck mass. Diagnosis is through radiographic and direct laryngoscopic study. Treatment includes intubation with repeated aspirations and, rarely, marsupialization. Emergency treatment by aspiration may be helpful with endoscopic excision at a later date. In patients with large laryngoceles, an external surgical approach is necessary.

F. Laryngeal Hemangiomas

These rare, benign, slow-growing masses are usually diagnosed between 6 and 12 months of age. Characteristically, the patient is asymptomatic at birth. Approximately 50% of patients have associated cutaneous lesions over the face, head, or neck. Endoscopically, the lesion appears as a smooth, compressible mass inferior to the posterior commissure. Treatment may require tracheotomy. Corticosteroids and radiation have been used, as well as surgical intervention.

G. Laryngeal Cleft

Patients with this disorder have respiratory obstruction, dysphonia, dysphagia with aspiration, or recurrent pneumonia. They frequently also have other congenital anomalies. Direct laryngoscopy and cinefluoroscopy establish the diagnosis, and surgical correction, if necessary, should be performed through a lateral pharyngotomy.

H. Neurogenic Lesions

Vocal cord paralysis is the second most common congenital laryngeal anomaly; bilateral recurrent laryngeal nerve paralysis is twice as common as the unilateral disorder. Bilateral paralysis or paresis is rare in an otherwise normal infant, but it is frequently associated with cerebral agenesis, mental retardation, meningomyelocele, and birth trauma. Treatment must be directed toward the underlying disease. Unilateral vocal cord paralysis often requires no treatment. Bilateral vocal cord paralysis may necessitate tracheotomy, with arytenoidectomy or arytenoidopexy. Such an operation is best delayed until the patient is 5 or 6 years old. Acquired vocal cord paralysis is discussed later in this chapter.

II. INFLAMMATORY CONDITIONS

These conditions usually produce stridor, wheezing, or hoarseness. Pain, swallowing difficulties, and respiratory obstruction may also accompany inflammatory conditions of the larynx.

A. Acute Laryngitis

This disorder may be secondary to vocal abuse, to inhalation of fumes, or to viral or bacterial infection. Voice rest, humidification, and administration of cough suppressants are frequently helpful. Throat culture should be done when infection is suspected, and appropriate antibiotics should be prescribed, to treat the underlying infection. Singers should be advised to allow the inflammatory process to subside before resuming singing. See Chapter 24.

B. Acute Laryngotracheal Bronchitis

This disorder usually causes subglottic edema resulting in a characteristic barking cough and hoarse voice. Eighty percent of cases are of viral origin; parainfluenza virus, respiratory syncytial virus, adenovirus, and measles virus are the most common pathogens. The disease typically occurs in children under 3 years of age and causes increasing cough and hoarseness. High fever is unusual, although inspiratory stridor, tachypnea, retractions, and diminished breath sounds are common. Restlessness, tachycardia, pallor, and cyanosis suggest hypoxia. The diagnosis is confirmed by a soft tissue roentgenogram of the neck showing subglottic narrowing. Therapy should include hydration and moisturization of the air. A short course of high doses of corticosteroids, 1 mg/kg every 6 hours, is usually attempted, but the efficacy of such a regimen has not been established. Bacterial infection, when present, is usually by gram-positive cocci. Therefore, patients are usually also treated with ampicillin, 50 to 100 mg/kg per day. Nasotracheal intubation in the operating room may be necessary, and tracheotomy should be performed if intubation is impossible. Indication for intubation is deterioration of the patient's condition in spite of humidification, antibiotics, corticosteroids, and rest.

C. Acute Epiglottitis

This rapidly progressive bacterial cellulitis of the superglottic airway puts the patient at risk of sudden total airway obstruction. It is a medical emergency, and its diagnosis must be followed by immediate intubation. The causative organism is Haemophilus influenzae type B, and the usual drug of choice is ampicillin, although chloramphenicol may be necessary in certain resistant cases. The patient's medical history suggests the diagnosis. One usually sees a rapid progression of symptoms, most often in children 3 to 6 years old. The patient has fever, malaise, dysphagia, inspiratory stridor, and an extended neck. These children are typically seen sitting up in bed, leaning forward, drooling. The swollen, cherry-red tip of the epiglottis may be visible when the child opens his mouth, but examination with a tongue blade is contraindicated and may precipitate immediate obstruction of the airway. Radiographs may be done; however, conservative management of epiglottitis demands prophylactic nasotracheal intubation to prevent sudden airway obstruction. This disease demands the complete co-operation of skillful anesthesiologists and otolaryngologists, who should carefully and deliberately ensure that the child, preferably carried by a parent, reaches the operating room safely. The child should not be harassed or agitated because this could precipitate total airway obstruction. Once the airway is secured, antibiotics should be continued for 7 to 10 days. The tube may be removed in about 48 hours, preferably in the operating room, where a direct laryngoscopy can ensure the safely of extubating the patient. In contrast to patients with acute laryngotracheal bronchitis, these children should not be merely observed, but rather should be intubated as soon as the diagnosis of acute epiglottitis can be established.

D. Acute Spasmodic Laryngitis

This disorder can be uncomfortable for both patient and physician. Episodes of acute spasmodic laryngitis usually follow an upper respiratory tract infection. This condition causes the larynx to become sensitive and to undergo repeated episodes of laryngospasm. A vaporizer is helpful; however, severe symptoms require hospitalization and observation. Antibiotics are not indicated, and the condition is self-limited. Because such episodes may be related to esophageal reflux, this association should be evaluated in the treatment of this condition, especially if it is recurrent. See Chapter 22.

E. Laryngotracheal Diphtheria

This entity must be considered in the differential diagnosis in any child with acute laryngotracheal bronchitis. Diphtheria is an acute infectious disease that may involve any part or all of the upper respiratory tract. The disease usually occurs in children over 6 years of age, but adults may be affected. Diagnosis depends on identification of the pathogenic organism, Corynebacterium diphtheriae, on smear or in culture. Treatment must include immediate administration of diphtheria endotoxin and penicillin. Tracheotomy is indicated because the characteristic thick, dirty-gray pseudomembrane, which is densely and tenaciously adherent to the underlying structures, may occlude the patient's airway.

F. Chronic Nonspecific Laryngitis

This disorder may be the result of vocal abuse, cigarette smoking, exposure to industrial fumes, or persistent mouth breathing, especially if the air is particularly dry or polluted. Treatment must involve a search for the irritant, as well as voice rest. Humidification is helpful, and any related treatable diseases such as chronic sinusitis should be considered. Corticosteroids may be useful in the short term, but one should not rely upon them. Smoking and excessive alcohol ingestion must be discontinued, and voice rest should be prescribed. Speech therapy is helpful. See Chapter 24.

G. Chronic Atrophic Laryngitis (Laryngitis Sicca)

This form of chronic laryngitis is characterized by atrophy of the mucosa and mucosal appendages of the larynx. It is frequently seen in patients who have undergone radiation therapy; it may follow simple, chronic nonspecific laryngitis. Laryngitis sicca also occurs in patients with Sjögren's syndrome and, occasionally, in pregnant women. The patient complains of a dry, tickly throat with persistent cough and thick, viscid secretions. Cough and hoarseness are more severe in the morning, and laryngeal crusting may be noted. The laryngeal mucosa has a dry, glazed, roughened appearance. As with chronic nonspecific laryngitis, the removal of irritants should be attempted, and humidification should be instituted. The administration of iodides, such as potassium iodide, 30 mg t.i.d., may be of value.

H. Chronic Hypertrophic Laryngitis

This form of laryngitis is usually the result of vocal abuse and excessive smoking. The vocal cords appear beefy red and occasionally demonstrate leukoplakia. The edema is mainly confined to the area of Rienke's space, but the vocal cords may have an angrier appearance. Voice therapy should be instituted, although one must be sure to rule out early carcinoma. Direct laryngoscopic examination with biopsy should be performed when one suspects the presence of a malignant lesion. Elimination of causative agents is important in this condition.

I. Mycotic Infections

1. Blastomycosis

a. ***North American blastomycosis*** is caused by Blastomyces dermatitidis. The larynx is involved in this infection, occasionally with a diffuse nodular infiltration that later ulcerates. Healing and fibrosis may result in vocal cord fixation or stenosis. Pseudoepitheliomatous hyperplasia may be present and may be confused with carcinoma. Although hoarseness is usually the most striking initial symptom, the patient may have cough or hemoptysis. The diagnosis can be made by identification of the organism in a biopsy specimen, but final identification requires cultures. Treatment is with intravenous amphotericin B for 8 to 10 weeks. A recommended total dose for an adult is about 2 g. If the infection extends beyond the skin and is associated with cavitary lung lesions, treatment should be extended to about 10 to 12 weeks, with a total dose of amphotericin B of 2.5 g.

b. ***South American blastomycosis*** is caused by Paracoccidioides brasiliensis. That this mycosis superficially resembles Blastomyces dermatitidis may lead to misdiagnosis. This disease, endemic to South America, causes painful, mucosal ulcerations in the upper respiratory tract. The laryngeal lesions resemble those of the North American disease. The diagnosis can be made by histologic section, although confirmation by culture is preferable. Mild cases may be cured with oral sulfonamide therapy; advanced cases should be treated with intravenous amphotericin B. Ketoconazole may also be useful in paracoccidioidomycosis.

2. **Histoplasmosis** is a systemic fungal disease that may produce laryngeal lesions. The larynx and the tongue are sites of predilection, and the lesions are granulomatous in nature. Although they are occasionally confused with tuberculous lesions, the lesions of histoplasmosis involve the epiglottis and the anterior portions of the larynx, whereas tuberculosis usually involves the posterior commissure. Amphotericin B is the drug of choice in the treatment of histoplasmosis.

3. **Candidiasis (Moniliasis)** Candida albicans is an oval, budding, yeast-like fungus frequently present in the mouth and respiratory tract. The number of candida organisms in the respiratory tract is increased in patients receiving antibiotics, especially the tetracyclines. Acute oral lesions usually respond to the application of 1% aqueous gentian violet or nystatin suspension. Disseminated candidiasis should be treated with intravenous amphotericin B, 0.4 to 0.5 mg/kg every day for several weeks. Ketoconazole, in an adult dose of 200 mg per

day, is the drug of choice for chronic mucocutaneous candidiasis.

4. **Actinomycosis** is a rare, chronic, suppurative disease caused by Actinomyces israelii or, less commonly, by A. naeslundii. This disease can become manifest in a number of ways, and the diagnosis may be difficult to establish. The tissues of the involved site are usually swollen, with a woody hardness and a dusky, red hue. A board-like infiltration of the tissues and, occasionally, draining sinuses are present. The presence of "sulfur granules" in a biopsy specimen is suggestive of the diagnosis; however, the organism must be isolated by appropriate cultures. Surgical intervention may be necessary. Abscesses should be drained, and bony sequestra should be removed. Prolonged antibiotic therapy is critical, and penicillin or tetracycline should be continued for 3 to 6 months after the infection has resolved clinically. Because penicillin and tetracycline are so effective, the more expensive agents are probably not necessary.

J. Perichondritis

This disorder may be associated with many acute and chronic laryngeal diseases. Trauma, surgical procedures, postcricoid ulceration from long-standing feeding tubes, the presence of foreign bodies, and radiation therapy may lead to the development of perichondritis. Tuberculosis, tertiary syphilis, and, of course, carcinoma can also lead to this disease. Symptoms depend on the extent of disease. Early in the course, one may see only redness and swelling; however, laryngeal edema, pain, hoarseness, and dyspnea may result as the disease progresses. Severe pain on swallowing that radiates to the ear is common in patients with perichondritis. Treatment must be directed toward the elimination of all further trauma involving the perichondrium, control of secondary infection, drainage of any abscesses that may be present, and maintenance of the airway. Antibiotics and corticosteroids are frequently helpful, depending on the cause of the disease. Cultures must be obtained, and appropriate antibiotic therapy must be instituted. Surgical intervention should be avoided if at all possible. Occasionally, however, the disease is so extensive that the nonfunctioning larynx must be removed.

K. Foreign Body

Foreign bodies in the larynx usually produce prompt and definite symptoms. Such patients frequently have localized pain, coughing, occasional dyspnea, and hoarseness or even complete aphonia. The foreign bodies can usually be visualized with a mirror, but they sometimes pass through the glottis and may become tracheal or bronchial foreign bodies. In general, foreign body removal should not be attempted at night, unless airway embarrassment is present or impending. One should try to obtain a facsimile of the foreign body and should practice removing it through the laryngoscope to be used. One must be careful to check the equipment before embarking on this potentially catastrophic procedure. At any point, a partial airway obstruction can be inadvertently converted to a total airway obstruction, and it is essential to be prepared to perform an emergency cricothyrotomy or tracheotomy. Great preparation and planning are necessary before one attempts to remove foreign bodies, especially in children (Otolaryngol. Clin. North. Am., *3*:395, 1970).

III. GRANULOMATOUS DISEASES

A. Tuberculosis

In most cases, tuberculous laryngitis is a complication of active pulmonary tuberculosis. Diagnosis is established with a biopsy and staining for the acid-fast bacillus. Hoarseness is usually the first and most common sign, although pain on swallowing is also noted. Referred pain to the ear is another early symptom. The interarytenoid space, the vocal processes, and the false cords may become involved before hoarseness, pain, dysphagia, or referred otalgia occurs. One must rule out the presence of syphilis or carcinoma in these patients. Treatment of laryngeal tuberculosis is essentially that of the pulmonary disease, with the addition of voice rest. Tracheotomy to relieve obstruction is rarely necessary; however, secondary stenoses may require surgical treatment.

B. Leprosy

This infectious disease is caused by Mycobacterium leprae. The skin and mucous membranes of the face and upper respiratory tract are insidiously involved by diffuse or nodular infiltration. These nodules ulcerate and become secondarily infected. In early involvement of the larynx, the voice becomes muffled because of lesions of the superglottic structures. Later, hoarseness and dyspnea occur when the vocal cords are affected. Pain, odynophagia, and referred otalgia are not usually signs of leprosy of the larynx. The supraglottic areas of the larynx are involved first. These diseased areas are a dull, gray color; the nodules later ulcerate and become covered with an exudate. Cervical lymph node enlargement is common, and one must rule out the presence of carcinoma before making this diagnosis. This disease must also be differentiated from syphilis and tuberculosis. Biopsy is necessary to establish the diagnosis. Although spontaneous arrests may occur, diaminodiphenylsulfone (DDS) is effective in 80% of cases. The drug must be given over a long period, from 1 to 4 years, before marked improvement occurs. Corticosteroids may be helpful in relieving respiratory obstruction, and tracheostomy may be necessary. Three types of leprosy are known: nodular or lepromatous, neural or anesthetic, and tuberculoid. The lepromatous variety is the most important to laryngologists and, unfortunately, has the poorest prognosis; pneumonia, tuberculosis, and amyloidosis are the common causes of death.

C. Sarcoidosis

Although sarcoidosis may involve the larynx, it must remain a diagnosis of exclusion, once other possible granulomatous diseases have been eliminated. When sarcoidosis involves the larynx, it causes a diffuse enlargement of the epiglottis, the aryepiglottic folds, or the arytenoid cartilages. This involvement is sometimes so extensive that the true vocal folds cannot be visualized. About 5% of patients with sarcoidosis have laryngeal symptoms, and tracheostomy may be necessary. Laryngeal sarcoidosis may occur as an isolated phenomenon, and biopsy is necessary for the diagnosis. Corticosteroids, both systemic and locally injected, have been used in the treatment of laryngeal sarcoidosis, and this therapy should be instituted if the patient is symptomatic.

D. Syphilis

Syphilitic laryngitis is a clinical rarity, but secondary syphilis may involve the larynx. The patient usually has coexisting lesions in the mouth and throat along with generalized lymphadenopathy. The gummatous tumor masses associated with tertiary syphilis can be of any size and may be located anywhere in the larynx. These lesions are reddened, firm, edematous masses, usually associated with a perichondritis. Early lesions may be small. Late syphilitic lesions are usually seen as ulcerated, nodular, gummatous formations. The ulcer may be superficial or deep, and arytenoid movement may be impaired. After healing, cicatricial fibrosis and deformity are common and leave the epiglottis scarred, twisted, notched, or even absent. Serologic testing, including the fluorescent treponemal antibody absorption test (FTA-ABS), should be performed to rule out the presence of syphilis. Penicillin G is the treatment of choice for this disease.

E. Scleroma (Rhinoscleroma)

This chronic infectious disease of the respiratory tract is characterized by lesions primarily involving the nose, but it may involve the pharynx, tongue, larynx, trachea, and bronchi. These indurated lesions are caused by Klebsiella rhinoscleromatis. These lesions undergo painless, slow, progressive enlargement and eventually cause symptoms of nasal and laryngeal obstruction. Biopsy is necessary to establish the diagnosis; complement fixation and agglutination tests are also helpful. The larynx is involved in about 15% of cases, and tracheostomy is occasionally necessary. Tetracycline, streptomycin, chloramphenicol, and cephalexin are usually advocated for the treatment of this disease.

F. Wegener's Granulomatosis

This disorder, which may involve the larynx, trachea, and bronchi, causes granulomatous lesions, vasculitis, and nephritis. The lesions in the respiratory tract frequently involve the paranasal sinuses and the lungs; however, the larynx is sometimes affected, with deep, ulcerative lesions. The earliest clinical manifestations are sinusitis and ulcerative rhinitis that do not respond to the usual therapy. Although the origin of the disease is unknown, it is suspected to be autoimmune. The use of cytotoxic agents has been gratifying in the treatment of this disease. The treatment of choice is cyclophosphamide, although azathioprine is effective in many cases. Chlorambucil may also be administered. Although cyclophosphamide is usually given orally, intravenous cyclophosphamide may be indicated when the disease is progressing rapidly. One must monitor the patient's white blood count carefully because treatment is usually continued for a year after the patient is in remission. Dialysis and adrenal corticosteroids are occasionally needed in these patients.

IV. ALLERGIC AND HEREDITARY ANGIOEDEMA

A. Allergic Laryngeal Edema

Allergic reactions in the larynx occur in varying degrees. Mild allergic reactions may produce hoarseness and are usually the result of edema of the contact surfaces of the true vocal cords. When more severe forms of allergic edema involve the larynx, a medical emergency may develop. It is necessary to distinguish allergic edema of the larynx from hereditary angioedema involving the larynx because treatment differs. The patient's medical history is important in the diagnosis of allergic edema of the larynx. One should suspect this disorder in a patient who has allergies or who has a family history of allergies. If one can establish the role of allergy in the patient's laryngeal edema, then one may place primary importance on avoidance of the offending agent. Desensitization is sometimes helpful, as are antihistamines. In patients with chronic allergies without airway compromise, steroids, both systemic and topical, should be withheld. Treatment of acute episodes of severe respiratory distress must be aggressive; one must be prepared to intubate the patient. Epinephrine, 1:1,000 dilution, may be given subcutaneously, or one may dissolve 0.5 ml 1:1,000 epinephrine in 10 ml saline solution, to be given intravenously for severe reactions. This dose may be repeated every 20 minutes for 2 to 3 doses. Relative contraindications include cardiac arrhythmias, a pulse rate over 140, and severe hypertension. One must maintain an adequate airway, and tracheostomy may be required. Aminophylline, 500 mg, infused at a rate no faster than 20 mg/min, should be given intravenously for bronchospasm. Antihistamines are probably of little value in treating the acute episode. They may block further histamine binding to target tissue, however, and diphenhydramine hydrochloride (Benadryl), 25 to 50 mg, should therefore be given intravenously. Hydrocortisone, 500 mg intravenously or its equivalent, should be given initially and every 6 hours for severe bronchospasm and prolonged respiratory distress. Corticosteroids do not replace epinephrine, but they are important in preventing recurrences.

B. Hereditary Angioedema

Hereditary angioedema is characterized by recurrent attacks of mucocutaneous swelling that frequently involve the face and may lead to airway obstruction. This disease is also associated with abdominal pain, nausea, vomiting, or diarrhea (Ann. Intern. Med., *84*:581, 1976). This inherited autosomal dominant trait is due to deficient activity of the inhibitor of the activated first component of complement. The patient may not have a positive family history. Such patients usually have recurrent peripheral edema. Allergic evaluation is frequently negative in these patients because the defect is a lack of C$\bar{1}$ inhibitor. These patients usually have low levels of C4 and C2 because no C$\bar{1}$ inhibitor is present to prevent excessive cleavage of C4 and C2 by activated C$\bar{1}$. When C$\bar{1}$ inhibitor levels are low and if C4 levels are low or normal, the diagnosis of hereditary angioedema is likely. If C4 levels are normal during an episode of angioedema, the diagnosis of hereditary angioedema is unlikely. These patients must have prophylactic therapy preoperatively because trauma often induces massive swelling. Fresh frozen plasma should be used if C$\bar{1}$ inhibitor or C4 levels remain low prior to surgical intervention. Long-term androgen therapy is effective in these patients. Danazol, a synthetic androgen, has few virilizing side effects and is also effective. The drug appears to bring about the reappearance of C$\bar{1}$ inhibitor in its functional form and thus stabilizes the complement cascade (Laryngoscope, *93*:749, 1983). Acute episodes of angioedema must be treated aggressively, and the patient's airway must be maintained as previously described for allergic swelling of the larynx.

V. CHRONIC NONSPECIFIC DISEASES

A. Pachyderma Laryngis

Pachyderma laryngis refers to a localized hyperplastic condition of the larynx. This condition is usually caused by vocal abuse, and chronic irritation by stuffy atmospheres, tobacco, and alcohol. The epithelium may be extensively thickened and cornified, and granular laryngitis may develop. The superior surface of the vocal cords may be studded with small, reddish granulations. Biopsy is indicated to rule out neoplastic lesions. The treatment of this condition is nonspecific. Removal of irritants is of primary importance, and speech therapy is sometimes helpful. See Chapter 24.

B. Keratosis of the Larynx

The normal epithelial covering of the larynx is nonkeratinizing squamous epithelium, except for the lining of the laryngeal ventricle and the subglottic areas. Although the term keratosis does not denote a definite or specific entity because its microscopic appearance varies, the term usually implies the presence of a whitish plaque. The lesion is not usually accompanied by an inflammatory reaction and is typically found in middle-aged men. The malignant potential of keratosis is difficult to assess; however, patients are advised to stop smoking and to decrease their exposure to other causative irritants. Direct laryngoscopy with excision is occasionally indicated, and periodic re-examination is also indicated. One usually recommends direct laryngoscopy with excision to rule out the presence of carcinoma in situ or invasive carcinoma.

C. Chronic Cicatricial Stenosis of the Larynx

This disorder can occur in patients with tuberculosis, scleroma, syphilis, leprosy, or glanders. One must determine the nature and severity of the patient's symptoms, as well as the exact level and extent of the stenosis. If the stenosis is a result of an inflammatory or neoplastic condition, one must, of course, ensure that the primary etiologic agent is no longer active. Symptoms usually consist of respiratory obstruction and hoarseness. It is difficult to improve the quality of the voice in patients with this disease, so major surgical intervention should be confined to patients with significant respiratory obstruction. In those with extensive stenosis, tracheostomy is frequently necessary. Supraglottic scarring of the epiglottis and false vocal cord may be approached through an external pharyngotomy. Glottic stenosis frequently demands insertion of a McKnaught Keel through a thyrotomy. Infraglottic stenosis may be a result of external trauma or a superiorly placed tracheotomy. Excision of the stenotic area, with anastomosis between the thyroid cartilage and trachea, may be helpful. Occasionally, infraglottic stenosis results from endotracheal intubation, and arytenoidopexy or laser excision with prolonged stenting may be indicated.

D. Arthritis of the Cricoarytenoid Joint

This disorder is usually seen in the acute stage, when the patient has hoarseness, odynophagia, pain on speaking and coughing, pain radiating to the ear, dyspnea, and tenderness. Chronic arthritis usually causes slight hoarseness, dyspnea, and, occasionally, stridor. Hoarseness may not be present in patients with fixation of only one vocal cord. Mirror examination reveals roughness and thickening of the mucosa over the arytenoid cartilages and narrowing of the vocal chink. Bowing of the vocal cords during inspiration with midline fixation of the arytenoid cartilages and fixation of the arytenoids to the cricoid cartilage suggest the diagnosis of this condition. The majority of these cases are usually associated with generalized rheumatoid arthritis, but this disorder may also be seen in patients with gout, Reiter's disease, and disseminated lupus erythematosus (Laryngoscope, *73*:801, 1963). The underlying arthritis should be treated with salicylates and sometimes corticosteroids. Arytenoidectomy or arytenoidopexy is the only satisfactory treatment when bilateral midline fixation occurs. Unilateral fixation rarely requires therapy.

E. Laryngeal Stenosis

The treatment of laryngeal stenosis must be individualized because narrowing of the lumen of the larynx occurs in many conditions. Treatment of the stenosis must therefore be directed toward the underlying cause. Laryngeal stenosis may be the result of the congenital abnormalities previously discussed, of inflammatory conditions also previously discussed, or of traumatic, neurologic, or neoplastic conditions. Available therapeutic options include dilatation, excision, direct reanastomosis, or even partial or total laryngectomy. Laser excision and stenting are helpful in treating subglottic stenosis.

F. Laryngeal Trauma

One must suspect contusion of the larynx in patients with neck injuries. Immediate diagnosis is the key to appropriate therapy. Mirror examination and a lateral roentgenogram may be helpful. If an arytenoid cartilage has been dislocated, it should be relocated by direct laryngoscopy. Of primary importance is the maintenance of the patient's airway. Tracheotomy or even cricothyrotomy may be indicated. One must suspect a laryngeal fracture even in a patient with minimal trauma to the neck. Patients with a bruise over the laryngeal cartilage, especially those with hemoptysis or a slight change in vocal quality, must be suspected of having a laryngeal fracture and must be treated aggressively. These patients should not be sent for roentgenograms unaccompanied because complete laryngeal obstruction can occur in minutes. Surgical exploration may be indicated if the patient has cervical emphysema or cartilage disruption. Open neck wounds should be debrided; laryngeal cartilage fracture should be reduced and immobilized, with repair within 7 to 10 days of the injury. A stent is usually necessary and is applied through a thyrotomy or an infrahyoid laryngotomy. It is fixed superiorly and inferiorly by stainless steel sutures passed through the skin, with the superior end at the level of the aryepiglottic fold and the inferior end superior to the tracheotomy site. These sutures are left in place for 4 to 6 weeks. Hyoid bone fractures should be treated expectantly because airway compromise is uncommon. In treating a thyroid cartilage fracture, tracheotomy should be performed under local anesthesia because intubation may compromise the remaining airway. Cervical spinal films must be obtained before extending the patient's neck, to rule out fracture. Fractures should be repaired as soon as the general medical status of the patient permits. Immediate surgical intervention reduces the possibility of stenosis secondary to fibrosis.

G. Intubation Granuloma

Intubation granulomas usually occur over the vocal processes of the arytenoid cartilages, located in the posterior third of the true vocal cords. These lesions cause hoarseness, but they can usually be successfully removed endoscopically with the operating microscope. Patients should be informed that these lesions may recur. Scattered reports note an improvement of this condition with the use of oral zinc sulfate.

VI. NEUROGENIC DISORDERS

A. Vocal Cord Paralysis

In evaluating vocal cord paralyses, it is important to distinguish among disturbances of supranuclear origin, those of nuclear origin, and those of infranuclear origin. **Supranuclear** contribution to the vagus nerve is bilateral, and hence unilateral interruption of these fibers does not produce unilateral vocal cord paralysis. The clinical symptoms are dysarthria and dysphonia, along with other manifestations of vagal dysfunction. The voice usually is monotonous, harsh, and overly loud at the beginning of a phrase, before becoming breathy and fading away. Articulation is slurred, and the patient has difficulty in making quick, repetitive sounds. Respiration may not be co-ordinated with the voice. Bilateral interruption of the supernuclear pathways may cause the vocal cords to lie in the abductive position. Although it is theoretically possible to have a unilateral paralysis of one functional muscle group in the **nucleus ambiguous,** in actual practice, most lesions overlap with other contiguous brain stem structures, and one therefore sees additional findings when lesions occur at the nuclear level. In evaluating **infranuclear** lesions, one must carefully rule out a pathologic process at the base of the skull and of the lateral pharyngeal space. The ninth, eleventh, and twelfth cranial nerves may be simultaneously involved with the tenth. These lesions may produce ipsilateral pharyngeal or hypopharyngeal paralysis, ageusia of the posterior third of the tongue, and paralysis of the shoulder girdle. Lesions of the lower neck and mediastinum are also associated with infranuclear lesions. At this level, one must look for involvement of the eleventh cranial nerve or the phrenic nerve. Lesions of the base of the skull that may produce vocal cord paralysis include nasopharyngeal tumors, cordomas, fractures, Arnold-Chiari malformations, or aneurysms. Lesions in the lateral pharyngeal space include tumors of the deep lobe of the parotid gland, neurilemomas, lymphangiomas, keratomas, leiomyomas, and rhabdomyosarcomas (Trans. Am. Acad. Ophthalmol. Otolaryngol., *73*:389, 1967). In a patient with a suspected lesion of the lower neck or mediastinum, trauma, especially surgical, must be considered. Thyroidectomy is the commonest cause of unilateral vocal cord paralysis. Neoplasms, such as bronchogenic carcinoma and carcinoma of the esophagus, thyroid, or breast, must also be considered. Mechanical factors, such as cardiovascular anomalies, hilar adenopathy, or even benign enlargements of the thyroid gland, may put pressure on or stretch the nerves and may thereby lead to vocal cord paralysis. Evaluation of these patients should include a complete blood count, urinalysis, roentgenograms of the chest, skull, and cervical spine, barium swallow studies, glucose tolerance test, sedimentation rate, thyroid scan, and viral titers. Occasionally, lumbar puncture is indicated. Computed tomographic (CT) scanning of the involved area should also be considered. Unilateral or partial bilateral paralysis may be asymptomatic for many years and may then gradually produce obstruction.

1. **Unilateral vocal cord paralysis** usually results in a brassy voice without loss of volume. The patient may have lessened abduction on inspiration, secondary contracture of the vocal cord in adduction, and finally, complete paralysis in which the vocal cord lies in the cadaveric position and the uninvolved vocal cord crosses the midline to compensate. The voice is usually coarse and husky, and the patient loses the ability to sing. Many patients recover in 6 to 12 months, and surgical intervention to improve cord motion is not indicated less than a year from the onset of the disorder. Vocal cord injections may be indicated for paralysis in the paramedial position, to increase bulk and to move the vocal cord medially. The underlying cause must be evaluated and treated. Voice therapy is sometimes helpful. See Chapter 24.
2. **Bilateral vocal cord paralysis** usually causes inspiratory stridor, and 50% of these patients require tracheostomy to relieve airway obstruction. The voice is strong, but the airway is obstructed. Placement of fenestrated tracheostomy tubes may be helpful in this condition. Arytenoidectomy or lateral positioning of the arytenoid cartilage usually improves the airway, although it compromises vocal ability. This procedure may also lead to aspiration. See Chapter 22.
3. **Superior laryngeal nerve paralysis** Sensation of the superior larynx is a function of the internal branch of the superior laryngeal nerve. Vocal symptoms include lowered pitch, limited pitch range, hoarseness, and vocal weakness. Usually, no therapy is necessary in patients with paralysis of the superior laryngeal nerve; however, voice therapy may be helpful. Surgical narrowing of the cricothyroid space is of benefit in rare instances. This procedure is accomplished by suturing the thyroid muscle to the cricoid cartilage, to elevate the cartilage during phonation.

B. Myasthenia Gravis

Myasthenia gravis can be seen at any age, although it usually occurs in young adults. A high percentage of patients with myasthenia gravis have some thymic enlargement, and about 10% may have a malignant tumor of the thymus. CT scanning should be used to rule out the presence of such a tumor. Patients usually have eye muscle or facial muscle symptoms or some difficulties with swallowing or speech. The characteristic weakness occurs after the use of a muscle group and shows a rapid fatiguing quality. Improvement is significant after rest. This disorder may first affect speech and may involve both the laryngeal and pharyngeal musculature. The weakness may respond either to neostigmine (Prostigmin) or to edrophonium chloride (Tensilon). Neostigmine, 15 mg orally, is of more help than edrophonium because edrophonium only gives one about 2 minutes to evaluate the laryngeal weakness. With neostigmine, one should examine the patient in 30 to 40 minutes to determine whether function is improved. At the present time, corticosteroids are the mainstay of treatment. The disease may progress rapidly; the usual cause of death is respiratory failure or inspiratory disorder. Because these symptoms are usually preventable if the patient is under treatment, one must not overlook the possibility of this diagnosis. See Chapter 22.

C. Parkinson's Disease (Paralysis Agitans)

This disorder usually occurs in middle or late life, with gradual progression and a prolonged course. Although the diagnosis may be unclear in its early presentation, the disorder is easily diagnosed in its fully developed form. The patient has a stooped posture, stiffness and slowness of movement, a fixity of facial expression and a rhythmic tremor of the limbs that subsides on active, purposeful movement or complete relaxation. The patient also has a monotonous, weak voice along with a general slowness and diminution of all motor activity. The tremor fluctuates, but it is usually most pronounced at rest and in the hands. It may involve the legs, lips, tongue, and neck muscles and has also been seen in lightly closed eyelids. Treatment of this disease should be prescribed by an internist or a neurologist and usually includes Artane, benztropine mesylate (Cogentin), amantadine (Symmetral), propranolol (Inderal), and levodopa. The side effects of these medications, particularly levodopa, are significant and include gastrointestinal symptoms such as nausea and orthostatic symptoms. When the disease is in remission and is effectively treated by these medications, the voice quality improves dramatically. As the disease progesses, however, the voice softens and may become little more than a whisper.

D. Amyotrophic Lateral Sclerosis

This disease of the nervous system causes a progressive loss of anterior neurons with resultant muscle weakness and wasting. A number of forms of this disease may involve progressive dysfunction of the tongue, pharynx, or vocal cords. Ultimately, the disease progresses and involves almost all voluntary muscles. The tongue, sometimes the earliest organ to demonstrate the disease, may manifest atrophy, fasciculations, and fibrillations. Paresis of the palate and a decreased gag reflex may soon follow. No specific treatment exists, but patients frequently profit in the early stages from speech therapy and counseling regarding communication aids.

VII. FUNCTIONAL DISORDERS

A. Psychogenic Aphonia

Patients with this condition undergo a psychogenic loss of the voice of abrupt onset, usually at the time of emotional crisis. The patient may have a complete loss of voice or may speak in a strained whisper. It is difficult to establish in each individual situation whether the disease is of a psychosomatic origin or whether it is the result of malingering. The patient usually complains of sudden voice loss unaccompanied by other symptoms. Typically, it occurs in young women and does not interfere with the patient's ability to laugh, cry, or cough. Examination with the laryngeal mirror is surprisingly easy. One must seek the assistance of a speech therapist or possible psychiatric or psychologic counseling. The prognosis is generally good, depending on the underlying disorder. See Chapter 24.

B. Dysphonia Plicae Ventricularis

This disorder, also called false cord voice, is caused when the patient uses the ventrical and false cords in phonation. The resulting voice is harsh or low pitched, with a rattling, cracking, rumbling sound. The origin of the condition is unclear, and the diagnosis can be easily made by indirect laryngoscopy. Speech therapy should be instituted, and psychotherapy may be considered. Some authors recommend removal of the false vocal cords by laser in difficult cases; however, this therapy seems to be extreme for a condition in which the prognosis is usually good if the patient undergoes voice therapy. See Chapter 24.

C. Spastic Dysphonia

This term refers to a condition in which the voice is alternately harsh and soft. This disorder is associated with excessive adduction of the vocal cords during phonation. The cause is not yet established, and these patients respond poorly to voice therapy or intensive psychotherapy. Recently, resection of the right recurrent laryngeal nerve has been advised for this disabling condition. Initially, the results were encouraging, but recurrences of spasticity have been documented. The current prognosis for this condition is guarded. The strained, creaking, choked vocal attack and the tense, squeezed voice sound appear to be accompanied by extreme tension of the entire phonatory system. Laughing, singing, and whispering are less affected, if at all. See Chapter 24.

D. Vocal Weakness

This term describes a condition of functional weakness of the voice despite a grossly normal vocal organ. It has also been called phonasthenia and is caused primarily by faulty use of the voice. This condition, which usually occurs in emotionally labile people, is accompanied by multiple, subjective complaints including unpleasant sensations around the neck, throat, or larynx. The symptoms typically improve with rest and are worse when the patient is under emotional stress. This type of condition is usually seen in people whose occupation requires much talking, such as teachers, doctors, lawyers, and telephone operators. Indirect laryngoscopic examination may reveal slight reddening of the vocal cord margins and tenderness of the cervical muscles. Therapy involves the removal of any precipitating causes. Speech therapy should be instituted, and psychotherapy may be indicated. See Chapter 24.

VIII. BENIGN TUMORS

A. Vocal Nodules

These lesions occur in children and in adults and are caused by using the voice too loudly and too long. The nodules are seen frequently in boys between 8 and 12 years of age who often yell out of doors. Vocal nodules also occur in inadequately trained singers who try to achieve special effects with their voices in an incorrect manner. Singing in an unnaturally low register is a major factor. The lesions occur at the junction of the anterior third and posterior two-thirds of the true vocal cords. This location is in the midline of the membranous vocal cord because the posterior third of the true vocal cord covers the vocal process of the arytenoid cartilage. The nodules produce hoarseness and give the voice a breathy quality. Speech therapy is indicated in these patients, although it is difficult to ensure that young children yell less. Endoscopic removal is rarely indicated, but it may be helpful in adult patients with hard nodules that are unresponsive to voice therapy.

B. Vocal Polyps

Polyps of the true vocal cord also develop in patients who use their voice too loudly and too long. Similar changes can result from chronic allergic exposure and chronic inhalation of irritants. The polyps interfere with the approximation of the true vocal cords, add mass to the true vocal cords, and cause hoarseness. They also produce a breathy quality to the voice. The patient must discontinue the misuse and abuse of the voice and must institute long-term therapy with a speech pathologist. Voice therapy should precede any surgical intervention, unless one suspects that these polypoid changes may be the result of a neoplasm. Once speech therapy has been undertaken, polyps may be removed by direct laryngoscopy with the use of the operative microscope. Care must be taken to prevent damage to the underlying musculature of the vocal cords. Voice rest is indicated, although it does not have to be absolute. Whispering is discouraged because it tenses the vocal cords; rather, the patient should phonate in a soft, natural tone of voice. Six weeks after the operation, voice therapy should be resumed and continued until maximum benefits are obtained. Surgical excision may be accomplished with the carbon dioxide laser or with microlaryngeal instruments. Smoking should be discouraged because of the risk of recurrence, especially if the underlying irritant is not discontinued. See Chapter 24.

C. Contact Ulcers

Contact ulcers are caused by vocal abuse and occur in the mucosa covering the vocal processes of the arytenoid cartilage in the posterior third of the true vocal cords. Patients with contact ulcers have a sensation of irritation of the larynx and clear their throats frequently. This clearing of the throat brings the vocal process of the arytenoid cartilages immediately and forcefully into contact. Speech therapy is indicated, and the prognosis is favorable. Biopsy may be indicated to reduce the amount of granulation tissue present and to rule out the presence of a malignant lesion. Voice rest must be stressed, and irritants must be removed. See Chapter 24.

D. Juvenile Papillomas

This lesion is the most common benign tumor in children. Historically, papillomas have been divided into juvenile-onset and adult-onset lesions. The adult-onset variety is much less aggressive than the juvenile tumor. Laryngeal papillomas most commonly occur on the true vocal cords, although any site on the larynx may be affected. The cause is unknown, although a viral origin is currently hypothesized. Simple endoscopic removal of these lesions is the most common treatment; however, the carbon dioxide laser is helpful in the management of this disease. Tracheostomy is occasionally indicated, but the procedure may be followed by seeding of the papilloma into the tracheal bronchial tree. Radiation is contraindicated. Many investigational forms of therapy are currently in use, such as vaccines, immunotherapy, cryosurgery, and ultrasound. Interferon may be helpful in the control of this disease.

E. Granular Cell Myoblastoma

Although formerly thought to be of muscular origin, this tumor has been shown by ultrastructural studies to be of neural origin. The tumor should more appropriately be referred to as a granular cell tumor. Symptoms are hoarseness, dysphagia, cough, and, occasionally, pain. The tumor has a 2:1 male predominance and usually occurs in the fourth decade. The majority of these lesions arise from the posterior third of the true vocal cord. The gross appearance is that of a small, nonulcerated sessile or pedunculated mass that ranges in color from white to yellow to gray. The treatment of this lesion is by endoscopic removal because recurrence is unlikely. The tumor itself is usually covered by pseudoepitheliomatous hyperplasia. This lesion must be distinguished from squamous cell carcinoma, which requires more aggressive therapy than granular cell tumor.

F. Chondromas

Chondromas most frequently occur in middle-aged men. The chief presenting symptom is hoarseness secondary to restriction of vocal cords and dyspnea secondary to obstruction. The cricoid cartilage is the site of 75% of the laryngeal chondromas, followed by the thyroid cartilage, epiglottis, and arytenoid cartilages. The treatment, surgical excision, depends on the size and location of the lesion. A thyrotomy may be indicated for tumors of the anterior aspect of the cricoid cartilage, and a lateral, external approach with or without pharyngotomy may be indicated for chondromas of the thyroid or posterior aspect of the cricoid or arytenoid cartilage. Because these lesions are hard, biopsy may be difficult, and distinguishing this tumor from a well-differentiated chondrosarcoma may be challenging.

G. Leukoplakia (Hyperkeratosis)

This term designates a whitish patch surrounded by normal or inflamed mucosa. Hyperkeratosis often develops into invasive carcinoma in the presence of associated cellular atypia. This lesion usually occurs secondary to persistent irritation, and its treatment includes endoscopic removal, careful follow-up, and removal of causative agents, such as smoking and drinking.

H. Pseudoepitheliomatous Hyperplasia

This phenomenon is unique to granular cell tumors. Unfortunately, it may mimic well-differentiated squamous cell carcinoma. These squamous cells show reactive and hyperplastic changes, but give no evidence of malignant change. The nuclei are small and lack mitotic activity. When the differential diagnosis of pseudoepitheliomatous hyperplasia is suggested in a patient with a laryngeal tumor, one must obtain deep biopsies to establish the presence of a granular cell tumor with overlying pseudoepitheliomatous hyperplasia. Once this diagnosis is established, endoscopic removal is usually adequate treatment.

I. Adenomas

Pleomorphic adenomas have been described in the larynx. Portions of the larynx and trachea are rich in mucous glands, and the adenomas arise from these structures. Treatment depends on the size and location of these tumors, although they usually can be removed perorally. Occasionally, thyrotomy is necessary.

J. Chemodectomas

Chemodectomas of the larynx are rare and have been reported under a variety of names including glomus tumor, paraganglioma, and apudoma. These tumors usually involve the aryepiglottic folds and ventricles in the superglottic larynx. Tumors involving the glottic or infraglottic areas are rare. These lesions have a potential for malignant change. Hoarseness is the most common chief complaint, followed by dysphagia, pain, dyspnea, and hemoptysis. Lateral pharyngotomy is occasionally needed for excision; however, laryngofissure and endoscopic removal have also been used. Surgical removal is the treatment of choice.

K. Lipomas

Although lipomas of the larynx are rare, they have been reported in association with generalized or systemic lipomatosis. These tumors occur most frequently in the epiglottis and aryepiglottic folds and grow slowly. The may become large prior to discovery and may obstruct the airway. These tumors appear as submucosal, smooth, yellowish masses. Treatment consists of total excision. Endoscopic removal is often feasible for small lesions, especially if they are pedunculated. Lateral pharyngotomy is usually recommended for submucous tumors.

L. Hemangiomas (Adult)

Biopsy is indicated for the adult laryngeal hemangioma, in contrast to the pediatric lesion. These tumors usually arise on or superior to the vocal cords, and patients have vague, often extended histories of hoarseness and dysphagia. These tumors are most often seen in males. The potential for hemorrhage during biopsy or excision is well documented. Occasionally, small lesions may be removed endoscopically, but lateral pharyngotomy is also successful. Treatment is complete surgical excision.

M. Retention Cysts

These cysts are formed by enlargement of a gland in the mucosal lining of the larynx. The cysts most commonly involve the epiglottis and the entrance of the larynx, although they may occur within the vocal cords. They appear as a smooth, round, yellowish, compressible mass. These cysts may resolve spontaneously, or they may be removed laryngoscopically. Marsupialization of these lesions is also acceptable.

N. Prolapse of the Ventricle

In this disorder, apparently normal mucosal tissue protrudes from the laryngeal ventricle. This condition is frequently seen in patients with chronic laryngitis. The mucosal protrusion occurs because of inflammatory infiltrate and tissue hypertrophy. Hoarseness is the most common presenting symptom, although it may be variable and intermittent. Occasionally, a nonproductive cough is present. The appearance is that of a smooth, pale, or purplish mass protruding from the ventricle. On direct laryngoscopic examination, the mass moves freely and is not attached to the true vocal cord. The mass may sometimes be pushed laterally into the ventricle. Treatment is by laryngoscopic removal with forceps or with the carbon dioxide laser.

O. Laryngoceles

The laryngocele is a dilatation or herniation of the laryngeal ventricle. The respiratory epithelium contains seromucinous glands, and an accumulation of secretion leads to progressive enlargement. Inflammation can also cause rapid enlargement. These lesions usually cause hoarseness and inspiratory stridor, and on physical examination, marked swelling of the false vocal cord in the aryepiglottic fold is noted. Laryngoceles may be internal, external, or both. Internal laryngoceles may be aspirated, incised, drained, or marsupialized. The external and combined varieties usually necessitate an external approach.

IX. MALIGNANT TUMORS

The most common malignant tumor of the larynx is squamous cell carcinoma. Malignant tumors of the minor salivary glands are rare. This section deals exclusively with the treatment of squamous cell carcinoma of the larynx.

A. General Principles

1. **Multiple primary sites** In treating patients with carcinoma of the larynx, one must look for a second primary site. Various reports have quoted the incidence of multiple primary carcinomas of the head and neck to range between 15 and 30%. These multiple primary sites are much more common in patients with a long history of smoking and drinking and in patients with alcoholic liver disease.
2. **Follow-up** Patients must be followed-up for life. They are usually seen monthly for their first year after treatment, bimonthly for the second year, trimonthly for the third year, and so on. Patients should then be examined every 6 months; one should obtain chest films at that time, especially if the patients continue to smoke.
3. **Small lesions** of the larynx are usually curable. All patients who are hoarse for more than 3 weeks should have their vocal cords visualized. X-ray therapy and surgical therapy probably carry equal cure rates for small lesions of the larynx.
4. **Larger lesions** probably need combined therapy. Currently, one hopes that some of the newer chemotherapeutic agents will improve the prognosis in patients with larger lesions of the larynx, especially if these drugs are used in induction fashion.
5. **Therapy** must be individualized. One should take into account life expectancy, personality, mental stability, family situation, and distance between home and treatment site. Recommending six weeks of radiation therapy to a patient who will be unwilling or unable to complete this therapy is inappropriate. Exact location, size of tumor, duration of symptoms, and of course the presence of cervical metastasis must be considered in treatment planning.
6. **Personal care** Patients must not be abandoned even after all reasonable hope of cure has dissipated. They should be seen regularly and comforted and assured that they will not have to die in pain. If the physician who assumes responsibility for

the management of this patient is unable to cure the cancer, he must nonetheless attempt to make the patient's remaining days as comfortable as possible and must not abandon the patient.

B. Partial Laryngeal Resection

1. **Vertical hemilaryngectomy** is usually indicated in patients who have normal vocal cord mobility with less than 30% of involvement of the anterior contralateral true vocal cord. Involvement of the ventricle or subglottic extension of the tumor of greater than 10 mm anteriorly should not be present. In patients who have undergone radiation therapy, one should hesitate to perform this procedure when contralateral vocal cord involvement or greater than 5 mm of anterior subglottic extension is present. Vocal cord fixation is a contraindication to vertical hemilaryngectomy.
2. **Supraglottic laryngectomy** may be performed for lesions of the supraglottic larynx that do not involve the ventricles. Pyriform sinus lesions that do not affect the depths of the pyriform sinus may be treated by supraglottic laryngectomy combined with neck dissection or radiation therapy, as indicated.

C. Specific Sites of Involvement

1. **Carcinoma of the epiglottis** Patients with carcinoma involving the laryngeal surface of the epiglottis not extending to the aryepiglottic fold or the base of the epiglottis are good candidates for supraglottic laryngectomy or radiation therapy.
2. **Carcinoma of the false cords** Small T_1 lesions are treatable by radiation therapy. Larger lesions may be treated by either surgical procedures or combined therapy, and as long as the lesions do not extend into the ventricle, conservation operations of the larynx should be considered.
3. **Carcinoma of the aryepiglottic fold** Radiation therapy should be considered for T_1 lesions. Larger lesions are probably better treated by operation or combined therapy. One of the risks of treating small supraglottic lesions with radiation therapy is that recurrences may not be diagnosed until the chances for performing a conservation operation have been lost.
4. **Carcinoma of the ventricle** is best treated with radiation therapy, or combination therapy for larger lesions.
5. **Carcinoma in situ of the membranous true cords** Vertical hemilaryngectomy has already been discussed and is applicable for small lesions of the membranous true vocal cords. When the diagnosis is carcinoma in situ and not invasive carcinoma, vocal cord biopsies carry a 75% rate of cure. More extensive biopsy procedures, such as vocal cord stripping, should probably be performed when the diagnosis is carcinoma in situ, to

rule out the co-existence of invasive carcinoma. Radiation is initially contraindicated in the treatment of carcinoma in situ, but it is effective against invasive carcinoma.

6. **Transglottic carcinoma** describes a situation in which the tumor crosses the ventricle or involves the larynx superior and inferior to the true vocal cords. This tumor must be treated aggressively because 5-year survival rates are generally quoted at about 50% following total laryngectomy and about 25% following radiation therapy. These lesions probably should be treated with combined therapy.
7. **Carcinoma of the pyriform sinus** has a poor prognosis. These lesions are limited inferiorly by the apex of the pyriform sinus, superiorly by the lateral glossoepiglottic fold, laterally by the thyroid cartilage, and medially by the aryepiglottic fold and arytenoid cartilage. These lesions should be treated with combined radiation and surgical therapy because of their poor prognosis.
8. **Nodal metastasis** Radical neck dissections should be performed in patients with palpable lymph nodes, and elective radical neck dissections are probably indicated for any given tumor with a 30% incidence of occult metastasis. This point is controversial because radiation therapy may be able to cure occult metastasis. Moreover, radical neck dissection may be just as effective once occult metastasis becomes clinically apparent in patients for whom radiation therapy is unsuccessful. Unfortunately, adequate data are not yet available; therefore treatment must be individualized.

24

HOARSENESS AND CARE OF THE PROFESSIONAL VOICE

APRIL E. TUCK

I. GENERAL PRINCIPLES

A. Definition of Functional Voice Disorders

The otolaryngologist is frequently confronted with a patient who has vocal hoarseness. Laryngoscopic evaluation may reveal the presence of a lesion, such as a nodule, polyp, or edema, or it may demonstrate no physical abnormality. The diagnosis is generally the all-encompassing "functional voice disorder." This section explores hoarseness, functional voice disorders, and the professional voice. Neoplastic lesions are not discussed in this chapter, but they must be ruled out in any patient who has been hoarse for more than 3 weeks. See Chapter 23.

B. Definition of Hoarseness

The term hoarseness, generally employed to describe particular acoustic characteristics of a pathologic voice, has become both specific and nebulous. Specifically, the term denotes a vocal quality that draws attention to itself because of its acoustic aberrance. Descriptions of the acoustic characteristics of hoarseness vary, however. Technically, hoarseness is a combination of harshness and breathiness. Despite specific terminology describing the acoustic patterns of a patient's voice, such problems may or may not be indicative of specific lesions.

C. Parameters of Functional Voice Disorders

Functional voice disorder is the common term for the aforementioned problem. The cause can range from a single traumatic incident, such as screaming, to prolonged, habitual misuse of the voice. Trauma to the voice may entail, for example, yelling, excessive loud laughing, or screaming. Habitual abuse includes inappropriate management of the breath stream, strained, tense phonation, detrimental compensatory mechanisms, poor laryngeal valve operation, and incorrect coordination of the respiratory, phonatory, or articulatory systems. Such vocal behavior becomes habitual and may eventually lead to a functional voice disorder. A third possible cause is a psychogenic disorder. These various voice disorders can affect any member of the population, although an individual whose voice is necessary to his vocation is especially at risk.

D. Definition of Professional Voice

The professional voice is owned and operated by a variety of individuals. Loosely described, a person for whom the voice is a major instrument for daily work has a professional voice. This group spans the realm of professions from teacher to businessperson, from lawyer to performer, from politician to cheerleader. Any problem with the voice can create serious difficulties for these individuals. For this reason, the professional speaker who has a functional voice disorder must be evaluated and treated immediately.

II. MEDICAL HISTORY

A crucial key to diagnosis and treatment of the voice disorder is an extensive medical history.

A. Patient's Description of the Problem

Frequently, one can gain much more information than expected by asking patients to describe their own voice problem. Questions should include the following.

1. **How severe is the problem, and does the severity vary?** If so, what changes occur as it varies? Is the voice different under various conditions?
2. **By whom and when was the problem first noticed?** Was the onset sudden or gradual?
3. **Under which circumstances does the problem occur?**

B. Patient's Home and Work Environments

1. **What are the patient's vocal requirements at work and at home?**
2. **Is there much tension at work or at home?** Where does the patient initially feel tension manifest in the body? How does he relax?

3. **What is a typical day for the patient?**
4. **Does anyone in the patient's family have similar problems?**

C. Individual Vocal Use

1. **Has the patient had any formal voice or speech training or therapy?** If so, what type, when, and where?
2. **How often is the patient required to talk or sing?** Is amplification provided? Under what conditions must he perform (large halls, smoke-filled rooms, competing noise)?

D. Home Remedies

It is also crucial to investigate the patient's own voice remedies. Most individuals treat their own voices according to what they think will work or what they have heard will work.

1. **Does the patient take any drugs to aid the voice?**
2. **Does the patient engage in vocal rest?** How does the patient define vocal rest? Whispering? For how long?

E. Personal Habits

Patient's habits often irritate any existing voice problems. Questions should probe the individual's use of alcohol, with or without cigarette or marijuana smoking, the use of prescription or nonprescription drugs, and the amount and type of any exercise taken.

III. SCREENING OF VOICE PROBLEMS

A. Respiratory Function

As alluded to earlier, functional voice problems may arise from a variety of poor respiratory habits. While the patient is seated and quiet, the physician should observe the overall breathing pattern. Good posture and diaphragmatic-abdominal breathing patterns are appropriate. Frequently, however, the otolaryngologist notes a significant thoracic or clavicular component in the breathing pattern, with or without poor posture. One must watch for similar patterns during conversation with the patient. Management of the breath stream can also be noted. One should determine whether the patient wastes air or speaks at residual volumes.

B. Pitch and Loudness Levels

One may perform a cursory evaluation of the patient's pitch and loudness levels simply by listening. One must listen to the patient during conversation, and one must perceive the patient's habitual loudness level, as well as pitch. It is also important to observe the degree to which pitch and loudness levels vary. Often, a correspondence between the two parameters can be found.

C. Rate of Speech and Articulation

One must note any perceptually abnormal articulatory gestures or rate of speech. Such features often contribute to the overall acoustic effects of a dysfunctional voice.

D. Tension

Habitually increased tension levels within the shoulder, laryngeal and neck, or facial regions may create or may aggravate a functional voice disorder.

E. Quality

The most apparent feature of a functional voice disorder is the quality of voice. Throughout the examination, it is imperative to listen critically to the ongoing status of the patient's quality of voice. Parameters include severity, variability, and presence of pitch breaks, glottal fry, periodic aphonia, and fatigue. Note the differences between conversational quality and the sustainment of "ah." The aforementioned screening procedure and the patient's medical history should give the physician a reasonable understanding of the patient's voice profile. This information should allow the physician to make an informed diagnosis.

IV. ETIOLOGIC CONSIDERATIONS

A. Nodules

Unilateral or bilateral vocal fold nodules are a frequent cause of vocal disorder. Generally found on the anterior third of the vocal fold near the commissure, a nodule may range in appearance from a small, pale fluid-filled sac to a larger, calloused, yellowish growth. The usual cause of nodules is vocal abuse or misuse. Research has shown that voice therapy frequently eliminates the need for surgical treatment, especially for patients with early nodules. Further, the recurrence rate for vocal nodules is significant when surgical procedures are performed without pre- or postoperative voice therapy. Because nodules may result from inappropriate behavior, it is necessary to eliminate the specific behavior and to retrain the voice.

B. Polyps

The presence of either sessile or pedunculated polyps cannot always be attributed to misuse or abuse of the voice. Voice therapy alone does not resolve well-developed polyps; however, instruction is useful for development of compensatory strategies.

C. General Abuse or Misuse

Frequently, vocal abuse or misuse is the primary cause of lesions. It can lead to functional disorders that have no overt physical symptoms. Misuse of the vocal mechanism may result from poor breathstream management during phonation, inappropriate pitch and intensity levels, poor laryngeal valving, use of strained vocalizations, or habitual laryngeofacial tension, for example. Individuals who consistently expose themselves to smoky, dusty environments while talking are at risk. Vocal abuse or misuse occurs when the respiratory, phonatory, and articulatory systems are not allowed to function appropriately under proper conditions. The individual who has no specific lesion is often most difficult to treat. A thorough reassessment of negative vocal behavior must be combined with subsequent retraining. See Chapter 23.

D. Edema

The patient with vocal fold edema and resultant hoarseness is often overlooked as a possible voice abuser. Edema may change vocal fold mass and may thus force the patient to engage in inappropriate compensatory vocal maneuvers. See Chapter 23.

E. Psychogenic Disorders

Subsequent to negative historical and physical findings, a physician is often perplexed about the cause of a patient's "hoarseness." In such cases, the possibility of psychogenic variables should be addressed. Frequently, the patient develops "sudden" hoarseness or aphonia with no other physical symptoms. Further gentle probing by the appropriate professional often unearths a history of prolonged, unmanageable stress, acute trauma, or conflict prior to the development of the voice problem. Once the emotional issue is resolved, the patient's voice often returns. Such cases warrant immediate consultation by a speech pathologist and psychologist.

V. TREATMENT

The aforementioned etiologic factors are among the more common. Subsequently, however, the well-informed physician should make the appropriate referral.

A. Referrals

Subsequent to laryngologic evaluation, referral to a certified speech and language pathologist trained in voice disorders should be made for a full assessment of vocal functioning and development of an appropriate treatment protocol. The most effective approach for individuals with functional voice disorders is one developed jointly by the speech and language pathologist and the otolaryngologist. Subsequent referrals to a psychologist, audiologist, allergist, or any other appropriate specialist may be required. Regardless of treatment approaches or referrals, however, the patient with a professional voice must understand and must implement a regimen of vocal hygiene.

B. Vocal Hygiene

All too often, functional voice disorders are precipitated by poor vocal habits. It is crucial that the patient understand the need for proper care and maintenance of the voice. Basic principles of vocal hygiene include the following:

1. **Avoidance of excessive loud laughing, cheering, or screaming.**
2. **Avoidance of strained throat clearing and coughing.**
3. **Avoidance of abrupt glottal attack or straining of voice.**
4. **Avoidance of speaking in noisy places without proper amplification.**
5. **Avoidance of speaking with an upper respiratory infection.**
6. **Reduction of acting, singing, and talking.** During speaking, use of a quiet, breathy voice without whispering.
7. **Use of correct posture when speaking,** without straining the facial and laryngeal musculature.
8. **Avoidance of mouth breathing in cold weather.** If possible, home and work environments should have filtered heat and proper humidity levels.
9. **Maintenance of good health habits.** Exercise that is regular but not too vigorous or noisy. Avoidance of smoke and dust. Monitoring of all medications to ensure that they do not adversely affect the voice.
10. **Avoidance of highly spiced food and substitution of skim milk and ice milk for whole milk and ice cream,** especially several hours prior to any speaking or singing rehearsals or engagements.
11. **If speaking without amplification, sitting in the center of a room,** to avoid having to strain to be heard.
12. **Prevention of potential laryngeal trauma,** by wearing automobile seat belts and shoulder straps.
13. **Curtailment in the use of alcohol, aspirin, depressants, and antihistamines.**
14. **Vocal and general rest.**
15. **Use of sugarless gum and sugarless candy,** to relax the system and to create saliva. Relaxation when vocalizing.
16. **For singers, singing only within one's pitch range.** Avoidance of all extremes of pitch and loudness.
17. **Ingestion of warm liquids,** such as herbal teas and water, regularly to keep the vocal system flushed and relaxed.

V.

HEAD AND NECK

25

FACIAL PAIN, NECK PAIN, AND HEADACHE

WERNER D. CHASIN

I. FACIAL PAIN

The diagnosis of facial pain is based primarily on knowledge both of the anatomic structures in the affected area and of their innervation.

A. Upper Third of Face

Structures to be considered are muscles, arteries, orbital contents and adnexa, paranasal sinuses, nasal cavity, teeth, and nerves.

1. **Frontal sinus** Pain may be due to acute infection, chronic sinusitis, intermittent blockage of the ostium by edematous mucous membrane, blockage of the duct by an osteoma, and, rarely, blockage by tumor.
   a. ***Acute frontal sinusitis*** is usually associated with an upper respiratory tract infection and is characterized by frontal pain that often begins 2 hours after arising from bed. The patient may note tenderness of the walls of the sinus. The nasofrontal duct is often occluded, and no intranasal pus is present. If the sinus is draining, pus will be seen in the anterior half of the middle meatus of the nose. The sinus may be opaque to transillumination. Treatment consists of administration of an oral antibiotic and a topical nasal vasoconstricting drop or spray preparation such as 0.25% phenylephrine (Neo-Synephrine). When the infection is recalcitrant, a nasal culture is taken from the middle meatus, to guide one in the choice of antibiotic. When an infection fails to respond to treatment and a patient de-

velops severe pain, or when swelling of the forehead or upper eyelid develops, it may be necessary to admit the patient to the hospital for intensive treatment with intravenous antibiotics and, probably, for trephination of the sinus. See Chapter 15.

b. ***Chronic frontal sinusitis*** is diagnosed on the basis of a history of recurrent sinusitis with frontal discomfort between episodes of infection. A mucocele or pyocele may erode through one of the walls of the sinus and may produce a mass of the orbital or of the anterior cranial fossa. The diagnosis is made radiographically. Chronic frontal sinusitis does not respond well to medication, and these patients require a surgical procedure. See Chapter 15.

c. ***Frontal osteomas*** may be a cause of facial pain. They are diagnosed by x-ray studies and can be removed surgically.

2. **Migraine,** both classic and common types, may produce frontal pain. The diagnosis is based on a typical history of migraine pain produced during periods of emotional tension and associated with nausea, photophobia, and sometimes scintillating scotoma. Treatment is with ergotamine tartrate, 1 tablet at the first sign of pain and, if necessary, 1 tablet every 30 minutes for a maximum of 6 tablets per episode.

3. **Frontal tension pain** Under ideal circumstances, patients with recurrent frontal muscle pain should undergo psychotherapeutic evaluation and management. For symptomatic relief, a tranquilizer such as chlordiazepoxide (Librium), 10 mg 3 times a day, is helpful.

4. **Supraorbital neuralgia** These severe pains in the distribution of the supraorbital nerve are of unknown origin. They may be treated either with carbamazepine (Tegretol) or by alcohol blockade of the supraorbital nerve. Severe cases require neurorrhaphy.

B. Middle Third of Face

This region includes the portion of the face between the eyebrows and the inferior edge of the nose.

1. **Orbital pain**

a. ***Infections and inflammatory disorders of the adnexa*** include such conditions as blepharitis and conjunctivitis. If evidence of such a disorder is present, the patient should be referred to an ophthalmologist.

b. ***Dacryocystitis*** The patient has pain and swelling just inferior to the medial canthus of the eye. One usually sees purulence in the medial corner of the eye, and epiphora may be present. This condition is best treated with antibiotics, chosen according to culture results, and with the application of warm compresses. Once the infection has subsided, the patency of the nasolacrimal duct and sac should be tested by saline irrigation through the inferior lacrimal punctum.

c. ***Orbital cellulitis and orbital abscess*** usually are complications of frontal or ethmoid sinusitis. The patient has orbital pain, possible swelling of the upper eyelid, and conjunctivitis with limitation of eye movement, in addition to signs of serious illness. The patient requires hospitalization for intensive antibiotic treatment and, possibly, sinus and orbital drainage. The diagnosis can be made accurately by computed tomographic (CT) scanning of the orbit.

d. ***Orbital tumors*** may produce pain as well as displacement of the eye and interference with vision. Such tumors may be primary in the orbit, for example, melanoma or rhabdomyosarcoma may represent extension of a malignant tumor of a paranasal sinus, or they may represent metastases from remote sites. These patients require extensive medical and radiologic evaluation including CT scanning of the orbit and sinuses. Treatment depends on the nature of the tumor.

e. ***Mucocele and mucopyocele*** are benign masses that originate in the frontal ethmoid or, rarely, the sphenoid sinuses with extension into the oribit. When infected (pyocele), they produce pain as well as swelling, displacement of the globe, and limitation of motion of the globe. After evaluation, these patients require surgical removal of the mass and an appropriate sinus operation.

f. ***Pseudotumors*** This inflammatory condition of the orbit mimics a tumor and may be localized to the orbit, or it may be part of a generalized disease such as Wegener's granulomatosis. Treatment is based on a diagnosis of the cause of the tumor; these patients often respond to corticosteroids.

g. ***Glaucoma*** must always be considered as a cause of facial pain in patients over 40 years of age. Intermittent narrow-angle glaucoma is an even likelier diagnosis when vision is altered without restriction of extraocular muscles. Ophthalmologic referral is indicated.

h. ***Iritis*** is usually characterized by steady, boring pain aggravated by light. The pain is usually located in or superior to the eye and is often associated with erythema in the circumcorneal area. Slit-lamp examination is indicated.

i. ***Ophthalmic division tic douloureux*** During the acute phase of this disorder, patients have painful bullous skin eruptions of the eyelids and the skin of the forehead on that side. In some individuals, pain persists when the skin lesions have completely disappeared.

2. **Nasal pain**

a. ***Traumatic and post-traumatic disorders*** When the pain is associated with an acute nasal injury that could include bone or cartilage fracture, treatment consists of reduction of the fracture and administration of analgesics. A septal hematoma, if present, must be aspirated to prevent loss of cartilage. Some individuals continue to have pain in the nasal area even after a fracture has healed. These individuals must be treated with mild analgesics and reassurance that the pain will eventually disappear. In patients expecting financial compensation, this pain can be expected to last until the claim has been settled.

b. ***Cellulitis*** The patient has redness and swelling of the skin of the nose. The condition may be due to an infection associated with an underlying skin disorder of the nose, or it may represent an extension of a furuncle of the nasal vestibule. The condition may be painful, and the patient may be at risk for developing cavernous sinus thrombophlebitis. Such patients should be treated intensively with antibiotics, usually against Staphylococcus aureus, and with hot compresses. They should be advised to report immediately if the infection spreads superiorly in the face or if orbital pain develops. These circumstances are indications for immediate hospitalization and intensive treatment with antibiotics for impending or actual cavernous sinus thrombophlebitis.

c. ***Infected septal hematoma*** occurs either after blunt nasal injury in which a hematoma of the septum becomes infected or after a septal operation in which the retained hematoma becomes infected. These patients require immediate incision and drainage of the septum and hospitalization for intensive antibiotic treatment. They are at risk for collapse of the external nose from dissolution of the septum and for cavernous sinus thrombophlebitis.

d. ***Wegener's granulomatosis*** This autoimmune disorder often begins in the nose and causes nasal stuffiness, crusting, and pain that soon spreads to involve the paranasal sinuses. This condition may be diagnosed by a small biopsy of the nasal mucosa in which the pathologist searches for evidence of granulomatous inflammation with vasculitis. Multiple biopsies may be necessary to obtain diagnostic samples. If the diagnosis of this disorder is made, the patient will require treatment with cyclophosphamide and corticosteroids.

e. ***Intranasal tumors*** Some, usually malignant, tumors produce nasal pain by invasion of sensory nerves in the nose. In all intranasal examinations, the nasal mucosa must be shrunk with a topical vasoconstrictor such as phenylephrine, to enable one to observe the interior of the nose adequately. Tumors may require biopsy, but only when roentgenograms demonstrate that the mass does not represent a herniation from the subarachnoid area, such as an encephalocele or meningocele. Treatment depends on the nature of the tumor.

f. ***Chondritis and relapsing polychondritis*** Patients may develop an infection of the cartilage and perichondrium of the nasal skeleton either postoperatively or from a systemic autoimmune disorder called relapsing polychondritis. The nose becomes red, swollen, and tender overlying the cartilages. If the condition is due to infection, it must be treated intensively with antibiotics, usually those sensitive to Staphylococcus aureus, and with warm compresses. If the condition is caused by relapsing polychondritis, the patient will require glucocorticosteroids in moderate doses.

g. ***Keratoacanthoma*** This skin tumor may clinically and histologically resemble a squamous cell carcinoma, but its behavior is self-limiting. It usually affects elderly Caucasians and appears as a dome-shaped tumor growing within 2 to 3 weeks from a small papule to a nodule 1 to 2 cm in diameter. The lesion usually disappears within 2 to 6 months, but it is frequently removed surgically for diagnostic purposes.

h. ***Malignant tumors of the nasal skin*** Patients may develop pain in the nose from malignant tumors of the external skin or the skin in the vestibule of the nose. The two most common such tumors are basal cell and squamous cell carcinomas. The diagnosis is made by observing the lesion and by performing a biopsy. Treatment is based on the nature of the tumor.

i. ***Septal perforation with crusting*** Occasionally, patients who have developed a septal perforation from trauma or nose picking, as a complication of a septal operation, from the prolonged intranasal use of cocaine, or secondary to Wegener's granulomatosis develop extensive crusting in the walls of the perforation. When these crusts become large and hard, they irritate the nasal mucosa of the septum as well as the middle and inferior turbinates. Treatment consists of removal of the crusts and the application by the patient of a nasal lubricant such as mineral oil or petrolatum if the perforation is accessible. In certain instances, surgical repair of the septal perforation is indicated, although the results of this type of operation are only partially satisfactory.

j. ***Foreign body and rhinolith*** Foreign bodies are most often found in children and in mentally retarded individuals. The foreign object itself may produce pain, or pain may be caused by the infectious reaction that usually develops. Rhinoliths represent the gradual accretion of salts and minerals in the nasal secretions. The rhinolith looks like a foreign body in the nose, but is formed in situ. Foreign bodies and rhinoliths require removal under local or, sometimes, general anesthesia. Packing or a plastic sheet should be placed between the nasal septum and the lateral wall of the nose on the side of the foreign body, to prevent the formation of adhesions, which commonly follow the chronic inflammatory reaction.

k. ***Cutaneous lymphoma of the nose*** This uncommon condition causes a red, painful swelling of the skin of the nose simulating cellulitis. The condition does not respond to antibiotics and warm compresses. Usually, after futile treatment with these measures for a few weeks, the physician suspects a lymphoma of the skin, which can be diagnosed by a small skin biopsy. These patients then require careful total-body evaluation and treatment according to the staging of the lymphoma. If the condition is limited to the nasal and facial skin, it may respond to radiation therapy alone.

l. ***Dacryocystitis*** This infection of the tear sac produces painful swelling lateral to the nose and inferior to the medial canthus of the eye. The condition may be confused with an infected cyst or localized cellulitis of the skin. An associated obstruction of the drainage system is present, with purulence in the corner of the eye and an overflow of tears onto the cheek. The condition requires treatment with antibiotics according to culture results and subsequent examination of the patency of the nasolacrimal duct system, to rule out an underlying or a pre-existing obstruction.

m. ***Nasoalveolar cyst*** is a congenital inclusion cyst in the lateral portion of the premaxilla between the superior alveolus and the pyriform aperture. These cysts occasionally become infected and cause painful swelling of the skin lateral and inferior to the ala of the nose extending into the substance of the upper lip. On intranasal examination, one may see a red swelling in the nasal vestibule or the anterior portion of the inferior meatus. These cysts require drainage either into the nose or into the superior gingivolabial sulcus and eventually require excision by a sublabial approach.

3. **Pain in the cheeks**

a. ***Maxillary sinus infection*** Patients develop infections of the maxillary sinus following upper respiratory tract infections and exacerbations of chronic maxillary sinusitis, from acute occlusion of the maxillary sinus ostium during allergic attacks, and sometimes as the result of apical or periapical maxillary tooth infection, usually premolar, extending into the maxillary sinus. The patient has pain and tenderness of the cheek that is best elicited by pressing on the anterior wall of the maxillary sinus with the index finger slipped underneath the upper lip, to exclude tenderness of the skin and the subcutaneous tissues. The patient may have drainage from the nose, and if this drainage is foul smelling and foul tasting, the focus of infection will be a maxillary tooth (dental antrum infection). Treatment consists of antibiotics given according to the results of nasal culture. If the infection fails to respond after suitable trials of antibiotics, sinus irrigation performed through the inferior meatus of the nose or through the natural ostium of the sinus may be helpful. If one suspects the focus of infection to be a tooth, the appropriate dental x-ray studies should be obtained, and the patient should be referred to a dentist. If the sinus infection does not clear after appropriate dental care, the patient may require a Caldwell-Luc sinus operation. See Chapter 15.

b. ***Maxillary sinus tumors*** Malignant and sometimes benign tumors within the maxillary sinus may produce cheek pain. Clues to the presence of a tumor, rather than an infection, include erosion of one or more of the walls of the sinus as seen on radiographs, swelling or expansion of the superior maxillary alveolus, and numbness and hypesthesia of the skin of the cheek and upper lip. These patients may have intranasal findings, possibly including blood-stained mucoid drainage. The diagnosis is made by biopsy of the tumor intranasally, if possible, or by open biopsy of the maxillary sinus through a Caldwell-Luc approach. Treatment is based on the nature of the tumor.

c. ***Pain of dental origin*** Frequent causes of midfacial pain are such conditions of the maxillary teeth as periapical abscess, gingivitis, and lesions of the maxillary alveolus. The condition may be diagnosed by the appropriate dental radiographs, which are superior to sinus radiographs for this purpose. If a dental problem is found, the patient should be referred to a dentist or an oral surgeon.

d. ***Cluster headaches (Horton's syndrome)*** This form of migraine is characterized by severe midfacial pain in the cheek and orbit associated with ipsilateral nasal stuffiness and clear rhinorrhea and with redness of the ipsilateral eye. The condition may develop alone, or, more typically, it may occur in association with other types of migraine in the same individual. The pain, which is extreme, may occur at any time of the day, but it characteristically awakens the patient in the middle of the night. The cluster headache gets its name from the tendency of the painful episodes to cluster over a period of 1, 2, or 3 weeks; the patient may be free of such attacks for variable periods of time between the clusters. The treatment is similar to that for migraine, although these patients may require referral to a headache specialist. In addition to medications, these patients frequently require psychotherapy.

e. ***Tic douloureux of the maxillary nerve*** is a painful, lightning-like pain in the distribution of one or more branches of the trigeminal nerve. Each episode lasts for only a moment, but the pain is severe. Before the diagnosis is made, irritative lesions such as tumors affecting the trigeminal nerve must be excluded. Treatment consists of carbamazepine (Tegretol) administration. Recently, increasing evidence has suggested that some cases of tic douloureux are due to vascular malformations that irritate the trigeminal ganglion and roots intracranially. In such patients, an appropriate decompression operation has a significant success rate.

f. ***Vascular facial pain*** Some individuals develop constant, aching discomfort in the midface that waxes and wanes in intensity, but is not severe and does not usually disturb sleep. The condition is due to an idiopathic disorder of the arteries of the soft tissues of the face and falls most closely into the category of migrainous diseases. The condition may be diagnosed by palpating the appropriate branches of the external carotid artery in the patient's face and finding them to be tenderer than the corresponding vessels on the asymptomatic side of the face. The vessels in the cheek that are amenable to palpation include the superior labial artery, the facial artery, the external maxillary artery in the notch of the mandible, and the greater palatine artery near the pterygoid hamulus. This condition usually responds to treatment with amitriptyline, 10 mg 3 times a day and 20 mg at night. The disorder is self-limiting and usually occurs during times of emotional stress.

g. ***Post-traumatic pain*** Patients who have had fractures of the maxilla and nasal bones, and some patients who have had dental extractions, may have persistent pain in the cheek. This condition usually abates in a number of weeks or months.

h. ***Myofascial pain*** In a few patients, persistent and puzzling facial pain results from long-term psychogenic contraction of the facial musculature. The condition is analogous to posterior cervical headaches due to continuous contraction of the posterior cervical muscles. The disorder is psychogenic, and the patient may respond to psychotherapy and sedatives or tranquilizers.

i. ***Tumors*** Intracranial and extracranial tumors that irritate the maxillary nerve may produce either constant or tic-like pain of the midface. Such lesions include schwannoma of the trigeminal nerve, meningioma, nasopharyngeal carcinoma, and metastatic tumors to the nerves. The diagnosis is made by appropriate x-ray studies; CT scanning is particularly helpful. Treatment depends on the location and type of tumor.

j. ***Atypical facial pain syndrome*** A number of entities

have been described to explain puzzling types of midfacial pain. These entities include vidian neuralgia, Sluder's syndrome, geniculate neuralgia, and atypical facial pain. It is unlikely that such conditions actually exist, and it is probable that these disorders can be categorized as vascular.

k. ***Septal spurs*** Occasional patients may have severe midfacial pain due to a sharp septal spur that makes contact with the lateral wall of the nose, particularly the inferior or middle nasal turbinate. If the pain can be abolished by anesthetizing the contact area with a topical anesthetic or with an anesthetic injection, then one may consider a septal operation to remove the spur.

C. Lower Third of Face

1. **Dental disorders** Various disorders of the mandibular teeth, gingival alveoli, and mandible may produce pain in the lower portion of the face. These conditions include abscessed and carious teeth, gingivitis, and tumors and cysts of the mandible. The patient should be referred to a dentist or an oral surgeon for management of this condition. See Chapter 18.

2. **Oral cavity carcinoma** Malignant tumors of the oral cavity, especially of the floor of the mouth and tongue, may produce pain of the lower third of the face by involvement by the tumor of the inferior alveolar, lingual, and mandibular nerves. In addition to newly discovered tumors, the physician must also obtain a past history of removal of, or radiation treatment for, malignant tumors of the oral cavity. Such patients may have an occult recurrence of the tumor that produces pain. These conditions must be managed by biopsy of the lesion, appropriate x-ray studies, and treatment according to the characteristics of the tumor.

3. **Intra- and extracranial tumors affecting the mandibular nerve** Benign and malignant tumors that irritate the mandibular division of the trigeminal nerve intracranially, in the infratemporal fossa, or in other portions of the floor of the mouth may produce pain in the lower third of the face. Such tumors may be diagnosed by neurologic evaluation, including a search for hypesthesia in the distribution of the mandibular nerve or branches of the mandibular nerve, as well as CT scanning of the intracranial and extracranial spaces. Management depends on the findings.

4. **Vascular pain** The same type of vascular pain that may produce midfacial pain may also cause pain in the inferior third of the face. The diagnosis may be made by palpating the external maxillary artery as it crosses the notch of the mandible and the inferior labial arteries and searching for tenderness on the involved side. Treatment consists of amitriptyline administration.

5. **Tic douloureux affecting the mandibular division** As with midfacial pain, patients may develop tic douloureux in the distribution of the mandibular nerve. This condition is treated either by carbamazepine (Tegretol) or, if unsuccessful, a neurosurgical procedure.

6. **Tumors of the skin** Malignant tumors, including basal cell and squamous cell carcinomas, of the skin of the face may produce pain locally or by invasion of sensory nerves. The diagnosis is made by clinical examination and biopsy, and treatment depends on the histopathologic characteristics of the lesion.

7. **Post-traumatic pain** Patients may develop pain in the inferior third of the face as a sequel to fractures of the mandible or severe contusions of the soft tissues of this area. This condition is usually self-limiting and is treated with simple analgesics.

D. Temple and Side of Face

1. **Temporomandibular joint disorders** are common causes of pain in the temple and the side of the face. Such dysfunctions include functional or myofascial disorders of the joint and surrounding muscles, true arthritis of the joint, recurrent dislocations of the joint, and cartilaginous disorders of the disc of the joint. These patients frequently complain of otalgia, with radiation of pain to the side of the face. They often have subtle or gross disorders of occlusion or evidence of bruxism. Some of these patients have missing molar and premolar teeth that have not been replaced with dentures. First-aid measures for the treatment of such pain consist of soft diet, avoidance of chewing, and warm applications to the tender joint and periarticular tissues. Long-term measures may include dental rehabilitation, and these patients may require referral to a dentist who has experience in disorders of the temporomandibular joint. Patients with true arthritis of the joint usually have systemic manifestations of arthritis, most often rheumatoid arthritis; treatment is similar to that for systemic arthritis. A patient with acute dislocation may require relocation of the joint; this is performed by pulling inferiorly on the mandible and pushing it posteriorly, so the mandibular condyle slips posterior to the articular eminence of the glenoid fossa. One should determine whether the patient is taking phenothiazines, which sometimes cause dislocations of the joint due to muscular rigidity. Such medications will have to be discontinued or replaced with agents that do not have this type of side effect.

2. **Dental disorders** Patients with disorders of the maxillary or mandibular molar and premolar teeth sometimes have pain in the side of the face. If the diagnosis can be made, then these patients should be referred to a dentist or an oral surgeon.

3. **Vascular pain** The same type of vascular pain that occurs in the midfacial and inferior facial regions can also produce pain in the side of the face when the external maxillary artery and superficial temporal artery are involved. Treatment consists of amitriptyline, 10 mg 3 times a day and 20 mg at night.
4. **Migraine** One of the common distributions of common and classic migraine pain is in the area of the temple and side of the face. These patients usually have a long history of such pain, sometimes associated with nausea, vomiting, scintillating scotoma, and a general malaise. The superficial temporal artery and its branches may be distended, tender, and pulsating. These patients are treated with antimigraine medications such as ergotamine tartrate or amitriptyline.
5. **Temporal arteritis** Patients with this inflammatory disorder of the temporal artery and its branches are usually 60 years old or older. The superficial temporal artery and its branches are painful, firm, tender, and nobby. The erythrocyte sedimentation rate is usually elevated in these patients, and they may have a low fever. The pain is severe and is caused by a specific granulomatous inflammation of the walls of the temporal artery. This disorder must be diagnosed and treated promptly because it may involve other arteries of the external and internal carotid system, sometimes leading to blindness. Treatment usually consists of prednisone administration.
6. **Parotid gland disorders** may produce pain in the side of the face. See Chapter 20.
   a. ***Calculi*** in the duct of the gland are not as common as calculi in the submandibular salivary gland. These ductal calculi obstruct the duct, distend the gland, and cause pain. The condition may be diagnosed by the appropriate radiographs, including lateral and anteroposterior views and an anteroposterior view with the cheek puffed out, to throw Stensen's duct into relief. Occasionally, a parotid sialogram may be required. If a calculus is diagnosed, an attempt may be made to remove it. If the stone is too far posterior in the duct, however, the patient may require an open operation on the parotid gland to remove the gland and the duct with the stone.
   b. ***Infections*** of the parotid gland occur most commonly in children with mumps and in debilitated adults, who are frequently in a postoperative and dehydrated state and who develop staphylococcal parotitis. In this condition, the gland is distended and tender, and the overlying skin is red. Fluctuance may not be felt because of the dense capsule of the parotid gland and because it may have subcompartments that prevent early coalescence of the abscess. This condition is a true emergency and requires intensive antibiotic therapy; it may also require incision and drainage of the parotid gland.

c. ***Sialectasia*** causes recurrent episodes of pain, pressure, and swelling of the parotid gland. In this condition, the ductal system of the parotid gland is ectatic, and as a result, a functional obstruction of the ductal system occurs, with periods of swelling caused by stagnation of parotid secretions. The condition is usually bilateral, although the clinical manifestations may occur on one side only. On physical examination, the parotid gland may be swollen and tender, but the skin is usually not inflamed. When the gland is compressed and Stensen's orifice is visualized, viscid, cloudy saliva is expressed. The patient is usually a healthy individual and is not as ill as a patient with true bacterial parotitis. The treatment for sialectasia of the parotid gland is not clearcut. One should avoid the frequent use of antibiotics because most of the episodes of the illness are self-limiting. The diagnosis can be made with certainty by obtaining a sialogram and looking for dilatation of the ductal system. In severe cases, the patient may require a parotidectomy for relief of symptoms.

d. ***Tumors*** Most tumors of the parotid gland are not painful. When a patient has a painful, noninflammatory swelling of the parotid gland and the physician suspects a tumor, the growth may well be malignant, especially if the patient also has weakness of the facial muscles indicating tumor involvement of the facial nerve. These patients require prompt diagnosis, and treatment consists of a combination of surgical intervention, radiation therapy, and possibly, chemotherapy, depending on the nature of the growth.

7. **Trigeminal and glossopharyngeal neuralgia**

a. ***Trigeminal neuralgia*** causes paroxysms of severe pain in the distribution of one or more of the branches of the trigeminal nerve. The patient usually has no neurologic findings, except some hyperesthesia of the skin after an episode. The condition is either idiopathic or is due to an abnormal vascular loop pressing on the trigeminal ganglion or on the roots of the nerve intracranially. When the patient has positive neurologic findings such as numbness of the skin or weakness of any of the masticatory muscles, another process, such as a tumor, should be suspected. Tumors affecting the trigeminal nerve occasionally also produce tic-like pain, but true trigeminal neuralgia has no positive neurologic findings. Treatment consists of the administration of carbamazepine (Tegretol). If this regimen is unsuccessful, then a surgical procedure of the trigeminal nerve will be indicated.

b. ***Glossopharyngeal neuralgia*** is similar to tic douloureux, except it occurs in the distribution of the glossopharyngeal nerve. These patients experience lightning-like, severe paroxysms of pain starting in the tonsillar area and the base of tongue and radiating into the ipsilateral ear. The pathologic features of this condition are similar to those of tic douloureux, and the disorder is treated in a similar fashion.

8. **Infratemporal fossa tumors** The infratemporal fossa is a deep-seated space inferior to the base of the skull and the pterygoid plates and medial to the zygoma. Patients with tumors that have invaded this space develop symptoms of irritation of the mandibular nerve. Such symptoms include pain in the side of the face, in the ear, and along the mandible. Tumors invading this space include nasopharyngeal carcinomas and carcinomas of the tonsil and retromolar trigone, and these patients should be evaluated carefully because treatment depends on the diagnosis. Infratemporal fossa invasion by tumors accounts for a small proportion of occult pain in the side of the face.

9. **Mandibular disorders** Patients who have tumors, cysts, and other disorders of the mandible such as eosinophilic granuloma may have pain in the side of the face. Diagnosis is made by appropriate radiographs, and these patients require surgical management. See Chapter 18.

10. **Ear conditions** Certain disorders of the ear may produce pain that radiates into the side of the face. The complete differential diagnosis of ear pain is covered in Chapter 6 of this book. Ear conditions that may cause widespread pain in the side of the face include external otitis, neoplasms of the ear canal and middle ear, histiocytosis affecting the temporal bone, and lesions affecting the nervus intermedius such as acoustic neuromas and meningiomas in the posterior cranial fossa. Treatment depends on the diagnosis.

11. **Bell's palsy** Pain is present in some patients with Bell's palsy, usually in and inferior to the mastoid tip and the ear. On occasion, this pain precedes the onset of clinical facial paralysis. If the patient has clinical paralysis, the diagnosis is clear. Otherwise, Bell's palsy should be considered in the differential diagnosis. Severe pain associated with Bell's palsy is sometimes considered a poor prognostic sign for spontaneous recovery of facial function. See Chapter 26.

12. **Masseter space infections** The masseter muscle is enveloped in a tight fascial compartment. As a result of dental infections and, sometimes, after injections of local anesthesia for dental and other types of intraoral surgical procedures, an infection gains entry into the masseter space. This disorder produces intense pain and trismus and, usually, swelling and tenderness of the tissues overlying the masseter muscle. The condition requires treatment with antibiotics and heat applications. Masseter space infection is to be differentiated from

benign hypertrophy of the masseter muscle, which may be either idiopathic or due to long-term clenching of the teeth. Patients with benign hypertrophy have swelling of the masseter muscle, but no signs of inflammation, such as tenderness or pain. See Chapter 28.

13. **Sphenoid sinus disorders** On occasion, disease processes including infections, mucocele, and tumors of the sphenoid sinus produce pain in the side of the face. The diagnosis is made on the basis of the patient's medical history, examination, and radiographs. Treatment is according to the disease process. See Chapter 15.

14. **Post-traumatic pain** Patients who have had injuries to the soft tissues of the side of the face and who have suffered fractures of the zygomatic arch or the side of the skull or mandible may have prolonged post-traumatic pain. Such pain finally subsides, and no specific measures are required other than the administration of analgesics.

15. **Muscular pain** Patients may develop chronic pain in the side of the face and temple as a result of prolonged contraction of the muscles. In most instances, this disorder is a result of chronic anxiety, and these patients demonstrate tenderness of the muscles including the temporal, masseter, and the pterygoid muscles. Treatment consists of psychotherapy by the primary-care physician, possibly supplemented by the administration of muscle-relaxing drugs. Patients with bruxism may require the fitting of a dental retainer to be worn between the teeth. Two specific conditions that may cause severe muscular pain in the side of the face are tetanus and extrapyramidal reaction to phenothiazine drugs.

16. **Parapharyngeal space tumors** Patients with deep-seated tumors in the parapharyngeal space may develop pain in the side of the face as a result of irritation of the branches of the glossopharyngeal and trigeminal nerves by these tumors. Diagnosis is made by careful physical examination and appropriate radiographs especially CT scanning, and treatment is based on the diagnosis.

17. **Intraoral tumors** Tumors that, by their location and extension, are likely to irritate the branches of the glossopharyngeal and trigeminal nerve may produce severe pain in the side of the face. Included are tumors of the tongue and all its portions, retromolar trigone tumors, which often invade the infratemporal fossa, tonsillar fossa carcinomas that invade the glossopharyngeal nerve, oropharyngeal tumors that invade branches of the glossopharyngeal nerve, and nasopharyngeal carcinomas, which may invade both the glossopharyngeal and the trigeminal nerve branches, as well as the infratemporal fossa. Patients with facial pain require careful examination of the head and neck, including examination of the oral cavity, for

occult tumors. Treatment depends on the nature and location of the tumor.

II. NECK PAIN

A. Cervical Spinal Disorders

Patients with a variety of disorders of the cervical spine, including arthritis, injuries such as whiplash trauma, and irritation of cervical nerve roots, may experience pain in the posterior portion and side of the neck. The diagnosis is made by a careful medical history, clinical examination, and radiographs. These patients should be referred to an orthopedist or a neurologist for treatment.

B. Lymphadenitis

Acute and, to a lesser extent, chronic lymphadenitis of the lymph nodes of the neck may produce pain and swelling of the nodes and the surrounding tissues. The source of the infection should be determined, and initial treatment consists of treating the primary focus of infection and the inflamed lymph nodes with the appropriate antibiotics and applications of heat. These patients should be observed periodically; they may require incision and drainage of the lymph nodes if coalescence and breakdown of the infection occurs. In trying to ascertain the source of the infection, the physician should ask the patient questions pertaining to cat scratches and tuberculosis exposure.

C. Postsurgical Pain

Patients who have undergone neck operations may experience prolonged pain in the side of the neck. This pain is usually due to injury to branches of the cervical plexus. Treatment consists of reassurance, if warranted, and the administration of mild analgesics. If a painful neuroma develops, however, these patients may require excision of the lesion.

D. Carotidynia

This idiopathic condition causes the common carotid artery, especially at the bifurcation, to become painful, tender, and distended. It is probably in the same family of disorders as facial pain of vascular origin. These patients often complain of a tender gland in the neck; the gland represents the distended carotid bulb. Patients sometimes hold the head and neck in a rigid position to the side of the painful carotid artery, to avoid stretching the vessel, and they may limit rotation of the neck for the same reason. In some of these patients, not only is the common carotid artery tender, but also the branches of the external carotid artery, such as the external maxillary and superficial temporal arteries. Treatment consists of either aspirin or amitriptyline. Warm applications may be helpful. The condition is most often associated with anxiety or depression.

E. Thyroiditis

Patients with acute autoimmune thyroiditis, as well as those with de Quervain's thyroiditis, develop swelling and tenderness of the thyroid gland and surrounding tissues that cause pain in the anterior and lateral portions of the neck. Once the diagnosis has been made, these patients should be referred to an endocrinologist for treatment. See Chapter 30.

F. Muscular Disorders

Contractions of the neck muscles, as well as post-traumatic irritation of these muscles, may produce pain in the neck. Treatment consists of reassurance, applications of heat, and administration of analgesics.

G. Disorders of the Parotid and Submandibular Salivary Glands

Painful disorders of the submandibular gland include calculus of the duct producing obstruction and distension of the gland, sometimes with secondary infection, infections of the gland unassociated with calculi, and malignant tumors of the gland that invade nerves. In patients with calculi and infections of the gland, swelling and tenderness are present. Treatment consists of the removal of any calculi and the use of antibiotics and warm applications. Tumors should be suspected when the gland is firm and when clear saliva can be milked from the submandibular duct. The majority of tumors of the submandibular salivary gland are malignant. The inferiormost portion of the parotid gland dips into the neck approximately to the level of the hyoid bone, although posterior to it. Painful conditions of this gland, including infection and tumors, may produce pain in the neck. Swelling of the gland is usual, and swelling in the superior portion of the neck that extends as far as the hyoid bone may represent a disease process in the parotid gland. Treatment is based on the diagnosis. See Chapter 20.

H. Branchial Cysts

These cysts represent embryologic remnants in the neck. When the cyst is simply distended without infection, it produces swelling with only slight pressure-related discomfort. These cysts often become infected and cause painful swelling with obvious evidence of infection. It is common for branchial cyst infections to occur for the first time in middle-aged individuals. Sometimes, the diagnosis can be made from the patient's medical history and the physical examination and can be confirmed by ultrasound or CT scanning. The acute infection is managed by incision and drainage and by the use of antibiotics, usually in a hospital. When the infection has subsided, the patient may require an open operation to the neck to resect the cyst.

I. Thyroglossal Cysts

These cysts are usually located at or near the midline of the neck between the base of the tongue and the thyroid gland. These patients have no symptoms as long as the cyst is simply distended with fluid, but because these cysts often become infected, patients can develop painful swelling of the anterior neck from an infected thyroglossal duct cyst. Treatment consists of heat and antibiotics and may require incision and drainage of the cyst. If the cyst is recurrent, then once the infection has subsided, the patient will require an open neck operation for removal of the cyst by the Sistrunk procedure.

J. Temporomandibular Joint Disorders

In some individuals, pain originating from disorders of the temporomandibular joint and periarticular tissues may radiate widely and may extend into the neck, sometimes toward the shoulder. The diagnosis is made by finding tenderness of the tissues around the temporomandibular joint. Initial treatment consists of heat, soft diet, and analgesics. If the problem is recurrent, however, it may require the attention of a dentist or other specialist with expertise in disorders of this joint. See Chapter 18.

K. Pharyngeal Infections and Tumors

Patients with pharyngeal infections such as peritonsillar cellulitis and abscess, retropharyngeal abscess, and paraesophageal abscess due to penetration by a foreign body or as a result of endoscopic examination, and individuals with malignant tumors in these areas may complain of pain in the side of the neck in addition to their throat symptoms. The diagnosis is made by a careful medical history, head and neck examination, and, if required, appropriate radiographs. Patients with infections require hospitalization; treatment includes incision and drainage, administration of appropriate antibiotics, and supportive care. Tumors require biopsy, staging, and appropriate management. See Chapter 28.

L. Foreign Bodies

Patients with foreign bodies in the hypopharynx, pyriform sinus, and esophagus may develop severe pain in the neck and, sometimes, the chest. The diagnosis is made on the basis of a careful medical history, appropriate x-ray studies, and extraction of the foreign body, usually by an endoscopic procedure in the hospital. Foreign bodies in the hypopharynx and pyriform sinus are sometimes removed in the clinic with a mirror or flexible bronchoscope and appropriate curved forceps.

M. Fasciitis of Neck

This rare clinicopathologic entity has been called nodular fasciitis, subcutaneous fibromatosis, pseudosarcomatous fasciitis, proliferative fasciitis, and infiltrative fasciitis. It is an unusual cause of painful swelling in the head and neck and may spontaneously regress. Surgical treatment of this condition is probably not necessary (J. Laryngol. Otol., *97*:973, 1983).

N. Grisel's Syndrome

This condition represents a subluxation of the atlantoaxial joint of the cervical vertebrae. These patients have pain and swelling in the superior portion of the neck and a tendency to cock the neck away from the affected side. The condition may be a sequel of severe pharyngitis, of adenoidectomy, or of severe upper respiratory tract infections. The swelling of the neck represents the prominence of the subluxated vertebra and should not be confused with an inflamed or infected cervical lymph node. Treatment consists of hot applications and analgesics. One may require the assistance of an orthopedist, who may prescribe a neck collar or even traction for the neck.

O. Laryngopyocele

When a laryngocele becomes infected, it is called a laryngopyocele. Patients with this condition develop painful and tender swelling in the anterolateral portion of the neck in the thyrohyoid membrane area or, sometimes, laterally in the anterior triangle of the neck. One usually notes hoarseness and, possibly, respiratory obstruction. Laryngoscopic examination reveals fullness of the false vocal cord and the supraglottic structures on the side of the lesion. The condition should not be confused with infection of a lymph node in the neck. Treatment consists of the administration of antibiotics and hot applications, and these patients may require hospitalization if the laryngeal airway is at risk. When the infection has subsided, these patients require an operation to remove the laryngocele.

P. Post-traumatic Pain

Patients who have suffered fractures of the hyoid bone and the laryngeal cartilages may have prolonged post-traumatic pain of the neck. If no need exists to reduce the fracture because of proper alignment of these structures, these patients should be treated with simple warm applications and analgesics. In some individuals, post-traumatic pain persists for many months.

Q. Thoracic Outlet Syndrome

Pain resulting from abnormalities of the thoracic outlet is usually felt in and around the shoulder in the supraclavicular region or between the shoulders. It is associated with tenderness of the structures superior to the clavicle. Subclavian artery aneurysms, tumors, or cervical ribs may be the cause and should be appropriately treated.

R. Ludwig's Angina

This serious infection of the floor of the mouth extends to the tissues in the submental triangles of the neck. These seriously ill patients have tender, brawny swelling of the tissues of the superoanterior neck and edema of the floor of the mouth with frequent elevation of the tongue. These patients require emergency admission to the hospital and treatment with intensive antibiotics and, possibly, incision and drainge of the abscess. Although the infection may be idiopathic, it is more often caused by dental infections or as a complication of intraoral, including dental, surgical procedures. See Chapter 28.

S. Lingual Abscess

This unusual infection occurs within the substance of the tongue. It produces severe pain in the mouth and tongue, sometimes radiating to the neck. Patients with a lingual abscess require admission to the hospital, intensive treatment with antibiotics, and possibly, incision and drainage of the abscess. These patients are at risk for airway obstruction.

III. HEADACHE

A. Tension Headache

This common type of headache is probably due to a combination of prolonged muscular contraction and irritation of the extracranial arteries of the scalp and neck. These headaches may be intermittent, associated with times of real or imagined stress, or they may be almost continuous. The headache is most typically located in the posterior portion of the neck and occipital area, but it may spread to involve the entire head. The patient may have a history of specific or nonspecific anxiety. The muscles and tissues of the scalp may be tender. Optimal treatment consists of psychotherapy; symptomatic treatment involves the judicious use of mild sedatives, tranquilizers, or combination drugs, such as Fiorinal, which contain a barbiturate as well as a mild analgesic.

B. Migraine Headache

Although the classic migraine is a unilateral headache, the headache may be generalized. These patients usually have a long history of recurrent, sick headaches associated with a general feeling of illness and sometimes nausea to the point of vomiting. Moreover, the patient usually has a family history of similar types of headaches. Objective findings may be absent, or the patient may note tenderness of some of the major branches of the carotid system. Treatment consists of ergotamine tartrate or amitriptyline. Psychotherapy is also useful.

C. Headache and Systemic Disorders

Many systemic disorders, such as hypertension, renal diseases, and endocrinopathies, are associated with headaches. The diagnosis is made by taking a thorough medical history and performing a physical examination of the patient. One should treat the underlying disorder.

D. Post-traumatic Headache

Headaches commonly occur after injuries to the skull and intracranial structures. Such pain may persist for many weeks or months and somtimes lasts indefinitely. The diagnosis is made by taking a careful medical history and performing a thorough examination, to rule out intracranial disorders and other causes of headaches. Treatment consists of reassurance and analgesics with periodic reexamination of the patient.

E. Cervical Spinal Disorders

Posterior and vertex headaches are often associated with disorders of the cervical spine. Such disorders include fractures, arthritis, degenerative disorders, and intervertebral disc problems of the cervical spine. The diagnosis is made by carefully taking the patient's medical history and by the physical examination, aided by appropriate radiographs. The headaches may be alleviated by managing the cervical spinal disorder.

F. Occipital Neuralgia

Patients may experience unilateral or bilateral severe pain in the occiput that may radiate over the top of the scalp on the same side. On physical examination, the physician may find spot tenderness of the greater occipital nerve as it crosses the posterior nuchal line. Some of these patients have ear complaints and believe that the occipital pain is due to an infection or other disorder of the ear. The diagnosis may be confirmed by blocking the nerve with an injection of lidocaine (Xylocaine). Treatment may consist of a trial regimen of carbamazepine (Tegretol). If this treatment is unsuccessful, the patient may require an alcohol blockade of the greater occipital nerve or a neurosurgical avulsion of this nerve. Occipital neuralgia may also be due to a disorder of the cervical spine.

G. Compensation Neurosis Headache

In certain individuals, headaches appear to persist after injuries to the skull and cervical spine. A careful medical history discloses that these patients are awaiting compensation for the injury. In such instances, treatment is not successful until the legal aspects of the case have been settled.

H. Intracranial Disorders

The physician evaluating a patient with headaches must not minimize the importance of this symptom. Headaches may be caused by serious organic disorders of the brain, meninges, and other intracranial structures. Examples of such disorders include cerebral edema, encephalitis, intracranial tumors including vascular malformations, hydrocephalus, meningitis and meningismus, intracranial abscess (epidural, subdural, or cerebral), hematoma of the brain and submeningeal spaces, osteomyelitis of the skull due to injuries or spread from sinus and ear infections, metastatic tumors to the skull or intracranial spaces, and a variety of bone disorders involving the skull such as Paget's disease of bone. The diagnosis is made on the basis of a careful medical history and complete physical and neurologic examination of the patient. An accurate diagnosis requires appropriate laboratory tests, especially x-ray studies, with CT scanning. The treatment of headaches due to intracranial processes is directed at the underlying disorder.

I. Temporal Arteritis

This disorder affects the extracranial and, sometimes, the intracranial branches of the carotid artery and occurs in individuals aged 60 years and over. It is a granulomatous inflammation of these vessels. Classic temporal arteritis causes the temporal artery to become tender, firm, swollen, and pulsating. These patients are ill, with a low-grade fever and an elevated erythrocyte sedimentation rate. They are at risk for developing arterial obstruction not only of the extracranial vessels, but also of the intracranial vessels, including the retinal artery, the obstruction of which results in blindness. The diagnosis must be made promptly on clinical grounds and confirmed by a biopsy of the superficial temporal artery. These patients require immediate treatment with corticosteroids, to prevent serious and irreversible complications.

26

DISORDERS OF THE FACIAL NERVE

ROGER L. CRUMLEY

I. ACUTE IDIOPATHIC FACIAL PARALYSIS (BELL'S PALSY)

A. General Considerations

Bell's palsy is the most common affliction of the facial nerve. Ideally, the diagnosis is made only by excluding all other causes of facial paralysis. In actual practice, this procedure is not cost effective, and the diagnosis is generally made if the palsy is of acute onset, if it has a duration of less than 3 months, and if it is unassociated with auditory, vestibular, or other neurologic phenomena. The clinician must, however, remain cognizant of the host of other disorders that produce facial paralysis (Table 26–1).

B. Diagnostic Evaluation

1. **Physical examination** must be meticulous to identify patients with incomplete paralysis; such patients need no treatment as long as the paralysis remains incomplete. Movement in any of the muscles of facial expression renders the paralysis incomplete. The inferior half of the orbicularis oculi muscle is the best place to look for fasciculation. Sometimes, the platysma is the only muscle with movement in a patient with incomplete paralysis. Relaxation of the levator palpebrae superioris muscle (oculomotor nerve) may be mistaken for orbicularis oculi contraction. Any such question can be resolved by examining eyelid closure when the patient is in the recumbent position, to prevent gravity from closing the eyelid. If complete paralysis is present, laboratory tests should be done.

TABLE 26–1

Causes of Sudden Facial Paralysis
Autoimmune disorders
Guillain-Barré syndrome
Demyelinating disease
Cerebrovascular accident
Granulomas
Sarcoidosis
Wegener's granulomatosis
Infections
Herpes zoster
Infectious mononucleosis
Leprosy
Meningitis (acute, tuberculous)
Otitis media
Poliomyelitis
Syphilis
Varicella
Rubella
Mumps
Neoplastic disorders
Acoustic neuroma
Facial nerve neuroma
Leukemia
Metastatic tumor
Parotid tumor
Pontine tumor
Skin cancer
Toxic and metabolic disorders
Diabetes
Uremia
Trauma
Facial laceration
Surgical complication
Temporal bone fracture
Vasculitis
Polyarteritis
Melkersson's syndrome

(Adapted from Otolaryngol. Clin. North Am., 7:358, 1974.)

2. Prognostic tests

a. ***Nerve excitability*** (square wave test, electrical stimulability) is tested using the Hilger or other electric nerve stimulator. When muscle contraction is elicited after 72 hours from the onset of the paralysis, the facial nerve fibers to that muscle are in a state of neurapraxia (first-degree injury). This finding means that the paralysis is potentially reversible. The stimulus should be delivered at near-pain threshold, or 10 ma on the Hilger nerve stimulator. The proximal trunk and all 5 peripheral branches should be tested, but in general, the buccal and zygomatic branches provide the best evidence of nerve excitability. This test has pitfalls, however. First, the test is meaningless in the first 3 days of paralysis. Second, at the levels of stimulus used (9 to 10 ma), masseter muscle contraction (trigeminal innervation) may be elicited. The unwary examiner may confuse this finding with facial muscle contraction. Patients with a stimulable nerve have a major portion of the nerve's fibers intact through the site of injury; a favorable prognosis is implied. In patients with a nonstimulable nerve, wallerian degeneration of most or all of the nerve's fibers has occurred; recovery will most probably be incomplete and characterized by spasms and synkinesis. If the nerve is stimulable, the test should be repeated daily until the paralysis resolves or becomes incomplete or until the excitability is lost.

b. ***Electromyography*** (EMG) can give helpful information at any time during the paralysis. Like the excitability test, EMG is unnecessary and excessive in patients with incomplete paralysis. If voluntary muscle action potentials can be elicited, partial innervation will still be present. When 14 days have elapsed, spontaneous denervation (fibrillation) potentials mean that degeneration has taken place. Later, between 3 weeks and 3 months, polyphasic potentials seen during attempts at voluntary movements herald the return of clinically evident movement.

c. ***Salivary flow*** is measured on both sides by placing a small or medium catheter (IntraCath) into Wharton's duct. In 5 minutes of collection, a volume on the paralyzed side of up to 25% of that on the normal side confirms the presence of neural degeneration. Because this test is tedious to perform, it is used ony when the foregoing tests show conflicting results.

3. **Topographic tests** The following tests enable the clinician to determine the site of neural injury within the nerve's bony fallopian canal:

   a. ***Salivary flow test,*** discussed previously, determines chorda tympani nerve function. If the involved side's volume is less than 25% of the volume of the normal side, then the site of the lesion will be proximal to the exit of the chorda in the lower mastoid segment.

   b. ***Acoustic reflex (stapedius muscle) test*** The absence of this reflex shows that the lesion is located proximal to the stapedius muscle, in the horizontal (tympanic) geniculate or labyrinthine segment.

   c. ***Schirmer's test*** compares lacrimal function in both eyes and hence measures the integrity of the greater petrosal nerve. Identical bands of filter paper are placed in each conjunctival sac. If the ipsilateral eye tears less than 40%

of normal, then the site of the lesion will be proximal to the geniculate ganglion area, that is, the labyrinthine segment.

4. **Other diagnostic tests** are indicated only in patients with complete paralysis.
   a. ***Temporal bone polytomograms or CT scans*** should be ordered to rule out the existence of a facial neuroma, an acoustic neuroma, or a congenital cholesteatoma.
   b. ***Complete blood count.***
   c. ***Cerebrospinal fluid studies*** are indicated if one suspects an infectious cause, such as meningitis or Guillain-Barré syndrome.
   d. ***Parotid sialography*** should be performed if any suspicion of a parotid mass exists. Adenoid cystic carcinoma may paralyze the facial nerve before becoming clinically apparent in the parotid gland.
   e. ***Posterior fossa myelography,*** glucose tolerance tests, and chest roentgenograms may help to exclude other causes of facial paralysis, but such tests are not ordered routinely.

C. Management

The two most common methods of treatment, corticosteroid administration and surgical intervention, remain controversial. The following protocol has been formulated to prevent overtreatment of patients with incomplete paralyses and to ensure that those with severe paralyses receive the attention they deserve.

1. **Incomplete paralysis** If the patient can move any portion of the muscles of facial expression on the involved side, no treatment will be necessary. The patient should be instructed to avoid cold and to call the physician's office daily regarding facial movement. Unreliable patients should be seen on a daily basis until the paresis clears or until it becomes a complete paralysis.

2. **Complete paralysis** These patients should be treated with prednisone, 60 mg orally each day for 10 days. If a patient does not respond to prednisone, surgical decompression of the nerve may be indicated. This procedure has been beneficial to a few patients with Bell's palsy. All patients with complete facial paralysis must be advised that the ipsilateral eye is in danger of desiccation. Patients should also be told that they have not suffered a "stroke" and that 80% of patients with this condition recover. The return to normal is usually noted in about 3 weeks, but it may take as long as 3 months. If facial nerve function does not return within 3 months, one must suspect another cause of the paralysis.

II. NEONATAL FACIAL PARALYSIS

A. General Considerations

The otolaryngologist must be able to distinguish between congenital facial paralysis or weakness and facial nerve injury from birth trauma. Evidence of birth injury should be sought; forceps delivery, unusual presentation, mastoid hematoma or contusion, forceps indentation over the mandibular angle, or unusual facial edema suggest the possibility. Facial skeletal asymmetry is seen in the presence of hemifacial microsomia. The presence of other congenital anomalies, such as abducens paralysis in Möbius syndrome, supports the diagnosis of a congenital lesion.

B. Diagnostic Tests

Facial nerve injury from birth trauma almost always involves the mastoid or parotid portions of the nerve. It is rare in infants delivered without forceps. The nerve excitability test shows the nerve to be normally stimulable. As in Bell's palsy, excitability testing is unnecessary and excessive in those with partial paralyses. The absence of nerve excitability in the first 3 days of life indicates that the nerve was abnormal or absent prior to birth. In these patients, EMG and facial muscle biopsy should be performed to confirm the diagnosis. In infants with no facial muscle, EMG electrodes fail to elicit any action potentials. Fibrillation potentials are seen in patients with birth injury paralysis with severe neural damage, but not until 14 days have elapsed. If, after excitability and EMG testing, questions still persist about the cause of the infant's paralysis, muscle biopsy of the orbicularis oculi or of the zygomaticus major muscle will determine whether muscle is present.

C. Treatment

In almost all instances of birth injury paralysis, lesions are due to contusion or stretching of the nerve. Complete return of function is expected. If the nerve excitability is absent on the fourth day, however, the nerve should be explored carefully in the area of the stylomastoid foramen. If nerve excitability is retained, but paralysis or paresis persists, a careful exploration of the nerve should be undertaken when the patient is a month old. If the physical examination, nerve excitability tests, EMG, and muscle biopsy all indicate the absence of facial muscle, treatment should be deferred for 1 to 3 years. Muscle or nerve transfers may be used to provide facial reanimation.

III. TRAUMA

A. Intratemporal Injuries

1. **Temporal bone fractures** are usually longitudinal relative to the axis of the temporal bone's petrous ridge. These fractures usually result in a torn tympanic membrane, bloody otorrhea, Battle's sign, and conductive hearing loss. Facial paralysis,

when present, is most often delayed and incomplete. These patients should be followed in the same manner as those with Bell's palsy. Only if the paralysis becomes complete is nerve excitability testing necessary. When nerve excitability is retained, the nerves recover. If nerve excitability is lost or if the return of function reaches a plateau, exploration should be done following topographic site-of-lesion testing. When the paralysis is immediate, daily nerve excitability testing determines appropriate candidates for exploration and decompression procedures. Patients with immediate paralyses who retain electrical stimulability usually recover with minimal sequelae. Those who lose nerve excitability should undergo nerve exploration and decompression 3 weeks after the injury. This time interval allows the neuronal cell bodies in the pontine facial nucleus to prepare for regeneration. This transformation is greatest at 3 weeks (J. Neurosurg., *30*:270, 1969). In traumatic facial paralysis following temporal bone fracture, site-of-lesion testing should be done to determine the region of injury. In most of these patients, the site of injury is at or near the geniculate ganglion, but exploration and decompression of the nerve should be performed throughout the entire temporal bone to the stylomastoid foramen, to avoid overlooking a second neural injury. See Chapter 3.

2. **Surgical injuries** The old dictum, "never allow the sun to set on a surgical facial paralysis," still applies. Any postoperative facial paralysis means that the nerve was seriously injured, anesthetized with local anesthetics, or rendered incapable of neural transmission by packing. This concept applies for all operations involving the middle ear or mastoid portions of the facial nerve. If local anesthetics were used, at least 6 hours from the last intraoperative application of these agents should pass before the wound is re-explored. This interval allows for absorption and resolution of such local-anesthetic paralysis. When surgical paralysis persists, all packing should be removed from the middle ear or mastoid cavity. If this procedure does not resolve the paresis, then the wound must be re-explored in the operating room. The nerve should be identified at a proximal or distal site and traced toward the injury. In the event of mastoid nerve exposure, it may be helpful to identify the tympanic segment of the nerve between the cochleariform process and the stapedial segment and to trace it distally. When the site of injury is found, the nerve should be fully decompressed, proximally and distally. Absorbable gelatin sponge (Gelfoam) pledgets may be placed against the nerve, but no packing should be used. If the patient is seen at the request of the surgeon who performed the prior otologic operation, polytomographic studies of the fallopian canal should be done to identify the site of injury. If several days or weeks have elapsed since the operation, the surgeon should be prepared

to perform nerve grafting at the time of re-exploration. Patients seen for facial paralysis following labyrinthine segment explorations or internal auditory canal procedures should be treated similarly unless the original surgeon believes that the proximal nerve was damaged or avulsed from the brain stem. In such an instance, hypoglossal-facial nerve anastomosis is advised.

B. Extratemporal Injuries

1. **Lacerations** Two world wars and hundreds of surgical repairs of the facial nerve have shown that a 3-week delay is unnecessary in most extratemporal injuries, including lacerations such as stab wounds. All 5 branches of the nerve should be tested in the emergency room or physician's office. The severed branch or branches may be predicted by the anatomic features of the wound's surface. The superior division of the facial nerve passes from a point 1 cm anterior to the tragus to the lateral end of the eyebrow. The buccal branch pursues a course parallel to that of Stensen's duct. The inferior division passes along a line from 1 cm anterior to the tragus to a point over the mandibular angle. The use of tiny skin hooks in the emergency room allows the examiner to identify the lacerated branches. All patients with lacerations of the parotid area should undergo probing of Stensen's duct, to verify and to treat such injuries prior to neurorrhaphy. These wounds should be explored immediately. If other injuries, prior ingestion of a meal, or intoxication require a delay, it is equally efficacious to perform such exploration the following day. Under no circumstances should more than 2 days be allowed to elapse before repair is performed; the distal branches will become nonstimulable by the nerve stimulator and may thereby be impossible to identify. Facial nerve lacerations medial (distal) to a line drawn between the lateral canthus of the eye and the lateral commissure of the mouth need not be repaired because distal regeneration will be satisfactory without the aid of surgical repair. All other lacerations of the extratemporal facial nerve, however, should be repaired with 10–0 monofilament nylon sutures and the operating microscope.

2. **Gunshot wounds and avulsion injuries** Facial nerve injuries secondary to gunshot wounds require steps additional to those mentioned for clean lacerations. Standard mastoid roentgenograms or polytomograms are essential to rule out injury of the mastoid portion of the nerve. Military rifle, close-range shotgun, or large-bore revolver injuries may cause intraneural damage to axons without apparent sheath disruption. Initial treatment should consist of exploration and debridement only. Immediate nerve grafting should not be done until the wound has cleansed itself and can be considered sterile once again.

For this reason, the 3-week rule is instituted for these injuries. At the time of initial exploration and debridement, the nerve may appear intact on inspection, even under a surgical microscope. Evidence of severe intraneural disruption, however, comes from clinical experience with such injuries and the demonstration of severe synkinesis in such patients. Nerve grafting, when necessary, should be performed 3 weeks after the injury. The greater auricular nerve may be used for such repairs if it was not involved at the time of the initial injury. The sural nerve from the lateral aspect of the lower extremity is an excellent alternative. It offers the advantage of long length and use of several segments as "cable" grafts between small branches.

IV. TUMORS

A. Facial Neuroma

This schwannoma may involve the facial nerve anywhere from the internal auditory canal to the stylomastoid foramen. These benign tumors often initially cause spasms and twitchings of the nerve in the distribution in one branch and then progress to a more complete facial spasm and, eventually, to total paralysis. Polytomograms or CT scans usually identify the location of tumor involvement because the fallopian canal is widened at that point. Removal of tumor and preservation of the nerve continuity are not possible in these patients, despite the presence of clinical nerve function. The entire nerve and tumor segment must be removed, and reconstruction by a "cable" graft of greater auricular or sural nerve must be performed.

B. Parotid Tumors

When associated with facial weakness or paralysis, such tumors are presumed to be malignant. The most effective control of such malignant tumors, including adenoid cystic carcinoma, squamous cell carcinoma, high-grade mucoepidermoid tumors, and malignant mixed tumors (see Chap. 20), involves radical parotidectomy with facial nerve sacrifice and grafting, followed by postoperative radiation therapy. The particular propensity of adenoid cystic carcinoma to invade the facial nerve or the perineural lymphatic vessels requires that intraoperative frozen sections or slices of the nerve be used to determine the adequacy of resection margins of the nerve itself.

V. ADJUNCTIVE MEASURES

In all forms of facial paralysis involving the ocular (zygomatic) branch of the facial nerve, the otolaryngologist must assume responsibility for the care of the eye. Loss of eyelid closure leaves the cornea unprotected and prone to drying and, ultimately, to ulceration. Lateral tarsorrhaphy is the best treatment in this situation because it allows the patient to see during the weeks or months necessary for resolution of the paralysis. For short-term eye protection, one may tape the eyelids or apply a central suture for apposition of the upper and lower lids. The use of plastic wrap and other similar occlusive material may abrade the cornea and are mentioned only to be condemned.

27

CLEFT LIP AND PALATE

CHARLES F. KOOPMANN, JR. AND
CHARLES J. KRAUSE

As the surgical specialty of otolaryngology and maxillofacial reconstructive surgery continues to advance, the practitioner-in-training will become ever more closely involved in the evaluation, counseling, and therapy of patients with craniofacial anomalies. Patients with clefts of the lip and palate have facial, oral, speech, and hearing problems. Over 250,000 persons in the United States have a cleft of the lip or palate or both. Because the parents of these patients frequently receive conflicting recommendations and because of the severe emotional stress placed on the family by the birth of a child with a craniofacial defect, the practitioner should be a source of emotional support and knowledgeable, consistent advice. The counseling physician must understand the repair of the cleft lip or palate and must be able to evaluate and appreciate associated problems related to the ears, dentition, and speech.

I. GENETIC CONSIDERATIONS

A. Etiologic Agents

In laboratory animals, cleft palates may be induced in numerous ways. Vitamin deficiency has produced cleft lip and palate in some swine models. In rats, posterior palatal clefts have been produced in 15% of animals deficient in riboflavin. Injection of large doses of corticosteroids (cortisone) results in cleft palates in the A-JAX mouse strains. Large doses of meclizine have produced cleft palates in rats. It is difficult to apply the results of these experimental models to the human embryo. In general, investigators have failed to establish a conclusive causal relationship between specific drug ingestion and cleft lips and palates in humans. Instead, most such evidence consists of isolated case reports.

B. Associated Abnormalities

A cleft of the palate is associated with other abnormalities 30 times more frequently than those associated malformations occur in the general population. These abnormalities are most commonly deformities of the ears and extremities and umbilical hernia. The association of cleft lip and palate with abnormalities in other organs has an incidence of 10 to 25%. These associated abnormalities include deformities of the fingers and toes, congenital heart disease, and mental retardation. In general, isolated cleft palates are more frequently associated with other anomalies than are isolated cleft lip and palate.

C. Sex Variations

Females are more likely to have isolated clefts of the palate than are males. Males more frequently have a combined cleft lip and palate than do females.

D. Laterality of Clefts

The occurrence of unilateral cleft lip and palate is more frequent on the left side. When a cleft palate is associated with a cleft lip, it is most likely associated with a bilateral, rather than a unilateral, cleft lip.

E. Racial Incidence

In the United States, the incidence among Blacks is 0.21 to 0.41 per 1000 live births, whereas among Caucasians, it is 0.77 to 1.40 and among Orientals, the incidence is 1.10 to 2.13 per 1000 live births.

F. Genetic Counseling

Cleft lip and palate is a multifactorial inheritance. It is affected by both genetic and exogenous factors. The risk varies from one family to another, depending on the number of patients in the family tree with cleft palate. Moreover, it matters whether the affected relatives are first-degree relatives, such as grandparents, aunts, uncles, nieces, or nephews, or third-degree relatives, such as first cousins. In general, if both parents are normal and if one sibling is affected, then the incidence of cleft lip with or without cleft palate is 4%, and that of cleft palate alone is 3 to 3.5%. The risk increases up to 50% if both parents and 2 of 2 siblings are affected.

II. CLEFT LIP

A. Timing of Repair

Some surgeons repair the cleft in the first 2 to 3 days of the patient's life. Certainly, this method is technically feasible and allows the parents to take home a more normal-appearing infant. At this time, however, the lip is poorly developed, and the vermilion border is not as distinct as it may be later in life. A more conventional time for repair is approximately 10 weeks of age, when the patient has a hemoglobin count of at least 10 g and weighs approximately 10 pounds (the rule of 10). Operation at this time has the advantages of an increased lip size, a more distinct vermilion border, and a more stable, well-developed infant.

B. Preoperative Maxillary Orthopedics

Preoperative maxillary orthopedics are designed to improve the alignment of the maxillary segment and, one hopes, to narrow the cleft deformity. Considerable debate currently exists on the effect of preoperative orthopedics on facial growth. To date, evidence suggesting that preoperative orthopedic treatment favorably influences long-term facial development is not conclusive. Most likely, the changes brought about are minor, although the technique may improve segment alignment to some extent and may facilitate lip repair. Moreover, by improving alignment, the degree of surgical undermining required may be reduced, and the effects on long-term facial growth may thereby be beneficial.

C. Lip Adhesions

1. **Purpose** In patients with wide cleft of the lip, a surgically induced lip adhesion may have an effect similar to that achieved by preoperative maxillary orthopedics. The role of the lip adhesion is to mold the underlying segments and to bring them into better alignment, to facilitate definitive lip repair.
2. **Advantages and disadvantages** Lip adhesions may be performed on the infant under local anesthesia with sedation and restraints. The disadvantage of a lip adhesion is that it may gradually become dehiscent or may create a scar that may later interfere with the definitive lip repair. If the adhesion is carefully designed, however, such scarring can be minimized. Although the inclusion of a lip adhesion in the management of such a patient does add another operation, in selected individuals with wide clefts, the benefits of improved alignment outweigh the disadvantages of the procedure.

D. Unilateral Cleft Lip

1. **Minimal cleft lip (notched vermilion border)** Some surgeons use the straight-line repair (so called Rose-Thompson operation) in patients with this entity. Because of the increased risk of postoperative scar contracture resulting in a recurrence of the notch, however, a Z-plasty may be performed. The authors prefer a Millard or a Bardach repair over a Rose-Thompson procedure.
2. **Partial or complete cleft lip** For patients with more extensive

clefts, the triangular flap or the rotation advancement repair of Millard is recommended.

E. Bilateral Cleft Lips

1. **Clinical features** The bilateral cleft lip may be either asymmetric or symmetric and may vary in degree from a minimal cleft on one side with a wide complete cleft on the other, to bilateral, severe, complete clefts. In general, as the extent of the cleft increases, the deficiencies of tissue and the resultant deformities, both of the reconstructed lip and of the alae and columella of the nose, also increase.

2. **Objectives of treatment**
   a. ***Preservation*** of the vermilion border of the prolabium.
   b. ***Augmentation*** of the vermilion border of the prolabium with muscle flaps from the lateral lip segments.
   c. ***Prevention*** of maxillary alveolar collapse.
   d. ***Repositioning*** of the protruded premaxilla.
   e. ***Reconstruction*** of Cupid's bow with the prolabial tissue.
   f. ***Symmetric alignment*** of the nasal alae.

3. **Timing of repair** in patients with bilateral cleft lips depends on the severity of the defect and on the necessity or availability of dental assistance in supplying presurgical orthopedic treatment. If definitive lip repair is possible, 2 modes of therapy may be considered. One is the single-stage bilateral repair. One may use either bilateral triangular flaps or bilateral rotation advancement flaps. Although some surgeons occasionally operate on patients in the first week of life for bilateral repair, the authors recommend waiting until the rule of 10 applies. A second approach is the use of staged repairs, again by one of the foregoing techniques. The first stage is performed when the patient is approximately 10 weeks of age, and the second stage is done approximately 4 to 6 weeks later. If the premaxilla protrudes excessively, definitive lip repair may be unfeasible without some form of premaxillary recession to relieve suture-line tension. The management of excessive protrusion of the premaxilla depends on the surgeon's experience with lip adhesions or surgical recession and with the availability of a prosthodontist skilled in the construction of presurgical orthodontic applicances. If such a dental colleague is available, an early trial of such a device will be optimal. The child should be observed bimonthly; if the recession is inadequate, then lip adhesions will be indicated. The advantages of a lip adhesion in this setting include the lack of necessity for revision of the dental appliance and the ease with which the parents may care for the child. The major risk of surgical recession of the premaxilla is impairment of subsequent anterior maxillary growth. Surgical resection of the premaxilla is not recommended.

F. Feeding

In general, infants with isolated cleft lip rarely present a feeding problem. The patient's parents may be instructed preoperatively to treat the patient with an isolated cleft lip as they would any normal infant. Should feeding problems exist, management is essentially that of the child with a significant cleft palate. The feeding of patients with cleft palates is discussed later in the chapter.

G. Dressings and Postoperative Care

1. **Bacitracin ointment** Although no dressings are required, the application of this ointment to the incision line after cleansing the sutures with hydrogen peroxide and cotton-tipped swabs keeps the wound clean and soft.
2. **Logan's bow** is of some benefit if one desires to use a protective dressing. This appliance probably does not relieve tension on the repair, but it does offer protection similar to that of a football face mask. It lessens the trauma that may occur on the suture line should the infant continually abrade the lip on the crib.
3. **Elbow splints** made from tongue blades and soft tape or cloth are useful to prevent lip trauma from the child's fingers.
4. **Postoperative feedings** should be given through a bulb syringe, a regular large medicinal syringe with rubber tubing for gavage, or a large medicine dropper for approximately 3 weeks. Pacifiers or other oral devices such as nipples from bottles are contraindicated.
5. **Suture removal** Approximately half the skin sutures may be removed as early as the third postoperative day, and the remainder of the sutures at key areas may be removed by the fifth or sixth day.

H. Postoperative Complications

1. **Wound infections** may develop as a result of any surgical procedure. Because of the bacterial flora of the mouth, however, the authors recommend that an antibiotic ointment such as bacitracin be applied to the incision site while sutures are in place. Prior to the application of bacitracin ointment, the wound should be cleaned with hydrogen peroxide and cotton-tipped swabs. This regimen should be performed two to three times a day.
2. **Widening of the scar** is most commonly due to tension or infection. This complication can be avoided by reduction of tension prior to the operation, either by premaxillary orthopedics or by creation of a lip adhesion.
3. **Retrusion of the premaxilla** rarely occurs today unless a surgical recession has been performed. In such a case, it appears

that resection of the vomer causes a failure of subsequent anterior growth.

4. **Whistle tip deformity** results from a thin prolabium. Frequently, whistle tip deformities occur in patients with severe, bilateral cleft lips. The severity of the deformity can be reduced by mobilizing lateral muscle flaps to augment the prolabium.

5. **Maxillary segment collapse** may be corrected or prevented by the use of dental devices that use a screw or spring to expand the segments. This technique requires an experienced prosthodontist and is not available to many practitioners. Thus, collapse of the maxillary segments in infants occasionally remains uncorrected until the child is old enough to allow more conventional methods of expansion, using dentures on deciduous teeth.

I. Deformities Secondary to Cleft Lip

1. **Flattening of the lip** on the repaired side is caused by a deficiency of tissue along the margins of the medial aspect of the cleft. It may also be caused by hypoplasia of the pyriform aperture of the maxilla along the cleft side. The deficiency may be corrected by a small graft in the region of the pyriform aperture using bone, cartilage, or dermis, or by the interdigitation of adjacent muscle tissue.

2. **Flattening of the prolabium** results from the vertical misdirection of the orbicularis oris fibers. The orbicularis oris muscle must be separated from the levator labii superioris muscle and rotated inferiorly, to create the normal oral sphincter.

3. **Excessive shortness or tightness of the lip** is found after the straight-line repair and may be corrected by Z-plasties or by a complete revision of the initial repair. The tight upper lip occurs if upper lip tissue is lost, and it may be corrected by the use of an Abbe flap or by maxillary advancement.

4. **Irregular alignment of the upper lip** may be corrected by excision and reapproximation or by Z-plasty. If a greater defect is present, it may be necessary to perform a vermilion advancement.

5. **Whistle deformity** is present when the patient has notching in the vermilion border of the upper lip. This defect may be corrected by a V-Y advancement of the vermilion border. Most often, however, if the lip is short, it is best to take down the previous closure and to elongate it.

6. **The long lip** results from excessive lengthening of the lateral portion of the lip during the initial repair. This defect may be corrected by excision of a portion of the existing scar and, possibly, by a small excision of excess tissue. This deformity may occur after a quadrangular or Z-plasty repair.

J. Unilateral Cleft Lip Nasal Deformity

This deformity includes an alar cartilage that is thin, distorted, and tipped caudally and a nasal aperture that is widened and flattened. The alar base is displaced laterally, and the entire inferolateral cartilage is flattened. One sees a rotation of the medial crus inferiorly and medially with a shortened columella. Moreover, the dome projection on the cleft side is decreased, and the dome has an appearance of a bifid nose. The lateral crus is displaced inferiorly. The bony and cartilaginous structures of the nose are distorted. The caudal edge of the cartilaginous septum is deviated toward the noncleft side, distorting the columella in a similar fashion. The midportion of the septum is deviated toward the cleft side and frequently causes nasal airway obstruction. Reconstructive surgeons disagree on when the cleft lip nose should be repaired. Some surgeons perform a primary nasal tip procedure during the primary lip repair. These surgeons contend that the nose may be made essentially symmetric during early infancy. The opponents of this view maintain that surgical revision will be required later, and therefore, early intervention in the nasal tip is not warranted. The authors recommend that, during the initial cleft lip repair, the surgeon strive to obtain both primary closure of the floor of the nose and a symmetric position of the alae on the cleft side. Secondary procedures should be deferred until later. Some authors recommend waiting until age 16 in females and age 18 in males for definitive repair, to ensure that nasal growth will be complete. Nasal tip revisions may be performed on patients between the ages of 6 and 8 years if the deformity is severe, however. The operative procedure should aim to repair any deformities in the nasal sill, to make the inferolateral cartilages symmetric, to support the nasal columella and tip by the use of cartilage implants, if necessary, and to establish symmetric alar base-columella relationships. Once the majority of nasal growth has occurred (early or midteenage years), the septal deviations may be corrected, and if necessary, osteotomies may be performed, to render the bony nose symmetric. Onlay grafts beneath the affected pyriform aperture may be performed at the time of the nasal tip operation, when the patient is 5 or 6 years old or older.

K. Bilateral Cleft Lip Nasal Deformity

The medial crura of the inferolateral cartilages are separated and cause a lowered dome and shortened columella. The lateral crura are inferiorly displaced, with the resultant appearance of a collapsed nasal tip. The alar domes and bases are displaced laterally, with a depression in the center, to give the appearance of a bifid nose with a flattened tip. Hypoplasia is usually present in the region of the pyriform apertures and leads to a flattened alar base. The timing of surgical correction of secondary bilateral cleft lip nasal deformities is similar to that for unilateral cleft repair procedures. In the primary operation, an attempt is made to repair the nasal floor, to establish a symmetric nasal aperture, and to attain a normal-sized nostril. When the patient is approximately 5 or 6 years old, a columellar lengthening procedure may be performed to elongate the columella. At this stage, the nasal tip cartilages may be revised and repositioned to give tip projection. If necessary, an onlay cartilage or bone graft may be placed inferior to the alar bases, to correct hypoplasia. Nasal tip operations and lip revisions may also be performed at this time. Again, bony nasal work is performed when patients are in the mid- and late teenage years. Nasal septal operations are performed at the same time as the bony corrections. If the upper lip is so deficient in tissue to require an Abbe flap, it may be performed after the midteenage years.

III. CLEFT PALATE

The primary palate includes the prolabium, the premaxilla, and the anterior septum. The secondary palate includes the incisive foramen and all hard palate posterior to the incisive foramen.

A. Classification

1. **Incomplete cleft of the secondary palate.**
2. **Complete cleft of the secondary palate,** extending as far as the incisive foramen.
3. **Incomplete cleft of the primary and secondary palates.**
4. **Bilateral complete cleft of the primary and secondary palates.**
5. **Unilateral complete cleft of the primary and secondary palates.**
6. **Cleft of the soft palate alone.**
7. **Submucous cleft palate.**

B. Incidence

Although counseling parents concerning the incidence of cleft palate is difficult because inheritance of the condition is multifactorial, one can state some general considerations. If one child in the family has a cleft palate, the risk of having another child with a cleft palate is 2%. If one parent has a cleft palate, the incidence of the offspring having a cleft palate is 7%.

C. Presurgical and Surgical Considerations

1. **Feeding** may become a problem in a patient with a wide cleft palate. Nasal regurgitation of milk and other liquids can cause respiratory problems as well as an increased incidence of otitis media. Therefore, if the patient has any difficulty with the standard nursery nipple, one should use a special type of nipple, much like the elongated shape of a lamb's nipple, available at most pharmacies, or a special cleft palate feeding kit, also commercially available. The parents must be counseled to pro-

vide slow, frequent feedings until the child becomes adapted to the new feeding device. Reassurance and diligent instruction by the physician and nursery personnel are essential.

2. **Facial growth** One problem encountered by all patients with cleft involving the hard palate, especially the maxillary alveolus, is distorted maxillary growth. This defect usually takes the form of arch asymmetry and deformity, varying from a crossbite in the region of the canine tooth on the cleft side to extreme midfacial retrusion or to a posteriorly displaced maxilla. The pertinent literature contains many articles on the effect of surgical procedures on the growth of the maxilla. Most workers agree that the oral mucoperiosteum is related to bone growth, and elevation or dislocation of this periosteum combined with fibrous tissue contracture in the postoperative period leads to malalignment of the maxillary segments. Parents must be apprised of the potential of midfacial growth abnormalities that may require extensive orthodontic treatment and, potentially, orthognathic surgical procedures.

3. **Surgical orthopedics** may be of some value in the patient with a complete bilateral cleft palate and protruding premaxilla, particularly in the expansion of the maxillary arch to provide room for the premaxilla to move into better alignment posteriorly. The efficacy of preoperative orthopedics is directly proportional to the skill of the prosthodontist, however. The average patient with complete cleft palate usually has minimal need for such prosthetic devices.

4. **Timing of repair** No unanimity of opinion exists with regard to the optimal time for repair of the cleft palate. Individuals concerned with facial appearance warn of an increased incidence in facial growth disturbances associated with early palatal operations. Speech pathologists frequently push for early surgical correction because they believe that such a procedure leads to better speech. If complete closure of the cleft is to be obtained by use of the von Langenbeck repair or the Wardill-Kilner pushback operation, the most common time for closure is when the patient is 18 to 24 months of age, once the deciduous dentition has erupted. An increasingly popular approach, however, is the closure of the soft palate at approximately 12 to 24 months of age, with closure of the hard palate cleft between the ages 4 and 6 years. The authors recommend that narrow clefts of the hard and soft palate or clefts on the soft palate alone be definitively closed when the patient is approximately 12 to 14 months of age. Wide clefts of the hard and soft palate are better closed in a 2-stage approach using soft palate closure at 12 to 14 months of age, followed by the closure of the hard palate at the ages mentioned previously.

5. **Cleft of the soft palate** The authors recommend that the cleft of the soft palate alone be closed by primary veloplasty

when the patient is 12 to 14 months old. Relaxing incisions may be made posterior to the maxillary tuberosity into the space of Ernst if necessary. A 3-layer closure of the nasal mucosa, muscle, and oral mucosa is then completed, using care to mobilize the levator sling posteriorly before approximating it in the midline.

6. **Submucous cleft palate**
   a. ***Diagnosis*** is based on one or more of the following findings: a bifid uvula, failure of the soft palate muscles to join in the midline, despite an intact mucous membrane, and midline depression or notch in the hard palate. The incidence of submucous cleft palate ranges from 1 in 10,000 to 1 in 20,000. Approximately 25% of patients found with a submucous cleft have abnormal speech due to velopharyngeal incompetence. Some authors believe that the patient with a submucous cleft palate has a short palate, although others deny that such an association is consistent.
   b. ***Treatment*** If the patient with the submucous cleft palate displays velopharyngeal incompetence, speech therapy may be the only treatment required. If a neurologic deficit or easy fatigability exists, however, a prosthesis, such as a palatal lift, may be used on a trial basis. If such a device fails, surgical management will be necessary. Mere apposition of the muscle fibers in the midline, even when combined with a pushback palatoplasty, is usually insufficient. These patients most commonly require a superiorly based pharyngeal flap, to achieve adequate V-P closure.

D. Problems Secondary to Cleft Palate

1. **Wide mobilization of palatal mucoperiosteal flaps** may predispose the patient to maxillary alveolar collapse. Such a deformity can be prevented by delaying closure of the hard palate cleft until the first molars are erupted, at 18 to 24 months of age. If a deformity exists, however, orthodontic appliances may be used to expand the maxillary segments.
2. **Orthognathic surgical procedures** If the patient has severe maxillary retrusion, maxillary advancement will be of benefit and may also be used as part of the cosmetic reconstruction in the cleft lip nose.
3. **Velopharyngeal insufficiency** or incompetence exists when functional valving between the oral and nasal cavities is inadequate and allows air to escape through the nose during speech (rhinolalia aperta). Other signs include facial grimaces, glottal stops, and articulation defects as compensatory mechanisms to correct velopharyngeal incompetence. In the patient with a cleft palate, the palatal motion may be diminished by scarring, or the palate may be foreshortened. A trial of speech therapy may be warranted. If this regimen is unsuccessful, a

pushback procedure may be all that is required, although more frequently, a pharyngeal flap is indicated. A more complete discussion of this topic follows in the next major section of this chapter.

4. **Eustachian Tube Dysfunction**
   a. ***Cause and incidence*** The eustachian tube dysfunction seen in individuals with cleft palate is secondary to failure of the tube to open, most likely from failure of the palatal muscles (tensor and levator veli palatini) to dilate the tubal ostium and lumen adequately. The reported incidence of hearing loss in individuals with cleft palates ranges from 0 to 90%. This hearing loss is nearly always due to middle ear effusion and, therefore, is only temporary in nature. When the effusion is chronic, myringotomy with placement of ventilating tubes should be performed. The incidence of effusion gradually declines with age until, just as in noncleft children, after 10 years of age nearly all have normal eustachian tube function and normal hearing.
   b. ***Effect of repair of palate*** After surgical closure of the cleft palate, over half the patients with ear abnormalities experience resolution of their signs and symptoms. Improvement in eustachian tube function following palatoplasty most probably is related to several factors, such as improved muscle action in opening the tubes by the midline anchor, diminished nasopharyngeal inflammation when food influx is prevented, and the improvement in eustachian tube function seen with advancing age, probably because of growth and development of tubal and peritubal structures.
   c. ***Ear disorders*** When middle ear disease in children with cleft palate is not properly managed, it may result in chronic middle ear disease, as in adults. Aggressive therapy to allow adequate ventilation of the middle ear space and to improve hearing during infancy and early childhood is indicated. Myringotomy and ventilating tubes at the time of cleft lip repair in a patient with a cleft lip and palate, or at a sign of chronic middle ear effusion in the patient with a cleft palate, are warranted in an attempt to reduce chronic middle ear problems in this high-risk group.

IV. VELOPHARYNGEAL INSUFFICIENCY (INCOMPETENCE)

A. Diagnostic Tests

1. **Speech sampling,** to demonstrate nasal escape.
2. **Neurologic evaluation.**

3. **Cephalometric studies,** to evaluate palatal motion and placement.
4. **Measurement of nasal air-pressure flow** during speech.
5. **Videoendoscopic examination** during speech.

B. Causes

1. **Congenitally short soft palate and normal pharynx.**
2. **Submucous partial or complete cleft of the palate.**
3. **Neuromuscular abnormality,** yielding partial or complete paresis of the soft palate.
4. **Normal soft palate but abnormally large pharynx.**
5. **Scarring,** secondary to injury or surgical procedures.

C. Treatment

1. **Speech therapy** may yield adequate results in patients with mild-to-moderate velopharyngeal insufficiency with minimal anatomic abnormalities. If the nasal escape is severe or if significant anatomic deviations are present, however, speech therapy should be considered as merely an adjunct to more effective forms of treatment.
2. **Dental prosthesis** A palatal lift prosthesis is useful in patients with slight velopharyngeal incompetence. This prosthesis simply elevates the soft palate to a superior carrying position and thereby reduces the amount of posterosuperior excursion necessary to achieve closure during speech. Far more common, however, are dental obturators. These adynamic dental prostheses extend around the soft palate posteriorly with an oval bulb to occlude the velopharyngeal port. The use of these prostheses is primarily limited to patients in whom surgical intervention is contraindicated.
3. **Posterior pharyngeal wall implants** have been used by numerous surgeons. Most recently, Proplast has had an excellent success rate. In patients with a gap of less than 3 mm between the soft palate and the posterior pharyngeal wall, Teflon injections have been successful. Because of rare vascular catastrophes, however, the United States Food and Drug Administration has temporarily withdrawn approval for injection into the posterior pharyngeal wall. Posterior wall implants are helpful in patients with a gap of 1 cm or less and who have adequate muscular function. The main risk in these implants is extrusion or inferior displacement.
4. **Palatal lengthening** Studies on the efficacy of the Wardill-Kilner type of palatal lengthening vary from marked speech improvement to the lack of speech improvement. Because of increasing evidence of significant risk associated with denuding

large portions of the palatal bone in the growing child, palatal lengthening procedures have become less common.

5. **Posterior wall pharyngeal flaps,** the most common surgical method of correctng velopharyngeal incompetence, may be either superiorly or inferiorly based. These flaps function by obturating the palatopharyngeal space. Lateral ports are fashioned on both sides to accommodate mucus and nasal air movement. During speech, the ports are closed by mesial movement of the lateral walls of the one pharynx. Some practitioners believe that the superiorly based flap is preferred in patients with large gaps between the soft palate and the posterior pharyngeal wall, when a long flap is needed, when a primary pharyngeal flap is part of the initial repair of the soft palate, and in patients who are excellent operative risks and in whom adequate exposure can be obtained. These surgeons use inferiorly based flaps in patients who are poor surgical risks, when exposure is difficult, when palatal motion is adequate, and in patients whose hypernasality is out of proportion to problems of articulation and nasal escape, that is, in older patients. Prior to placement of the superiorly based pharyngeal flap, a meticulous examination of the nasopharynx is necessary to evaluate the adenoid tissue. If a large adenoid pad is present, adenoidectomy is advisable prior to the placement of the flap. Adenoidectomy should not be performed in a child with cleft palate unless it has already been determined that a pharyngeal flap is necessary, however, because adenoidectomy may itself lead to velopharyngeal insufficiency.

28

DEEP INFECTIONS OF THE HEAD AND NECK

MARIE G. GAUTHIER

To diagnose and treat deep infections of the head and neck most expeditiously, one must be familiar with the anatomic features of the cervical fascia. Unfortunately, the terminology used in describing these layers is confusing, and many names have been given for the same potential spaces lined by this fascia. These spaces are clinically important and remarkably constant, however, and should be thoroughly understood by a surgeon attempting to treat abscesses involving these deep spaces.

I. NOMENCLATURE OF CERVICAL FASCIA

The fascia consists of a superficial and a deep layer. The deep cervical fascia has superficial, middle, and deep layers, as listed in Table 28–1.

A. Superficial Cervical Fascia

This loose layer in the neck has variable amounts of fat enclosing the platysma muscle. Superiorly, it extends to the tight fascia sur-

TABLE 28–1

Fascial layers of the neck
Superficial cervical fascia
Deep cervical fascia
Superficial layer
Middle layer
Deep layer
Alar layer
Prevertebral layer

rounding the mimetic muscles of the face, and inferiorly, it is continuous with the superficial fascia of the shoulder, chest, and axilla.

B. Deep Cervical Fascia

The study of the deep cervical fascia is controversial and confusing because of the multiple names applied to the same layers (Surg. Clin. North. Am., *54*:1297, 1974). In general, however, it is most useful to consider this fascia to have three layers: superficial, middle, and deep (Am. J. Anat., *63*:367, 1938).

1. **Superficial layer** This layer is best remembered by "the rule of twos" (Otol. Clin. North. Am., *9*:561, 1976). This sheet of fibrous tissue surrounds the neck and encloses two glands, two muscles, and two spaces. The two glands on each side of the neck are the parotid and submandibular glands. The two muscles are the trapezius and sternocleidomastoid muscles, and the two spaces are the suprasternal space and the space of the posterior triangle. Inferiorly, this fascial layer attaches to the sternum, the clavicle, and part of the acromion. Laterally, it attaches to the spines of the cervical vertebrae. Superiorly, it attaches to the hyoid bone and then to the body of the mandible. Continuing superiorly, the layer encloses the parotid glands and attaches subsequently to the zygoma and occiput, to form the temporalis fascia.
2. **Middle layer** This structure is also known as the visceral fascia because it surrounds the larynx and trachea, the esophagus, and the thyroid gland. This layer also encloses the strap muscles and forms part of the fascia surrounding the vascular space. Superiorly, the fascia attaches to the hyoid bone anteriorly and the skull base posteriorly. In this superoposterior area, it includes the buccinator muscle and has therefore been called the buccopharyngeal fascia. Posteriorly, the fascia forms the anterior boundary of the retropharyngeal space (Fig. 28–1).
3. **Deep layer** This layer consists of two divisions, the alar and the prevertebral layers.
   a. ***The alar layer*** lies posterior to the middle layer of the deep cervical fascia (visceral portion) and anterior to the prevertebral layer. It forms the posterior wall of the retropharyngeal space and the anterior wall of the "danger" space. To add to the confusion, the retropharyngeal space is sometimes called the postvisceral space. The alar layer contributes to the vascular space and extends from the vertebral transverse processes. This contribution by the alar layer to the vascular space fascia allows one to say that the three layers of the deep cervical fascia all contribute to the fascia surrounding the vascular space. The alar layer then fuses with the middle layer of the deep cervical fascia inferiorly at T1 and T2 posterior to the esophagus, inferiorly closing off the retropharyngeal space.

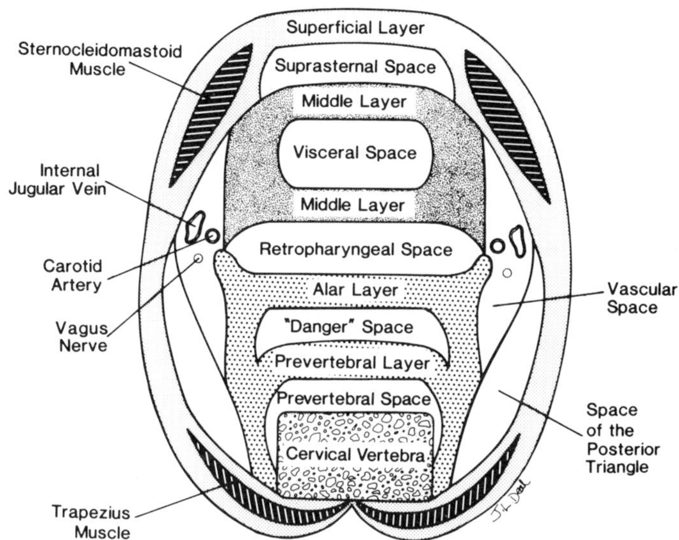

Fig. 28–1. The deep cervical fascia and the spaces inferior to the hyoid bone.

b. ***The prevertebral layer*** forms the anterior wall of the prevertebral space, also known as the vertebral space, and the posterior wall of the "danger" space. It encloses the deep muscles of the posterior triangle, and the phrenic nerve passes deep to it. This layer extends from the base of the skull to the coccyx.

II. GENERAL CONSIDERATIONS

A. Classification

To determine which space is involved with suppuration, it is most helpful to divide these spaces into three groups:

1. **Length of neck** This group comprises spaces involving the entire length of the neck.
2. **Suprahyoid** spaces are those found superior to the hyoid bone.
3. **Infrahyoid** The anterior space inferior to the hyoid bone is termed the infrahyoid space. These spaces are so classified in Table 28–2.

B. Medical History

Obtaining an accurate history is the single most important step in establishing the cause of infection and the site of involvement.

1. **Portal of entry** One must try to determine whether the ab-

TABLE 28–2

Classification of Deep Head and Neck Spaces
Spaces involving the entire length of the neck
Retropharyngeal space
"Danger" space
Prevertebral space
Vascular space
Suprahyoid spaces
Submandibular
sublingual
submaxillary
Masticator space
Temporal space
Peritonsillar space
Lateral pharyngeal space
Parotid space
Infrahyoid space
Visceral space

scess is of dental, oral, tonsillar, or pharyngeal origin. Unfortunately, in 50% of cases, no specific source of infection can be identified.

2. **Previous operation** A week is usually required for abscess formation. Computed tomographic (CT) scanning is especially helpful not only in locating the abscess, but also in determining whether an abscess has formed. Cultures, both aerobic and anaerobic, must be done, and the wall to the abscess cavity should undergo biopsy at the time of the surgical procedure.
3. **Previous medical treatment** The use of antibiotics can mask abscess formation.
4. **Systemic diseases** Nephritis, syphilis, and diabetes are often associated with deep neck infections and must be suspected in patients with these conditions.

C. Clinical Presentation

1. **Pain and limitation** of jaw or neck movement are present in all patients with deep neck infections and abscesses.
2. **Absence of fluctuance** Fluctuance of the neck is rarely noted because of the deep location of the process. Pitting edema of the skin is usually present when an abscess is ready to be drained, however.
3. **Diffuse, brawny swelling** is present in all infected spaces, except the prevertebral space. CT scanning is helpful in identifying and locating the abscess.

D. Bacteriologic Features

1. **Hemolytic streptococci** are the most common pathogenic organisms in head and neck infections.

2. **Staphylococcus aureus** is the most common pathogen in abscesses of the head and neck.
3. **Anaerobic bacilli** are significant pathogens in deep neck abscesses. Clues to anaerobic infection include dental infections and infections following surgical procedures or trauma to the oral cavity, foul-smelling discharge, and gas formation.

III. SUBMANDIBULAR SPACE INFECTIONS

A. Anatomic Features

1. **Digastric triangle** This space consists of the area of the digastric triangle, which has the following boundaries: superiorly, the mucosa of the floor of the mouth; superolaterally, the mandible; and laterally and inferiorly, the superficial layer of the deep cervical fascia, to the attachment on the hyoid bone.
2. **Mylohyoid muscle** incompletely divides the submandibular space into two connected subspaces: the sublingual or supramylohyoid space; and the submaxillary or inframylohyoid space. Dental infections anterior to the second molar tooth are first to involve the sublingual space. Usually, the roots of the second and third molars extend inferior to the mylohyoid attachment, so apical root infections of these teeth can directly involve the inframylohyoid space.

B. Ludwig's Angina

1. **Description** This disorder causes a rapidly spreading, indurated cellulitis beginning in the sublingual space and later involving the submaxillary space. Abscess formation is unusual, but an indurated cellulitis without lymphatic involvement causes massive swelling of the tongue and the floor of the mouth.
2. **Incidence** The disease occurs with equal frequency in both sexes, usually between the ages of 20 and 50 years.
3. **Causes** Dental caries and pyorrhea are the commonest sources, but the disorder may also be caused by trauma to the tongue and floor of the mouth and lingual tonsillitis. The bacteriologic features are discussed previously in this chapter.
4. **Clinical picture**
   a. ***Malaise*** The patient is in acute distress.
   b. ***Fever*** may rise to 41° C.
   c. ***Dysphagia*** is a prominent symptom, resulting from swelling of the tongue and the floor of the mouth that pushes the tongue superiorly and posteriorly toward the palate.
   d. ***Swelling of the floor of the mouth*** progresses to board-like firmness.
   e. ***Severe trismus and pain*** are present.

f. ***Dyspnea*** causes the patient to sit up. This symptom is due to laryngeal edema and swelling of the tongue.
g. ***Hard edema*** of the submental and anterior cervical region is present.
h. ***Leukocyte count*** is usually 10,000 to 25,000, with 80% polymorphonuclear leukocytes.
i. ***Absence of regional lymphadenitis*** is noted.

5. **Treatment**
   a. ***Early treatment*** includes close observation for early detection of airway compromise, antibiotics to abort early cases, and adequate nutrition, which may require tube feeding.
   b. ***Late treatment*** includes tracheotomy prior to surgical drainage in the presence of respiratory distress and at the first sign of dyspnea, surgical drainage by means of a horizontal incision inferior to the mandible over the area of swelling and induration with insertion of a drain, and general supportive measures such as antibiotics, intravenous fluids, and oral hygiene.

6. **Complications**
   a. ***Respiratory tract obstruction*** is possible.
   b. ***Aspiration pneumonia*** may occur.
   c. ***Dehydration*** is a potential complication.
   d. ***Mediastinitis*** The infection may travel to the lateral pharyngeal space and down the carotid sheath to the superior mediastinum.

C. Submental Infections

1. **Description** Suppuration is confined to the inframylohyoid space.

2. **Causes** Dental disorders in the mandibular incisor region or breakdown of submental lymph nodes may cause such an infection. Oral anaerobes are the pathogens.

3. **Clinical picture**
   a. ***Minimal respiratory distress*** and only moderate dysphagia are noted.
   b. ***Marked external induration*** in the midline resembles true Ludwig's angina.
   c. ***No swelling*** of the soft tissues of the floor of the mouth occurs. This structure is moderately elevated, however.

4. **Treatment** includes the administration of antibiotics and surgical drainage, by a horizontal incision made over the region of the greatest swelling when the infection is localized.

IV. MASTICATOR SPACE INFECTIONS

A. Anatomic Features

The masticator space is formed as the deep cervical fascia covers the masseter muscle laterally and the pterygoid muscles medially.

B. Description

Cellulitis and abscess formation involve the subperiosteal region of the mandible and may involve the masseter and pterygoid muscle fascia and the deep and superficial temporal muscle pouches.

C. Causes

1. **Infected tooth root** of a mandibular second or third molar or their extraction may result in a masticator space infection.
2. **Nonaseptic technique in local anesthesia** of the inferior alveolar nerve may also cause such an infection.

D. Clinical Picture

1. **Pain and fever** are of acute onset.
2. **Brawny induration** over the area of the angle and ramus of the mandible is seen externally. The swelling can extend to the inferior portion of the neck, as with a lateral pharyngeal infection.
3. **Marked trismus** develops.
4. **Severe dysphagia** is present.
5. **Pharyngeal swelling** over the medial aspect of the angle and ramus of the mandible is obvious. The tonsil is pushed toward the midline, but the lateral pharyngeal wall posterior to the tonsil is not swollen, as in lateral pharyngeal space involvement.

E. Treatment

1. **Roentgenograms** of the involved mandible and teeth should be obtained to reveal a possible focus of infection.
2. **Intravenous antibiotics** are indicated.
3. **Surgical drainage** External drainage is done if the swelling is mainly external; an incision is made at the angle of the jaw extending through the periosteum. Internal drainage is preferred for cosmetic reasons. Delaying surgical treatment beyond 10 days can lead to osteomyelitis and bone necrosis.

V. PTERYGOPALATINE AND TEMPORAL FOSSA INFECTIONS

A. Anatomic Features

The boundaries of the fossa are as follows:

1. **Superior** The sphenoid and orbital process of the palatine bone form the superior boundary.

2. **Posterior** This boundary is formed by the bases of the pterygoid processes and the inferior part of the anterior surface of the greater wing of the sphenoid bone.
3. **Anterior** The posterior wall of the maxillary sinus forms this boundary.
4. **Medial** This boundary is formed by the vertical portion of the palatine bone.
5. **Lateral** The temporalis muscle and other soft tissue structures form the lateral boundary.

B. Causes

1. **Dental extractions** of maxillary molar teeth may precipitate such infections.
2. **Nerve blocks** may be causative factors.

C. Description

A fulminating cellulitis develops progressively and involves the maxillary molar gingiva and the pterygopalatine, infratemporal, and temporal fossae. Abscess formation follows.

D. Clinical Picture

1. **Cellulitis** develops over the entire side of the head including the nose, the auricle, and the superior portion of the neck and extends over the mandible, the face, and the temporalis muscle.
2. **Proptosis of the globe** and abducens paralysis on the involved side are noted.
3. **Severe trismus** develops.
4. **Optic neuritis** may develop.

E. Treatment

1. **Immediate surgical drainage** should be initiated if signs of sepsis are present.
2. **Parenteral antibiotics** are indicated.
3. **Oral hygiene** is helpful.

VI. PERITONSILLAR ABSCESS

A. Anatomic Features

The peritonsillar space is a potential space lying between the fibrous capsule of the palatine tonsil medially and the superior constrictor laterally. The plane of least resistance in this space is that adjacent to the soft palate; 70% of abscesses localize to the superior tonsillar pole. Abscess formation in the midportion of the peritonsillar space may penetrate the superior constrictor muscles and may enter the lateral pharyngeal space. See Chapter 21.

B. Description

The suppuration extends beyond the tonsillar capsule, but it is still limited by the fascia of the superior constrictor muscle.

C. Incidence

The highest incidence is in older children and in young adults.

D. Causes

Gram-positive organisms are common pathogens. Streptococcus is the most common pathogenic organism in this condition.

E. Clinical Picture

1. **Trismus** is present in all cases. It is not as severe as in lateral pharyngeal space infections.
2. **Severe dysphagia** makes it difficult for the patient to swallow saliva.
3. **Unilateral swelling** of the peritonsillar area occurs, with deviation of the uvula to the uninvolved side.
4. **Speech abnormality** The patient speaks with a "hot potato" voice.

F. Treatment

1. **Surgical drainage** includes careful palpation for pulsations and fluctuation and needle aspiration with an 18-gauge needle, in an attempt to localize the pus. An incision is then made at the superior pole in the anterior tonsillar pillar, and a hemostat further opens the abscess. Suction must be immediately available to prevent aspiration of pus. Abscess formation in the midportion of the peritonsillar space (posterior and inferior to the tonsil) may require tonsillectomy for drainage.
2. **Parenteral antibiotics and fluids** are usually necessary because the patient cannot maintain an adequate oral intake.
3. **Oral hygiene** with saline washes is helpful.
4. **Relief of painful trismus** may be achieved by local anesthesia of the ipsilateral sphenopalatine ganglia by the intranasal application of cocaine.
5. **Immediate or delayed tonsillectomy** is indicated.

VII. LATERAL PHARYNGEAL SPACE ABSCESS

A. Anatomic Features

This cone-shaped space has the following boundaries:

1. **Base (superior)** The base comprises the petrous portion of the temporal bone.
2. **Medial** The superior constrictor muscle with its covering of buccopharyngeal fascia is the medial boundary.

3. **Lateral** The pterygoid muscles, mandible, and parotid gland comprise this boundary.
4. **Anterior** The pterygomandibular raphe forms the anterior boundary.
5. **Posterior** The apposition of the buccopharyngeal and prevertebral fasciae forms this boundary. It is therefore possible for infection to extend into the retropharyngeal space.
6. **Inferior** This space extends to the hyoid bone, where it connects with the submandibular space.
7. **Subdivisions** The styloid process divides the lateral pharyngeal space into two compartments. The posterior compartment contains the internal jugular vein, the carotid arteries, the ascending pharyngeal artery, cranial nerves IX to XII, and the sympathetic trunk. The anterior compartment contains fat, connective tissue, muscle, and lymph nodes.

B. Causes

1. **Peritonsillar abscess** can extend into the superior constrictor muscle.
2. **Deep parotid abscesses** may rupture into this space.
3. **Third-molar extractions** can lead to involvement of this space.
4. **Penetrating injuries** to the lateral pharyngeal wall may cause such an infection.
5. **Petrositis** may rupture into this space.
6. **Introduction of infection by local anesthesia** may occur, such as in tonsillectomy performed under local anesthesia.

C. Clinical Picture

1. **Sudden onset of chills and fever** occurs in an acutely ill patient.
2. **Marked trismus is evident,** as compared to the lesser trismus seen in patients with peritonsillar abscess.
3. **Swelling of the lateral pharyngeal wall,** especially behind the posterior pillar, helps to distinguish this infection from peritonsillar and masticator space infections.
4. **Displacement** The tonsil is usually pushed anteriorly as well as medially.
5. **Swelling** occurs at the angle of the jaw and in the submandibular region, as well as in the lateral neck with torticollis.
6. **Sepsis** may be present, especially with the onset of complications.

D. Treatment

1. **Antibiotic therapy** may abort abscess formation.
2. **Sepsis or hemorrhage** is a surgical emergency. External drainage is preferred because of the easier access to the carotid artery in case of hemorrhage. Intraoral approaches to this space are deplorable because of the risk of uncontrollable hemorrhage.

E. Complications

This infection has a high potential for life-threatening complications.

1. **Asphyxia** Respiratory distress demands a tracheotomy prior to any surgical procedure.
2. **Extension into the carotid sheath** is possible because the abscess may rupture into the vascular space with resulting massive hemorrhage.

VIII. PAROTID SPACE INFECTION

A. Anatomic Features

This space is bounded by the fascia that encloses the parotid gland, the seventh cranial nerve, and the lymph nodes. This fascia is frequently dehiscent medially.

B. Causes

Coagulase-positive Staphylococcus aureus causes most of the abscesses. This bacteriologic feature is an exception to the other space infections. Specific types of infection are as follows:

1. **Salivary calculus** is the most common cause of parotid space infection.
2. **Stomatitis,** systemic infections such as typhoid, scarlet fever, and smallpox and poisoning from heavy metals are all possible causes.
3. **Severe external otitis** can reach this space through the fissures of Santorini between the cartilaginous and bony ear canal.

C. Clinical Picture

1. **Tense painful swelling** occurs over the parotid area.
2. **Turbid fluid or pus** may or may not be expressed from the duct.
3. **Absence of early fluctuation** is noted because the fascia covering the lateral aspect is dense.

D. Treatment

1. **Antibiotics** should be administered.
2. **Adequate hydration and oral hygiene** are indicated.

3. **Surgical drainage** The abscess should be drained before fluctuation occurs. Needle aspiration reveals the presence of pus and guides the incision. One must rupture the partitions of multilocular abscesses. See Chapter 20.

E. Complications

This abscess can rupture into the lateral pharyngeal space because the medial portion of the parotid fascia is weak and is frequently dehiscent.

IX. RETROPHARYNGEAL SPACE INFECTIONS

A. Anatomic Features

This space lies anterior to the alar fascia and posterior to the posterior pharyngeal wall. It extends from the base of the skull to the level of the tracheal bifurcation. Because of a midline raphe, abscesses usually form lateral to the midline, whereas a Pott's abscess involving the prevertebral space is more apt to be in the midline (see Fig. 28–1).

B. Description

Pyogenic involvement of the retropharyngeal lymph nodes and the rich regional lymphatic plexuses is usually seen only in children because these retropharyngeal lymph nodes atrophy with age.

C. Causes

1. **Infections** in the regions draining to the retropharyngeal nodes, such as the nasopharynx, the eustachian tube, the nose, and the sinuses, are the most common cause in children.
2. **Trauma** is the most common cause in adults.

D. Incidence

This infection is essentially a disease of early childhood because the lymph nodes of this space atrophy by 3 to 4 years of age.

E. Clinical Picture

1. **Odynophagia and dysphagia** Young children refuse to eat. They may not complain of a sore throat.
2. **Fever** Moderate elevation of temperature is noted.
3. **Moderate neck rigidity** can usually be appreciated.
4. **Muffled voice** is frequently striking.
5. **Inflammation** The mucosa of the oropharynx is inflamed.
6. **Lateral impingement on the larynx** results in partial obstruction of the airway with noisy breathing.
7. **Fluctuance** may not be present, and palpation for this sign carries the risk of rupture of the abscess and aspiration.
8. **Roentgenographic evidence** Lateral neck roentgenograms

obtained during full inspiration reveal widening of the retropharyngeal soft tissues. At the level of C2, widening of greater than 7 mm is pathologic in children and adults. At C6, widening of greater than 14 mm in children (15 years and younger) and 22 mm in adults is considered abnormal.

F. Treatment

1. **Surgical drainage** The abscess should be drained as soon as it is diagnosed. Drainage without anesthesia, with the patient in the head-low position, is best.
2. **Preliminary tracheotomy** is necessary if respiratory distress does not allow the patient to lie in the head-low position.
3. **Low-lying abscesses** are opened through a lateral neck incision.

X. "DANGER" SPACE INFECTIONS

This space lies between the two layers of the deep cervical fascia. The alar layer forms the anterior wall of the space, and the prevertebral layer of the deep cervical fascia forms the posterior layer (see Fig. 28–1). The "danger" space deserves its name because, unlike the prevertebral and vascular spaces, which are dense and tight, this space is only filled with areolar tissue that can allow rapid spread of any infection from the base of the skull to the diaphragm. Infections may reach this space by lymphatic extension from the nose and throat or by direct extension from the retropharyngeal or prevertebral spaces. Treatment of abscess in this space is similar to that for an abscess in the retropharyngeal or prevertebral space because of their close proximity.

XI. PREVERTEBRAL SPACE ABSCESS

A. Anatomic Features

The prevertebral space runs from the base of the skull to the diaphragm.

B. Description

An abscess in this space is called cervical Pott's abscess and lies posterior to the prevertebral fascia. That it usually forms in the midline distinguishes it from the more lateral retropharyngeal abscess.

C. Causes

This infection is almost always caused by tuberculous caries of the vertebral bodies.

D. Diagnosis

The diagnosis is confirmed by lateral roentgenograms of the neck and cervical spine.

E. Treatment

Surgical drainage and the administration of antituberculous drugs are recommended.

XII. VASCULAR SPACE (CAROTID SPACE) ABSCESS

A. Anatomic Features

The carotid sheath lies within the vascular space. Infection can dissect to this space from any other space along shared fascial sheaths (see Fig. 28–1).

B. Causes

1. **Lateral pharyngeal space infection** most frequently extends to the carotid sheath.
2. **Breakdown of deep cervical lymphadenitis** is another cause.

C. Clinical Picture

1. **Marked swelling** of the anterolateral neck occurs with torticollis.
2. **Pitting and doughy feeling** of the swelling are noted.
3. **Hard, plum-colored swelling** results from hemorrhage.
4. **Sudden onset of shaking chills,** spiking fevers, and profound prostration announces internal jugular vein thrombophlebitis, associated with Horner's syndrome.

D. Treatment

1. **Antibiotics** should be given.
2. **Surgical drainage** The diagnosis of abscess formation makes immediate drainage imperative. Drainage should be avoided in patients with cellulitis.
3. **Ligation** Thrombophlebitis of the internal jugular vein may require ligation.

E. Complications

1. **Massive hemorrhage** The danger signs are:
   a. ***Spontaneous hemorrhage*** obviously not arising from a minor vessel.
   b. ***Hemorrhage from the external auditory canal,*** a rare and ominous complication.
   c. ***Hematoma*** of the surrounding tissues.
   d. ***Increasing pain and swelling*** locally and in the neck.
   e. ***Pulsation*** in the retropharyngeal or peritonsillar area.
   f. ***Cranial nerve deficits*** or Horner's syndrome.
2. **Mediastinitis** is a possible complication.
3. **Lateral sinus thrombosis** may occur.

4. **Disseminated abscesses** may be noted.
5. **Meningitis** is a possibility.

XIII. VISCERAL SPACE ABSCESS

A. Description

One notices suppuration just deep to the pretracheal fascia.

B. Causes

1. **Pharyngitis** One may see this type of abscess in a patient with pharyngitis with extension by the lymphatic vessels.
2. **Acute pyogenic thyroiditis** may also cause a visceral space abscess.

C. Clinical Picture

1. **Sore throat** is present.
2. **Redness and swelling in the hypopharynx** are noted.
3. **Dyspnea** occurs, secondary to compression.
4. **Tender swelling of the anterior cervical lymph nodes and of the thyroid** is seen. Pitting indicates pus.

D. Treatment

1. **Antibiotics** should be administered.
2. **Surgical drainage** is performed using the same approach as for tracheotomy.

XIV. CHOICE OF ANTIMICROBIAL THERAPY

A. Bacteriology

Deep neck abscesses are most commonly caused by mixed infections. Possible aerobic organisms usually include Streptococcus viridans, pyogenes, and pneumoniae (pneumococci), Staphylococcus aureus, Haemophilus influenzae, Escherichia coli, and Klebsiella. Anaerobic organisms are probably even more common and include peptostreptococci, peptococci, and Bacteroides species. Culturing of anaerobic organisms is difficult and may require 4 to 5 days. Smears for Gram staining should be obtained at the time of drainage.

B. Initial Choice of Antibiotics

Aqueous penicillin G (20 million Units) intravenously daily plus clindamycin (450 to 600 mg) intravenously q6h or chloramphenicol (1 gm) intravenously q6h are usually the drugs of choice.

29

NECK MASSES

W. FREDERICK McGUIRT

The differential diagnosis of a neck mass covers a spectrum of diseases (Table 29–1), and treatment is as varied as in any area of medicine. Although the possible diagnoses and the means of differentiating them are too numerous to list in this chapter, most neck masses represent inflammatory, congenital or developmental, or neoplastic conditions. This chapter takes a flow-sheet approach, to help the clinician to arrive at the most logical diagnosis and to give viable options in the management of each problem.

I. GENERAL CONSIDERATIONS

A. Age

When examining a patient with a neck mass, the first consideration should be the patient's age group, whether pediatric (0 to 15 years), young adult (16 to 40 years) or late adult (40+ years). In general, neck masses in children are more commonly inflammatory than congenital or developmental and more commonly congenital than neoplastic. This frequency is similar to that in the young-adult group (Table 29–2). In contrast, the first consideration in the older adult should be neoplasia, with less emphasis on inflammatory masses and even less on congenital masses, even though some congenital lesions may first manifest themselves late in life.

B. Location of the Lesion

After age, with its appropriate pathologic grouping of frequency and incidence, the next consideration should be the location of the neck mass (Table 29–2 and Fig. 29–1). This factor is particularly important in the differentiation of congenital and developmental

TABLE 29–1

Common Neck Masses

Neoplastic	Congenital and Developmental	Inflammatory
Metastatic	Sebaceous cyst	Lymphadenopathy
Unknown primary epidermoid carcinoma	Branchial cleft cyst, first and second	Bacterial
Primary head and neck epidermoid carcinoma or melanoma	Thyroglossal duct cyst	Viral
Adenocarcinoma	Lymphangioma or hemangioma	Granulomatous
Primary	Dermoid cyst	Tuberculous
Thyroid tumor	Ectopic thyroid tissue	Catscratch
Lymphoma	Laryngocele	Sarcoid
Salivary gland tumor	Pharyngeal diverticulum	Fungal
Lipoma	Thymic cyst	Sialadenitis
Angioma		Parotid
Carotid body tumor		Submaxillary
Rhabdomyosarcoma		Congenital cyst
		Thorotrast granuloma

masses because such lesions are consistent in location. The locations of neoplasms are both diagnostically and prognostically significant. The spread of head and neck carcinoma generally follows an orderly lymphatic pattern, and the appearance of a metastatic neck mass may be the key to identification of the primary tumor (Fig. 29–2).

C. Individual Approach

Beyond these general considerations, each patient must be evaluated on an individual basis. Specific aspects of the medical history and physical findings that reduce the list of possible causes should be sought, to limit the number of diagnostic tests needed in the differential diagnosis.

II. DIAGNOSTIC STEPS

A. Physical Examination

The most important diagnostic step is the physical examination. Many neck masses have physical findings that are specific and diagnostic in nature; those are described later in this chapter under the discussion of individual entities. A complete physical examination of the head and neck must be performed on every patient with a neck mass. Even the most thorough physical examination may leave the clinician unable to make a firm diagnosis, but with the patient's medical history, the physical examination may direct one to a general grouping such as vascular, salivary, or nodal, and inflammatory, congenital, or neoplastic conditions.

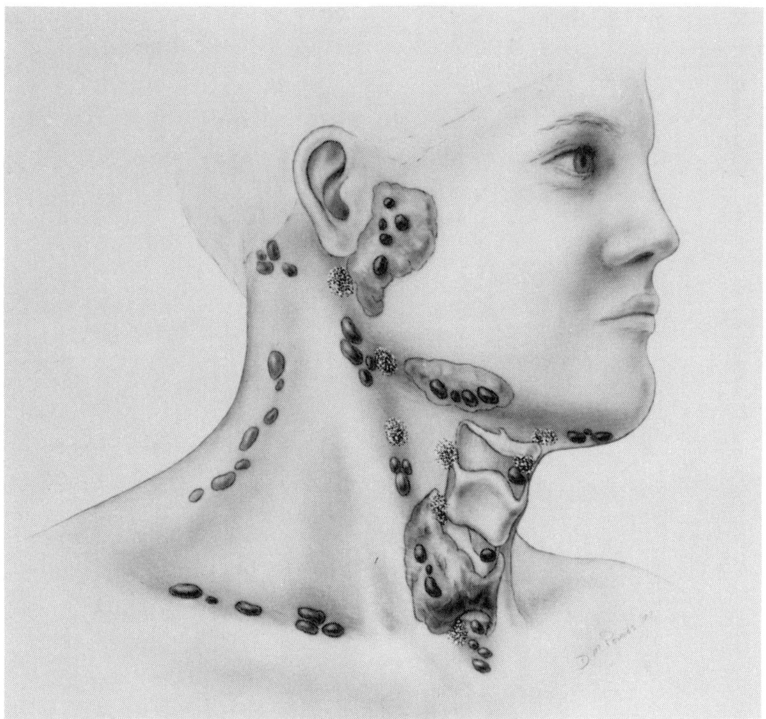

Fig. 29–1. Location of common lymphatic and glandular masses of the head and neck; stippled areas represent congenital masses.

B. Diagnostic Tests

At this point, various diagnostic tests may be helpful (Table 29–3).

1. **Pulsatile and compressible masses** For a patient whose mass is pulsatile, compressible, or has a palpable thrill or audible bruit, angiographic or ultrasonographic tests may be ordered. These tests differentiate degenerative vascular problems, such as aneurysms, from neoplastic conditions, such as glomus and carotid body tumors.
2. **Solid versus cystic masses** Ultrasonography may also be used to differentiate a solid from a cystic mass and is particularly helpful in distinguishing congenital branchial and thyroglossal cysts from solid lymph nodes, neurogenic tumors, and ectopic thyroid tissue (Am. J. Surg., *134*:369, 1977). The

TABLE 29–2

Diagnostic Flow Sheet			
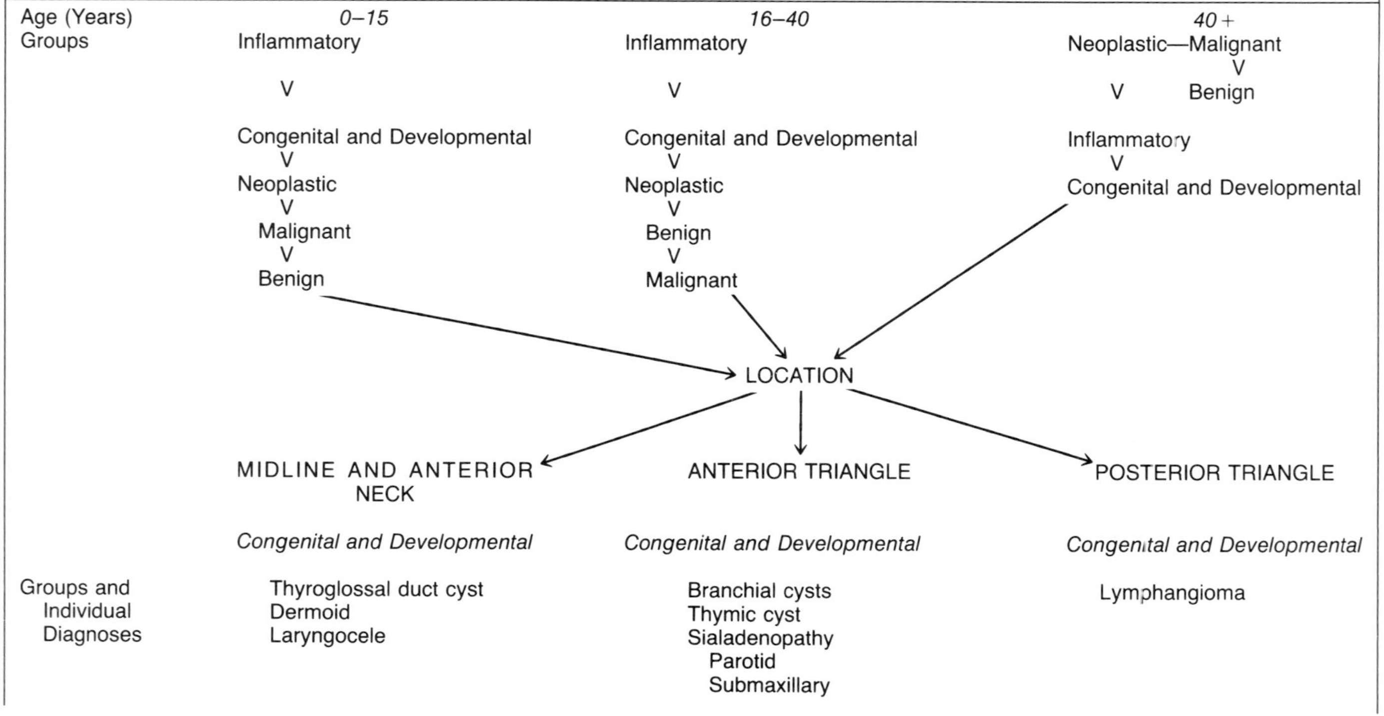 Age (Years)	*0–15*	*16–40*	*40+*
Groups	Inflammatory V Congenital and Developmental V Neoplastic V Malignant V Benign	Inflammatory V Congenital and Developmental V Neoplastic V Benign V Malignant	Neoplastic—Malignant V Benign V Inflammatory V Congenital and Developmental
		LOCATION	
	MIDLINE AND ANTERIOR NECK	ANTERIOR TRIANGLE	POSTERIOR TRIANGLE
	Congenital and Developmental	*Congenital and Developmental*	*Congenital and Developmental*
Groups and Individual Diagnoses	Thyroglossal duct cyst Dermoid Laryngocele	Branchial cysts Thymic cyst Sialadenopathy Parotid Submaxillary	Lymphangioma

Inflammatory	*Inflammatory*		*Inflammatory*
Adenitis	Adenitis		Adenitis
Bacterial	Bacterial		Bacterial
Viral	Viral		Viral
Granulomatous	Granulomatous		Granulomatous
	Sialadenitis		
	Parotid		
	Submaxillary		
	Thorotrast granuloma		
Neoplastic	*Neoplastic*		*Neoplastic*
Thyroid	Lymphoma	Primary vascular	Lymphoma
Lymphoma	Metastatic	Carotid body	Metastatic
	Upper jugular	Glomus	Superior
	Oropharynx	Hemangioma	Nasopharynx
	Oral cavity	Neurogenic	Scalp
	Lower jugular	Neurilemoma	Supraclavicular
	Hypopharynx	Salivary	Primary infraclavicular
	Larynx	Parotid	
	Submaxillary	Submaxillary	
	Oral cavity		
	Nasal-sinus		
	Face		

Key: V indicates "greater than."

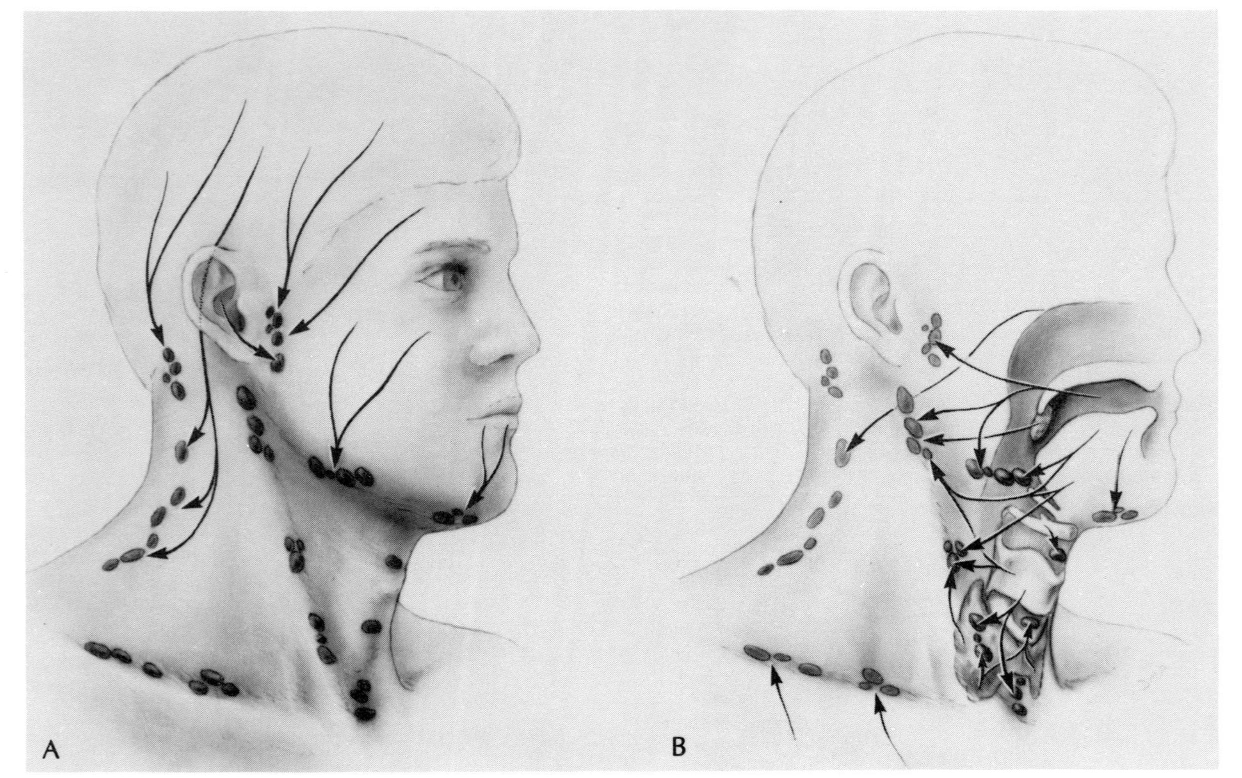

Fig. 29–2. Lymphatic drainage of external *(A)* and internal *(B)* areas of the head and neck.

TABLE 29–3

Diagnostic Examinations for Head and Neck Masses

Test Technique	Purpose and Value
Physical examination	Most important diagnostic technique; to be repeated
Endoscopy and biopsy	Identification of primary tumor as source of metastatic node; for all patients with suspected neoplasia
Radionuclide scanning	Identification of lesions of anterior neck compartment; helpful in diagnosing thyroid lesions and in localizing salivary gland lesions
Ultrasonography	Differentiation of solid from cystic masses, especially congenital and developmental cysts; a useful noninvasive technique for diagnosis of vascular lesions
Angiography	Diagnosis of vascular lesions and tumors fixed to the carotid artery
Sialography	Diagnosis of diffuse sialadenopathies or location of a mass within or outside of gland
Plain radiography	Rarely of help in differentiating neck masses
Computed tomographic (CT) scanning	Single most informative test, but questionably cost effective
Skin and serologic testing for fungi	For suspected chronic or granulomatous inflammatory lesion
Open biopsy	Confirmation of diagnosis, indicated only after workup is complete and if diagnosis is not evident; involves specimen for histologic frozen section and preparation for simultaneous radical neck dissection
Needle biopsy (fine needle; No. 25 Vim-Silverman contraindicated)	Confirmation of diagnosis at time of panendoscopy if panendoscopic examination results are negative; requires expert head and neck cytopathologic assistance; indications and appropriateness still evolving
Cultures with sensitivities	For inflammatory tissue only

accuracy of differentiating solid, complex, and cystic lesions by ultrasound ranges from 90 to 95% (Can. Med. Assoc. J., *115*:35, 1976). A complex mass with irregular cystic centers or a solid mass with low echogenic centers indicates a necrotic tumor node or an abscess.

3. **Salivary gland lesions** For lesions of the salivary glands, radionuclide scanning, sialography, and ultrasonography are all of value (Trans. Am. Acad. Ophthalmol. Otolaryngol., *84*:750, 1977). In questionable cases, the radionuclide scan or the sialogram or both can usually indicate whether the mass is within or outside the salivary gland, and thus whether it is of glandular origin. This fact alone has important therapeutic implications; however, sialography is probably more valuable in the identification of various causes of diffuse salivary in-

volvement with sialadenitis and other sialadenopathies. Treatment decisions based on findings from ultrasonography or radionuclide scanning alone are fraught with danger, however. The use of those tests should not alter the time-proved approach of superficial lobectomy or total gland excision, with pathologic examination of the specimen to determine the proper treatment of salivary gland disease (Ann. Otol. Rhinol. Laryngol., *86*:247, 1977). In general, plain roentgenograms are of little help in differentiating masses in the neck. Computed tomography (CT) scanning of the neck may give much of the same information, but it is expensive and should be used only for the diagnostically difficult cases.

4. **Suspected inflammatory adenopathy** For the patient with suspected inflammatory adenopathy whose examination is otherwise negative, a clinical trial of antibiotics and observation, not exceeding 2 weeks, is acceptable. If the mass resolves, no further workup will be needed; if the mass persists or increases in size, additional investigation will be necessary. Serologic or skin tests for fungal disease are especially useful in the pediatric patient; in the adult patient with an outdoor occupation or hobby or with no history of usage of the usual carcinogenic agents who has a bilateral and symmetric enlargement with a palpable, soft consistency, in the patient with a mass that fluctuates in size, and in the patient with systemic toxic symptoms.

C. Nodal Mass Workup

If the foregoing considerations do not confirm the diagnosis, any neck mass, particularly a unilateral asymptomatic mass corresponding to the location of known lymph node groups, must be considered to be a metastatic neoplastic lesion until proved otherwise.

1. **Search for the primary lesion** must include a second, thorough examination of the oral cavity, nasopharynx, hypopharynx, larynx, thyroid, salivary glands, and skin of the scalp and face (Table 29–4). If that examination reveals no source of primary neoplasm or infection, the aerodigestive tract must be examined panendoscopically, with special attention to the region from which primary lymphatic drainage to the area of the mass occurs (see Fig. 29–2). Roentgenographic studies should be obtained, including chest films and a contrast study of the upper digestive tract only if the mass is supraclavicular in location. An obvious lesion should undergo biopsy. When no lesion is seen or palpated, "guided" biopsies from the most logical areas of primary tumor, based on known lymphatic drainage patterns, are indicated. These areas usually are the nasopharynx in the area of Rosenmüller's fossa, the tonsil (in which case, a tonsillectomy rather than an incisional biopsy is performed), the base of the tongue, and the pyriform sinus. The rationale for the "guided" biopsy when an obvious lesion is not present is that the primary tumor is often submucosal

TABLE 29–4

Diagnostic Workup of Asymmetric Unilateral, "Nodal" Masses of the Head and Neck		
1. Complete repeated physical examination of:		
	Oral cavity	Thyroid
	Nasopharynx	Salivary glands
	Hypopharynx	Skin of head and neck
	Larynx	
2. Roentgenograms before open biopsy of cervical mass:		
	Nasal sinuses	Upper aerodigestive tract
	Chest	
3. Roentgenograms after open biopsy, if positive for adenocarcinoma:		
Gastrointestinal tract		
Genitourinary tract		
Mammograms		
Salivary scans and sialograms		
4. Panendoscopic examination		
5. "Guided" biopsy of:		
	Nasopharynx	Base of tongue
	Midline Rosenmüller's fossa	Pyriform sinus
		Tonsils (tonsillectomy)
Fine needle biopsy of neck mass		
6. Open biopsy of cervical mass with frozen-section diagnosis if no primary lesion is found:		
	Epidermoid carcinoma or melanoma (simultaneous radical neck dissection)	
	Lymphoma (close and stage before radiation therapy, chemotherapy, or both)	
	Adenocarcinoma (close; further pursue primary lesion)	
	Granuloma or inflammation (culture and close)	

or arises deep in the crypts of the palatine tonsil or the folds of the lingual lymphoid tissue.

2. **Biopsy of the lesion** If none of the foregoing measures allows diagnosis of the neck mass, then open excisional biopsy is the next step. Some workers advocate a fine-needle aspiration biopsy to precede an open biopsy; if desired, the needle biopsy can be done at the time of the panendoscopic examination if panendoscopy yields negative findings. Biopsy with a Vim-Silverman needle may seed the needle track with tumor, however, and is thus contraindicated. The technique of obtaining multiple aspirations with a No. 25 fine-gauge needle is finding favor in many medical centers, and it is the recommended method for those who wish to perform a needle biopsy before an open biopsy. The operator who uses this technique should be experienced in the proper procedures for collection and slide preparation to guarantee maximal information. One also needs a skilled cytopathologist who not only has extensive experience in cytopathologic examination, but also has great familiarity with the various disorders of the head and neck re-

gion. At present, fine-needle biopsy has some limitations. Only the pathology departments of larger hospitals have competent cytopathologists, and only rarely are those persons also skilled in differentiating the various types of salivary tumors, lymphomas, and other solid tumors of the head and neck, which are often difficult to diagnose correctly even when the entire mass is available for study. Although it is important to be able to differentiate between neoplastic and nonneoplastic lesions, the diagnosis of a specific cell type is even more important because treatment of the neck mass varies by specific diagnosis. In addition to the problems of diagnosing the less-common tumors of the head and neck, difficulties in diagnosing the easily recognized squamous cell carcinomas often arise because of problems with sampling. Some workers also argue that a negative needle biopsy still requires open biopsy for confirmation if the clinician has a high index of suspicion, and a positive needle biopsy with a negative physical examination still dictates an open biopsy for confirmation and radical neck dissection. Other uses for needle biopsy include the provision of information on known thyroid nodules and the confirmation of an ultrasonic diagnosis of a cystic lesion. Fine-needle aspiration is indicated when the physician wants to avoid violating the lymphatic drainage of the neck in a patient with a known or suspected malignant neck mass that needs confirmation for staging or for the planning of nonoperative therapy and in the rare patient who is a poor candidate for operative therapy. Fine-needle aspiration is not without its risks, however. Hematoma, recurrent laryngeal nerve paresis, and tumor seeding along the needle tracks following needle puncture of thyroid nodules have all been reported.

III. INDIVIDUAL NECK MASSES

A. Neoplastic lesions

1. Metastatic Lesions

a. *Unknown primary lesion* Because of the obvious implications, any mass in the neck must be approached with the thought that it is neoplastic and possibly malignant (N.C. Med. J., *39*:299, 1978; Am. J. Surg., *134*:517, 1977). In fact, the fear of cancer usually brings the patient to the physician. In 1950, in a review of 1300 primary tumors of the head and neck, a cervical lump was the presenting symptom in 12.4% of cases (Ann. Surg., *132*:867, 1950). These authors stated that "asymmetric enlargement of one or more cervical lymph nodes in an adult is almost always cancerous and usually is due to metastasis from a primary lesion in the mouth or pharynx." That principle remains sound today. The key to the validity of the statement lies in the words "enlarged lymph node," "asymmetric," and "adults." If one remembers that primary cervical malignant tumors are rare and that practically all malignant cervical tumors, exclusive of lymphomas, are metastatic, and if the history taking and physical examination are thorough, one should not confuse metastatic malignant cervical tumors with inflammatory lymphadenopathy, cysts, and benign tumors of the neck. That an asymmetric neck mass in the adult must be considered malignant until proved otherwise is well documented (Mich. Med., *69*:581, 1970). Biopsies of neck masses in 163 patients seen consecutively in a community hospital showed that 29.4% of patients over 40 years of age had carcinoma and 21.4% had lymphoma. Those figures agree closely with the 50% incidence of neoplasia previously reported in neck masses (Lancet, *70*:420, 1950); the incidence of malignant disease in a neck mass rose to 80% in one series when benign thyroid nodules were excluded (Surg. Clin. North Am., *36*:3, 1956). A second principle is that the immediate removal of an enlarged lymph node for diagnostic purposes is a disservice to the patient with metastatic cervical carcinoma. Distant metastases and late regional recurrence are more common in patients who have pretreatment biopsies than in patients with the same stage of disease who do not undergo such a procedure (Table 29–5). The group with pretreatment biopsy also has a higher incidence of local wound complications. These findings suggest that disruption of lymphatic drainage and manipulation of metastatic tumor decrease the chances for clean surgical excision and cure. This alteration of the normal lymphatic drainage pattern by incisional therapy has been well documented by lymphadenography of the neck. Probably, no surgical condition is more easily detected in early physical examination and is more difficult to diagnose and to treat definitively than a malignant tumor of unknown

TABLE 29–5

Correlation of Wound Necrosis, Local and Distal Recurrence, and Time of Biopsy

	Biopsy before Definitive Treatment	Biopsy at Time of Definitive Treatment	No Biopsy
Variable Examined	No. of Patients (Incidence)	No. of Patients (Incidence)	No. of Patients (Incidence)
	(%)	(%)	(%)
Wound necrosis	13/64 (20.3)	5/46 (10.9)	98/605 (12.9)
Regional neck recurrence	21/64 (32.8)	11/46 (23.9)	116/600 (19.5)
Distant metastasis	25/63 (39.7)	11/46 (23.9)	131/598 (21.9)

primary origin located in the neck. Diagnosis and cure must be attempted, however, starting with a careful examination of the oral cavity, nasopharynx, hypopharynx, larynx, thyroid, salivary glands, and skin of the head and neck. In a series of 128 patients with cervical carcinoma diagnosed by excisional node biopsy, 65% had an obvious primary lesion of the head or neck (Ann. Surg., *132*:867, 1950). These findings correlate well with a more recent report, which stated that 52% of 259 patients had obvious primary lesions of the head or neck (Cancer, *51*:854, 1973). If the results of physical examination of the head and neck are negative, an otolaryngologist should be consulted to survey the less-accessible areas of the upper digestive and respiratory passages (see Table 29–4). If the results of that examination are negative, then direct panendoscopic examination should be done, roentgenograms should be obtained, and a thyroid scan should be considered, as noted earlier. If panendoscopic study provides no evidence of a primary lesion, the sites most likely to contain an occult tumor should undergo biopsy. The location of the involved lymph nodes should suggest the sites for biopsy (see Fig. 29–2). Enlarged lymph nodes in the superior portion of the neck or in the posterior triangle suggest a nasopharyngeal lesion, whereas enlarged jugulodigastric nodes point more to the tonsils and the laryngopharynx, including the base of the tongue. When the enlarged lymph nodes are in the supraclavicular area or in the inferior third of the neck, the whole length of the digestive tract, the tracheobronchial tree, the breast, the genitourinary tract, and the thyroid gland must be considered as the potential location of the primary lesion because such primary lesions metastasize to the inferior portion of the neck. Because of consideration of cost, only a thorough physical examination is usually done to screen the areas of the lower gastrointestinal and genitourinary tracts and the breast before proceeding to the next step of biopsy if these areas are negative. If the diagnostic workup is thorough and if the site of the primary lesion is still not apparent, an open excisional biopsy of the cervical lymph node should be performed; the patient should be aware that a complete neck dissection may be necessary. The biopsy must be done through an incision lying along a previously marked-out incision line for a radical neck dissection, and it is performed only if the surgeon is able and prepared to do a radical neck dissection if the frozen section sample indicates epidermoid carcinoma or melanoma. Other findings dictate a course as outlined previously in this chapter. Open biopsy is indicated only in approximately 5% of all cancer patients with an initially unknown lesion who undergo this diagnostic workup. For the patient with an unknown primary tumor and metastatic squamous cell carcinoma, postoperative irradiation of the nasopharynx, the ipsilateral tonsil, the base of the tongue, and the contralateral side of the neck is sometimes advocated following radical neck dissection. Others advocate only local nodal excisions with full-course irradiation of both sides of the neck and the pharynx from the base of the skull to the clavicles. This practice of prophylactic irradiation is still controversial. Arguments against it include the following: a high percentage of unknown primary lesions are from infraclavicular sites or are metastases of a previous small skin lesion that cannot be proved or assumed to be the source of the malignant process, and these lesions simply do not benefit from such a course of irradiation; prophylactic radiation therapy may compromise treatment of, and may even induce, later mucosal carcinoma; and postoperative radiation therapy may also cause major prolonged morbidity in the form of xerostomia, dysphagia, and dental caries. These factors must be weighed against the increases in cure rates observed from such a postoperative regimen. Jacques stated that, in 75% of patients whose lesions are diagnosed as unknown primary lesions or are histologically classified as undifferentiated after these patients have undergone a diligent workup, the primary source is not revealed, even when the follow-up period is extensive (American College of Surgeons Postgraduate Course No. 10, 1979, p. 51). The best argument for postoperative irradiation can be made for the patient whose lesion is staged N_2 or N_3, with operation alone reserved for the patient with N_1 disease without capsular extension. Clinicians who do not support the practice of postoperative irradiation prefer to rely on careful follow-up examination and treatment of the primary lesion when it is found. Patients with malignant metastatic cervical lymph nodes and unknown primary lesions must be followed-up closely at monthly intervals for the first year, every 2 months for the second year, and every 3 months for the third year. Only by such careful follow-up can early detection and treatment of the primary tumor be ensured. In the past, the most common site of a late-appearing primary lesion was the nasopharynx because it is the most difficult area to examine and biopsy was not routinely done. Today, the most common locations of primary tumors that later become evident are the hypopharynx, the tonsil, and the base of the tongue.

b. ***Known primary lesion*** The neck mass in a patient with a known primary neoplasm of the head and neck should be treated in accordance with the principles described for each primary site in other chapters of this book. In general, when clinically positive cervical lymph node metastases are present, a complete cervical lymphadenectomy by radical neck dissection should be performed. When the primary lesion is not in the head or neck, excisional biopsy of the metastatic cervical mass for confirmation and staging is indicated, with further treatment dictated by the primary lesion. One should follow the suggestions given previously for patients with unknown primary lesions, to be certain that the mass in question is not a manifestation of a second, independent primary lesion of the head or neck. The incidence of second, concomitant, independent primary lesions is approximately 15% in patients with a head or neck neoplasm. An incidence of 6% for second silent aerodigestive tract tumors is found only if a full panendoscopic examination is performed (Laryngoscope, *92*:569, 1982). Knowledge of a second lesion may affect treatment decisions and may allow better prognostic counseling of the patient. Correlations of concomitant tumor sites include larynx with lung, tonsil with esophagus, and oral cavity with oral cavity.

2. **Primary lesions**

   a. ***Thyroid neoplasms,*** both benign and malignant, are a leading cause of anterior-compartment neck masses in all age groups and, along with malignant tumors of the lymph nodes, are the most common neoplastic lesions in the young and young adult groups. The young group frequently shows a male predominance as well as an increased incidence of malignant disease, in contradistinction to the young adult and older groups, which show a greater incidence of benign conditions and a female predominance. Lymph node metastasis is the initial symptom in about 15% of patients with papillary carcinoma, and up to 40% of patients with malignant thyroid nodules have a positive lymph node in the neck when first seen or at operation. Although the majority of thyroid nodules are hyperplastic goiter nodules or adenomas, they must be considered malignant until proved otherwise. Sonic scanning, isotopic scanning, thyroid function tests, and tests to detect thyroid antibodies are in order. Correlation of the nodule to hot or cold areas on the thyroid scan locates the source of the mass, and a peripheral area of uptake separate from the normal gland indicates ectopic or metastatic thyroid disease. Functioning nodules may be treated medically, but all nonfunctioning, cold nodules should be explored surgically with appropriate measures taken, depending on the cell type (frozen section) and extent of disease. For specific thyroid tests and treatment, see Chapter 30.

   b. ***Lymphomas, Hodgkin's disease, and lymphosarcomas,*** like thyroid neoplasms, are seen in all age groups, but they are statistically more likely to occur in, and to form a greater percentage of all neoplasms in, the young and young adult age groups (Ear Nose Throat J., *57*:136, 1978; South. Med. J., *71*:277, 1978). These lesions alone account for up to 55% of all pediatric malignant diseases. Local head and neck symptoms, except for progressive enlargement of lymph node tissue, are usually absent, but systemic and other complaints and findings, such as fever, diffuse adenopathy and hepatosplenomegaly, should be sought. Lymphomas are usually discrete, rubbery, and nontender, as opposed to squamous nodes, which are hard, tender, and often matted. Lymphomas may involve multiple groups of lymph nodes, as well as being multiple within a single group of nodes. Up to 40% of children with lymphosarcoma and 80% of children with Hodgkin's disease have a neck mass. In the youth and young adult with an enlarging neck mass, after examination of appropriate peripheral blood smears and chest films, one should perform an open biopsy with histologic examination, followed later by appropriate staging procedures. The immediate biopsy in these younger patients, following complete physical and laryngopharyngoscopic examination but preceding the full head and neck workup advocated previously in this chapter, is permissible because of the rarity of mucosal primary carcinoma in these age groups. If routine physical or laryngopharyngoscopic examination reveals an abnormality of Waldeyer's ring, that abnormality should undergo biopsy for staging purposes at the time of neck node biopsy.

c. ***Salivary neoplasms*** must be considered whenever an enlarging solid mass lies anterior and inferior to the ear, at the angle of the mandible, or in the submandibular triangle. Benign salivary lesions are asymptomatic, except for their presence, but symptoms of seventh-nerve (parotid), twelfth-nerve, and lingual nerve (submaxillary) involvement or skin fixation should suggest a malignant disease. Diagnostic tests, such as radionuclide scanning and sialography, indicate whether the mass is salivary in origin, but they do not help in the histologic classification of the lesion. The diagnostic test of preference is open biopsy, either by complete gland removal or by superficial parotidectomy, depending on the location of the lesion. Preoperative neurologic involvement or an intraoperative finding of nerve involvement by the tumor should dictate tumor resection with nerve resection and grafting. As with unknown primary lesions of the neck, in which the surgeon planning to do a lymph node biopsy must be prepared to perform an immediate radical neck dissection, the surgeon approaching masses in and around the ear should be prepared to perform a total parotidectomy and facial-nerve dissection. Any less radical approach diminishes the patient's chance for a complete cure. For further discussion of salivary gland disease, see Chapter 20.

d. ***Lipomas*** are ill-defined soft masses occurring in various neck locations, usually in patients over 35 years of age. They are asymptomatic, have no specific diagnostic characteristics, and are confirmed only by excisional biopsy.

e. ***Angiomas,*** in the form of lymphangiomas and hemangiomas, whether capillary, cavernous, or mixed, are considered congenital lesions when they occur in children and are discussed later in this chapter. Angiomatous masses occurring in middle-aged and older persons are usually aggressive lesions, such as hemangiosarcomas, lymphangiosarcomas, and hemangiopericytomas. For both benign and malignant angiomatous masses, the physical findings of compressibility, increased warmth, bruit, thrill, and bluish purple coloration are suggestive of the type of lesion; angiography both confirms the diagnosis and allows preoperative evaluation of the extent of tumor.

f. ***Carotid body and glomus tumors*** are rare or nonexistent in the pediatric patient (Arch. Otol., *101*:58, 1975). In adults, either tumor classically occurs in the superoanterior triangle at the carotid bifurcation as a pulsatile, compressible mass that rapidly refills on release and is movable from side to side but not superiorly or inferiorly. A bruit and thrill are present and, in glomus vagale tumors, the ipsilateral tonsil may pulsate and may be deviated toward the midline. The diagnosis is made by angiographic study. A carotid body or glomus tumor is resected in young adults and in elderly patients showing rapid tumor growth, impingement of the tumor on vital structures, or obstructive symptoms in the oropharynx or hypopharynx. Resection should be done under hypotensive, hypothermic anesthesia. Before the tumor is manipulated surgically, catecholamine production must be measured, to prepare for the dysrhythmias and the hypertensive crisis that may result from catecholamine release. Biopsy before resection is contraindicated. Carotid artery aneurysm may be mistaken for a carotid body tumor, but angiographic study distinguishes between these disorders.

g. ***Schwannomas or neurilemomas*** are solid neurogenic tumors that may occur anywhere in the neck, but are most common in the parapharyngeal space (Surg. Gynecol. Obstet., *111*:211, 1960; Trans. Am. Acad. Ophthalmol. Otolaryngol., *80*:459, 1975). They have no diagnostic characteristics, although origin from the vagus nerve may cause hoarseness accompanying the mass, and origin from the sympathetic chain may be associated with Horner's syndrome. Routine evaluation for an unknown primary tumor is indicated before surgical exploration and excision are performed.

h. ***Rhabdomyosarcoma*** may cause a metastatic neck mass in children, but the primary lesion is almost always evident elsewhere, usually in the orbit, the pharynx, or the ear. No specific prebiopsy test aids in the diagnosis.

B. Congenital and Developmental Disorders

1. **Sebaceous and epidermal cysts** are common in the older age group. Each cyst appears as a variably sized, slowly increasing, firm, smooth, nontender, painless mass, often exhibiting a corresponding dimple in the overlying skin. The lesion usually elevates the skin and moves with it. No specific diagnostic tests exist; diagnosis is by excisional biopsy and observation of "cheesy" keratin within the cyst. Pathologic examination confirms this diagnosis.
2. **Branchial cleft cysts** most commonly occur in late childhood or early adulthood (Laryngoscope, *79*:30, 1969; *82*:1581, 1972). These cysts frequently follow an upper respiratory tract infection, appearing as initially inflammatory lesions with symptoms of pain, swelling, tenderness to palpation, and local and systemic temperature elevation. After treatment with appropriate antibiotics, they may resolve, but more often they persist as soft, doughy, variably sized masses in several characteristic locations in the anterior triangle of the neck. The more common second branchial cleft cyst occurs deep to and along the anterior edge of the sternocleidomastoid muscle. The less common first branchial cyst occurs along the inferior mandible, at the angle of the mandible, or just inferior to the ear lobule. Ultrasonic scans can be helpful in identifying the lesions as cystic rather than solid. Aspiration of the contents reveals a milky, mucoid, or brownish fluid that often contains cholesterol crystals. Treatment involves initial control of local infection followed by surgical excision. For first branchial cleft cysts, one must be prepared and able to do a total parotidectomy with facial-nerve dissection and preservation. The lesion recurs unless the entire branchial tract to its most medial extent is removed. In general, incision and drainage of a lesion believed to be branchiogenic should be avoided because such a procedure complicates the later dissection. Should the cyst drain spontaneously or undergo incision and drainage preoperatively, with a resultant fistula, injection of methylene blue into the sinus tract 24 hours before excision may facilitate its removal.
3. **Thyroglossal duct cysts** Like branchial cysts, these midline structures in the anterior neck often appear after an upper respiratory tract infection (Am. J. Surg., *102*:494, 1961). Once the acute infection has been controlled by antibiotics, ultrasonography can be used to differentiate the persistent mass from a lymph node, a dermoid cyst, or thyroid tissue. Physical examination documents the diagnostic finding of vertical mo-

tion of the mass during swallowing and tongue protrusion. Radionuclide scanning should be done to ascertain whether the mass contains ectopic tissue that constitutes the only functioning thyroid tissue. The cyst's tract should be removed totally with the midportion of the hyoid bone (Sistrunk procedure). On occasion, lateral extension of the thyroglossal tract tissue can be identified and should be removed to prevent recurrence.

4. **Lymphangiomas** usually occur in the youngest age group; most are present at birth, and over 90% are evident within the first year of life. Those lesions in the neck most commonly appear in the posterior triangle. The cervical lymphangioma is a fluctuant, diffuse, soft, spongy mass, often with indiscrete margins. It may enlarge when upper respiratory tract infections are present. It is believed to arise from incomplete development and obstruction of the normal lymphatic system, and its extent is often much greater than is apparent. Transillumination is diagnostic, along with the physical appearance and the characteristics on palpation. Treatment is by surgical excision if the lesion is easily accessible or affects vital functions. Removal should not be attempted if it requires a mutilating procedure for limited benefits. Often, surgical treatment precipitates further manifestations of the disease in areas not clinically visible, and recurrence is thus common.

5. **Hemangiomas** Like lymphangiomas, hemangiomas are usually considered congenital because, in almost every instance, they are either present at birth or apparent within the first year of life (Postgrad. Med., *19*:262, 1956). These lesions are also classified as capillary, cavernous, and mixed. Although more common in the facial than in the cervical area, these lesions may occur in any area of the neck or in salivary gland tissue. Their bluish purple coloration, warmth, compressibility followed by refilling, bruit, and thrill help to identify them. Angiographic study is diagnostic, but it is rarely indicated. Treatment involves observation only, unless rapid growth, thrombocytopenia, or involvement of vital structures occurs; most of these congenital lesions resolve. Those that do not may later be resected or tattooed for cosmetic effect.

6. **Dermoid cysts** occur most commonly in childhood and early adulthood in the cervical areas corresponding to branchial and thyroglossal cysts (Arch. Surg., *109*:822, 1974). These cysts slowly enlarge because of accumulation of the sebaceous content, but unlike sebaceous cysts, they lie deep to the cervical fascia with the skin freely movable over them. No specific diagnostic tests exist, other than pathologic examination after surgical excision. These lesions can be differentiated from other cystic lesions by ultrasonography.

7. **Ectopic thyroid tissue** may occur in any age group and usually

appears as a midcompartment, anterior neck mass corresponding to the embryologic descent of the thyroid gland from the foramen cecum to the inferior portion of the neck. Occasional lateral neck masses appearing as normal thyroid tissue occur and, although classified as ectopic thyroid tissue, are best treated and explained as metastatic thyroid carcinomas. Thyroid scanning, which should be done in every patient with a midline lesion, confirms the presence of thyroid tissue.

8. **Laryngocele** can be either a developmental or a degenerative cyst. It is rare, but once it is present and attains considerable size, it typically appears just lateral to the thyroid cartilage. When it contains air, this lesion decompresses on palpation. Frequently, a history of voice changes and a Valsalva maneuver type of activity in the patient's occupation or hobby may be elicited, as in musicians or glassblowers. Soft tissue films of the neck or CT scans may show an air-containing cyst or an air-fluid level. Surgical excision is the treatment of choice.

9. **Pharyngeal diverticulum (Zenker's)** results from a congenital weakness or deficiency in the fibers of the inferior constrictor muscle just superior to the cricopharyngeus muscle, known as Killian's triangle. The mass is usually ill-defined, soft, and compressible and is associated with a burping sound on compression. The lesion occurs in older persons and produces dysphagia due to a lump in the throat, regurgitation of undigested food, and aspiration. Barium contrast studies are diagnostic, and treatment is by surgical excision (Arch. Otol., *105*:254, 1979). See Chapter 22.

10. **Thymic cysts** These rare cysts occur most often in boys between 4 and 7 years of age (Laryngoscope, *87*:1645, 1977; J. Pediatr. Surg., *10*:141, 1975). They form a painless swelling in the neck that occasionally enlarges during the Valsalva maneuver. These cysts lie within the carotid sheath and parallel to the sternocleidomastoid muscle. No specific preoperative tests are available for diagnosis, which must be confirmed by excisional biopsy.

C. Inflammatory Disorders

1. **Lymphadenitis** occurs in nearly every person at some point in life, especially during the first decade. Lymphadenopathy in response to bacterial or viral infections of the upper respiratory tract is so common that it is expected. Frequent sites of primary infection are the tonsils, pharynx, ears, scalp, teeth, and gums. The medical history and physical findings of infection of those primary sites are covered elsewhere in this text. In general, the source of the reactive lymphadenopathy is easily identified. Antibiotic therapy directed against gram-positive and anaerobic organisms is recommended, unless specific culture and sensitivity tests indicate the presence of other

organisms. In general, the enlarged lymph nodes occur in both the anterior and posterior triangles in patterns consistent with infection in the primary sites indicated in Figure 29–1. The lymph nodes are usually tender and mobile. Multiple nodal involvement may cause the lymph nodes to become matted together and to appear as a single, irregular mass. These nodal masses often persist for days, weeks, or years, and their rubbery consistency gives way in time to fibrosis. The mass does regress in size or, more important, does not grow larger, once the primary viral or bacterial infection is controlled, however. No specific diagnostic test exists, other than excisional biopsy with pathologic examination and culture. Biopsy should be limited to patients with progressively enlarging multiple lymph nodes; a single asymmetric nodal mass; a persistent nodal mass without antecedent active signs of infection; and actively infectious conditions that do not respond to conventional antibiotics and in which routine bacteriologic determinations are unsuccessful in identifying the infecting organism. A tissue sample is needed for further bacteriologic studies. Biopsy should only be performed after a complete head and neck examination has been done by a clinician using indirect, direct, endoscopic, and radiologic methods. This indication is especially applicable to adults because the incidence of mucosal malignant disease is high in that age group and biopsy of such a malignant nodal lesion may alter the prognosis.

2. **Granulomatous lymphadenitis** This inflammatory condition in the neck may result from infection with typical or atypical Mycobacterium tuberculosis, actinomycosis, histoplasmosis, sarcoidosis, and cat-scratch fever. Lymphadenitis from atypical tuberculosis is more likely to occur in children and to involve discrete lymph nodes in the anterior triangle of the neck. True tuberculous involvement, on the other hand, is more common in adults and in the posterior triangle and causes large, matted groups of lymph nodes. Actinomycosis most often occurs in the submandibular and superior jugular lymph nodes and results from dental infections. Cat-scratch fever lymphadenitis is seen predominantly in the pediatric age group as a single, tender, inflamed lymph node in the preauricular or submandibular area that may develop suppuration. Unlike other granulomatous disorders, this lesion often undergoes spontaneous resolution without treatment. Although results of skin or serologic tests are often positive in some of the granulomatous diseases, bacteriologic study is usually necessary for confirmation. Surgical intervention is employed for obtaining material for culture and microscopic examination to confirm the diagnosis. Biopsy of the nodal masses in the form of complete excision is usually curative as well. Incisional biopsy generally causes chronic drainage from the site and thus should

be avoided (J. Laryngol. Otol., *89*:933, 1975; J. Pediatr. Surg., *10*:419, 1975).

3. **Sialadenitis** of either the parotid or the submaxillary gland may present as a preauricular or a submandibular mass. Pain, the most common symptom, is made worse by eating; it may be associated with a "bad" taste. Signs of systemic toxicity, such as fever and leukocytosis, are present, as are local tenderness and warmth. The diagnosis is confirmed by expressing pus from the appropriate ducts. Antibiotics, hydration, and removal of any obstruction in the duct allow rapid resolution. Sialadenopathy, or diffuse noninflammatory enlargement of the salivary glands, may appear as symmetric, bilateral, neck masses and can usually be diagnosed by medical history, location, and sialographic study. Occasionally, open biopsy is necessary for diagnosis. See Chapter 20.
4. **Thorotrast granulomas** These inflammatory lesions are rare, but are usually easily diagnosed by roentgenograms and a history of prior contrast roentgenographic studies (Laryngoscope, *86*:1633, 1976).

30

THYROID DISEASE

ROBERT M. BUMSTED AND ARNOLD E. KATZ

Diseases of the thyroid gland result from qualitative or quantitative alterations in hormone secretion or enlargement of the thyroid gland. When hormone secretion is insufficient, hypothyroidism or myxedema results. Excessive secretion of thyroid hormones causes hypermetabolism. Enlargement of the gland may be diffuse or focal and may be associated with either of the foregoing syndromes. Treatment of thyroid disease must be preceded by a full evaluation of the cause of the disorder and the metabolic state of the patient. In patients with thyroid gland enlargement, one must rule out the presence of malignant disease.

I. EVALUATION OF THYROID FUNCTION

The synthesis and release of thyroid hormones have extra- and intrathyroidal controls. The hypothalamus releases thyrotropin-releasing hormone (TRH), which stimulates the pituitary gland to release thyroid-stimulating hormone (TSH). TSH stimulates the thyroid gland to increase iodine uptake and to synthesize and release the biologically active thyroid hormones, thyroxine (T_4) and triiodothyronine (T_3). These hormones, in turn, exert a negative effect at the pituitary gland to decrease the amount of TSH released and thereby slow the uptake of iodine and the production of thyroidal hormones by the thyroid gland. Although T_4 and T_3 are almost entirely bound to plasma proteins, specifically thyroxine-binding globulin (TBG), regulation of thyroid function is directed toward maintenance of a normal concentration of free or unbound hormone rather than the total amount of protein-bound and free hormone. The free or unbound hormone is the only one available to the tissue and therefore correlates most closely with the metabolic state of the patient. This factor leads to difficulties in the laboratory analysis of thyroid disease because the measurement of free hormone is more difficult than the measurement of total hormone in the blood. In some clinical situations, the total amounts of T_4 and T_3 in the blood are elevated, although the absolute concentration of free hormone may be normal and the metabolic state of the patient is normal. Because of these and other difficulties, several different techniques have been devised in an attempt to evaluate thyroid function accurately.

A. Radioactive Iodine Uptake (RAIU)

This direct test of thyroid function varies directly with the functional state of the thyroid gland and inversely with the plasma idodide concentration. The test does not distinguish well between normal and hypothyroid states; however, values above the normal range (5 to 30% of the administrated dose) indicate thyroid hyperfunction. This test is only valuable in distinguishing among different types of thyrotoxicosis. Iodine-induced hyperthyroidism, thyrotoxicosis factitia, painless, chronic thyroiditis, and the painful subacute thyroiditis are all associated with a low value of the RAIU test. It is important to differentiate these conditions from a gland that is actively producing and secreting large amounts of thyroid hormone because treatment of these conditions varies. Currently, this test is used only in evaluating thyroid hyperfunction.

B. Serum Protein Bound Iodine (PBI)

This test was once used as an indirect means of assessing serum T_4 and serum T_3 concentrations. The results of this test were frequently misleading because they were largely reflections of the amount of iodine-binding proteins in the blood and not reflections of the amount of thyroid hormone, a closer representation of the metabolic state of the patient. This test as well as the basal metabolic rate (BMR) is rarely used at present for evaluating thyroid function because the following tests are more accurate.

C. Quantification of Thyroid Hormones

The most commonly used test for evaluating the level of serum thyroid hormone is the competitive protein-binding displacement assay (Murphy-Patee). Radioimmunoassay is the most sensitive and accurate method of evaluating levels of T_4 and T_3 separately.

D. Triiodothyronine (T_3) Uptake

This test is used to measure the amount of thyroid binding proteins in the serum. Radioactive labeled T_3 is added to the serum and then a resin sponge is added that absorbs the non-protein-bound labeled hormone. The percentage of the radioactive hormone absorbed by the resin is reported as the result. Thus, the level of thyroid binding proteins varies inversely with the percent level of the test result. The higher the protein level, the lower the percent uptake. Combining the results of the serum hormone levels and the T_3 uptake provides the most accurate assessment of thyroid function. The free hormone (metabolically active) level is reflected by a mathematically derived result of these two tests (serum hormone and thyroid binding proteins). This is often referred to as the free thyroxine index or T_7. This is currently the best method of evaluating thyroid function.

E. Serum Concentration of Thyroid-Stimulating Hormone (TSH)

This valuable test aids in the diagnosis of overt and subclinical hypothyroidism. The normal range of TSH is less than 5 μU/ml, as measured by radioimmunoassay. Current sensitivity does not allow one to distinguish between normal and low values; however, elevated levels of TSH are invariably present in untreated hypothyroidism of thyroid origin. When the hypothyroidism is of pituitary or hypothalamic origin, values are either undetectable or normal. In thyrotoxicosis, serum TSH levels are undetectable, except in rare patients with a pituitary tumor that produces TSH-induced hyperthyroidism. The only other rare possibility is that if the TSH produced by the pituitary gland is not biologically active, one will note hypothyroidism with elevated rather than depressed serum TSH concentrations. In general, however, when TSH levels are increased in the hypothyroid patient, the hypothyroidism is of thyroid origin and is not induced by defects of the hypothalamus or pituitary gland.

F. Thyrotropin-Releasing Hormone (TRH) Stimulation Test

Following the injection of TRH in normal subjects, the pituitary secretes TSH and reaches its maximum 20 to 45 minutes after the initial injection. This level rapidly declines. When pituitary function is impaired, responses to TRH are abnormal. In a patient with hypothyroidism, one expects vigorous response of the pituitary to the TRH, whereas little or no response is expected in patients with thyrotoxicosis. Responses to TRH are also decreased in elderly individuals, especially men. A subnormal or absent response to TRH is usually an excellent confirmatory test for thyrotoxicosis. If hypothyroidism is induced by malfunction of the pituitary gland, the patient will have no response to TRH, except the rare patient who secretes biologically inactive TSH. Currently, this test is best used to detect early or borderline hypothyroidism and to evaluate the possible suppression of TSH production by thyroid hormone replacement (oral ingestion) therapy. In both of these situations, the administration of TRH will not produce an increase in serum TSH levels.

G. Cytomel (T_3) Suppression Test

This test is based on the observation that exogenous thyroid hormone normally suppresses pituitary TSH secretion, with a resulting decrease in the RAIU. A normal response is a decrease in the RAIU to less than half of control value and a decrease in the serum T_4 level because triiodothyronine is employed in the test (.075 to .1 mg daily for 10 days). An abnormal suppression test result is seen in hyperthyroidism, irrespective of the underlying cause, and may indicate either hypersecretion of TSH, the presence of an abnormal stimulator, or the autonomy of thyroid function. A normal suppression test result is incompatible with hyperthyroidism, but an abnormal suppression test result is not pathognomonic of hyperthyroidism because it may occur in seemingly euthyroid patients. Extreme caution must be used in testing elderly patients, in whom severe cardiovascular disease may be induced.

H. Technetium or Iodine Scanning and Ultrasonography

A radioactive scan is used to determine whether a thyroid nodule is functioning. A functioning nodule takes up the radioactive material and is considered to be "warm" or "hot" (malignancy less likely), while a nonfunctioning nodule fails to demonstrate uptake on the scan and is "cold" (malignancy more likely). Technetium is slightly less accurate than iodine but has the advantage of exposing the patient to a lower dose of radiation and allowing the scan to be obtained 1 hour after administration rather than 6 to 24 hours if iodine is used. It is also helpful in defining areas of increased or decreased function within the thyroid and in detecting ectopic thyroid, partial agenesis of the thyroid, functioning metastasis of thyroid carcinoma, and retrosternal goiters. Ultrasonography may also be useful in the evaluation of thyroid nodules. One should be able to differentiate solid from cystic lesions of the thyroid accurately 80 to 90% of the time.

I. Thyroid Antibody Tests

It is now possible to detect many antibodies involved in a variety of thyroid disorders. These antibodies are common features of autoimmune (Hashimoto's) thyroiditis (massive elevations). More moderate elevations are present in Graves' disease, acute thyroiditis, and in some types of thyroid cancer.

J. Fine-Needle Aspiration or Biopsy

In the hands of experienced pathologists and cytologists, this technique is over 90% accurate. It may be helpful in the diagnosis of diffuse thyroid enlargement thought to be thyroiditis or other nodules considered to be benign. Some workers believe that this technique should not be used if one suspects a differentiated malignant tumor. Open biopsy should be performed in patients with suspected thyroid carcinoma. Recent growth of a thyroid nodule or mass especially if painless; hoarseness; a history of X-ray therapy to the head, neck, or upper mediastinum in infancy or childhood; or demonstration by physical examination of a nodular mass fixed to the surrounding structures indicates that an open biopsy will probably be necessary unless an experienced thyroid cytologist is able to diagnose the lesion with fine-needle aspiration.

II. DISEASES OF THE THYROID

A. Nontoxic Goiter

Nontoxic or simple goiter may be defined as any enlargement of the thyroid gland that does not result from a neoplastic or inflammatory process. The condition is not initially associated with hyper- or hypothyroidism. When one or more factors impair the ability of the thyroid gland to secrete sufficient quantities of active hormones, the thyroid gland increases in mass and cellular activity to overcome this mild or moderate impairment of hormone synthesis. The patient remains metabolically normal, and laboratory findings demonstrate essentially normal thyroid function. If the underlying disorder is severe, however, compensatory responses may be inadequate, and the patient may develop hypothyroidism. It is also possible in this process for the gland to have a multinodular stage, often accompanied by the development of functional autonomy. At this point, hyperthyroidism may ensue spontaneously, or it may be induced by large quantities of iodide (Jod-Basedow phenomenon).

1. **Clinical symptoms** In simple goiter, the clinical manifestations arise solely from enlargement of the thyroid gland. Mechanical sequelae may include compression and displacement of the trachea or esophagus or the development of superior mediastinal obstruction in patients with large retrosternal goiters. Sudden hemorrhage into a nodule may lead to acute, painful swelling. The incidence of cretinism is increased in the children of parents with goiter.

2. **Therapy** The object of treatment is to reverse the thyroid hyperplasia either by promoting normal hormone function or by providing sufficient quantities of exogenous hormone to inhibit the TSH secretion and to put the gland at rest. If the cause is decreased thyroid iodine stores, small doses of iodine may prove helpful. More commonly, however, no specific etiologic factors can be demonstrated, and the patient is treated with sodium levothyroxine (Synthroid). In the younger patient, .1 mg daily is given, and the dose is increased over the next month to .15 to .2 mg daily. The TSH should decrease to a very low level. Special care must be used in initiating thyroid hormone replacement therapy in patients with severe myxedema and cardiac disease. If the thyroid deficiency is secondary to panhypopituitarism, then adrenal corticoid replacement must be initiated prior to thyroid replacement. In these patients, doses are initially low and are slowly increased. Surgical therapy of simple goiter is not usually necessary.

B. Hypothyroidism

This disorder is caused by a deficiency of thyroid hormone production that may result from any of three different disorders. Primary hypothyroidism is caused by malfunction of the thyroid gland itself. Although the gland is stimulated appropriately by the pituitary, which in turn is stimulated by the hypothalamus, the gland is unable to perform its function. Secondary hypothyroidism, a result of pituitary malfunction, can be diagnosed by the TRH stimulation test. When the hypothalamus is not producing TRH, a tertiary hypothyroidism is said to exist.

1. **Cretinism** is caused by hypothyroidism dating from birth; however, the manifestations are more commonly evident within the first several months of life.
   a. ***Clinical presentation*** Signs and symptoms include dwarfism, mental retardation, failure to thrive, umbilical hernia, enlarged tongue, and hyporeflexia. Abnormally long persistence of physiologic jaundice, hoarse cry, constipation, somnolence, and feeding problems should call attention to the diagnosis. X-ray examination reveals retarded bone age and epiphyseal dysgenesis along with delayed dental development. Mental development is retarded; however, eventual intellectual accomplishments depend on how soon full replacement therapy is instituted.
   b. ***Therapy*** involves replacement of thyroid hormone as soon as possible. Neonatal hypothyroidism can be diagnosed from measurements of serum T_4 or serum TSH in either umbilical cord blood or infants' blood. One in every 5000 infants is estimated to be hypothyroid. Therefore, every newborn should undergo screening for this disease, so treatment can be instituted as soon as possible. Sodium levothyroxine (Synthroid), 0.025 mg/day, is employed initially, and the dosage is gradually increased over the following 8 weeks. Most infants require 0.05 mg/day until they are a year old. If goiter is present, the degree of respiratory obstruction must also be evaluated.
2. **Adult hypothyroidism** is an insidious disease with many nonspecific symptoms such as lethargy, constipation, cold intolerance, and menorrhagia. Slowing of intellectual and motor activity may occur, and the patient usually has a modest weight gain in spite of a declining appetite. Otolaryngologic manifestations may include thyroid gland enlargement, hearing loss, tongue enlargement, nasal obstruction, and hoarseness due to edema of the vocal cords. If the disorder remains untreated, the patient with severe, long-standing hypothyroidism may pass into a hypothermic, stuporous state (myxedema), which is frequently fatal. The serum TSH level is increased in the thyroprival variety of hypothyroidism and is usually normal or undetectable in pituitary or hypothalamic hypothyroidism. One usually finds an increased serum cholesterol level in hypothyroidism and increased concentrations in serum levels of creatine phosphokinase, glutamic oxaloacetic transaminase, and lactic dehydrogenase. Electrocardiographic changes are common and include bradycardia, low-amplitude QRS com-

plexes, and flattened or inverted T-waves. Pernicious anemia is present 10% of the time, and histamine-fast achlorhydria is also common. Treatment should involve replacement of thyroid using synthetic hormones such as sodium levothyroxine (Synthroid). The average daily dose .15 mg. Restoration must be undertaken gradually in adults, and an initial daily dose of .025 mg levothyroxine is recommended. This dose can be increased by .025 to .05 mg 2- to 3-week intervals until a normal metabolic state is attained. In cretinism and juvenile hypothyroidism, it is essential to begin full replacement therapy as soon as possible. In patients with known or suspected pituitary and hypothalamic hypothyroidism, thyroid replacement should not be instituted until treatment with hydrocortisone has been initiated.

C. Hyperthyroidism

When the tissues of the body are exposed to an excess supply of active thyroid hormone, the clinical syndrome of hyperthyroidism results. Symptoms include weakness, nervousness, restlessness, weight loss with increased appetite, heat intolerance, excessive sweating, tachycardia, warm, moist skin, tremor, inability to sleep, oligomenorrhea and amenorrhea, dyspnea, palpitations, and enhancement of angina or the development of cardiac failure. The nervous symptoms dominate the picture in younger individuals, whereas cardiovascular problems predominate in older patients. Palmar erythema is often found, and the hair becomes fine and silky. Fine tremors of the fingers and tongue are characteristic, along with hyperreflexia. One observes widening of the palpebral fissure, infrequent blinking, lid lag, failure to wrinkle the brow on upward gaze, and a characteristic stare. Also present are the following: a wide pulse pressure, sinus tachycardia, atrial arrhythmias, systolic murmurs, cardiac enlargement, and occasionally, overt heart failure. The most common cause of hyperthyroidism is Graves' disease (diffuse, toxic goiter), which usually produces hyperthyroidism, ophthalmopathy, and localized or pretibial myxedema. Other causes include autonomous toxic nodules, thyroiditis, excessive thyroid hormone ingestion, or tumors inappropriately secreting TSH. Hyperthyroidism is also seen in T_3 toxicosis, T_4 toxicosis, and in the Jod-Basedow phenomenon. The Jod-Basedow phenomenon occurs in a previously euthyroid patient as a result of exposure to increased quantities of iodine.

1. **Medical therapy** depends on the cause of the disease. The following regimen applies to most patients with hyperthyroidism. Treatment of thyroiditis, thyroid carcinoma, and iodine-induced thyrotoxicosis must, of course, be individualized.
   a. ***Iodide*** promptly inhibits thyroid hormone release from the hyperfunctioning gland. It also inhibits thyroid hormone synthesis, but this effect usually lasts only 3 or 4 weeks. Because therapy does not control hyperthyroidism

for long periods, it should be confined to the treatment of thyroid storm or to the preparation for thyroid operations. A regimen of 1 to 2 drops of supersaturated potassium iodide (SSKI), given 3 times a day in water or juice, provides sufficient iodide and is associated with toxic side effects less frequently than higher-dose regimens. Such side effects include skin rashes, salivary gland swelling, and gynecomastia.

b. ***Thiourea derivatives*** Propylthiouracil inhibits hormone formation, but because these drugs mainly act by preventing the formation of thyroid hormone, they have no effect for about 2 to 3 weeks. The usual starting dose for propylthiouracil is 150 mg 3 to 4 times a day. Methimazole can be given 2 to 3 times a day, and its usual starting dose is 20 to 60 mg/day. Propylthiouracil is available in 50-mg tablets, and methimazole is available in 5- and 10-mg tablets. A normal metabolic state is usually obtained within 6 weeks. Toxic effects include skin rash, fever, arthralgia, diarrhea, salivary gland enlargement, and hepatitis. Agranulocytosis has been reported, but it is usually reversible. Periodic white blood cell counts should be done because leukopenia may occur suddenly and, if not detected early, may lead to lethal infection.

c. ***Propranolol*** is a beta-adrenergic blocking agent that can control the peripheral manifestations of hyperthyroidism. The agent improves or abolishes tremor, tachycardia, nervousness, and excessive sweating. Propranolol is usually contraindicated in patients with low-output congestive heart failure; however, its use may improve the cardiac status of the patient in high-output congestive heart failure and tachycardia caused by thyrotoxicosis. Propranolol should only be used as an adjunct and not as sole therapy because the underlying metabolic abnormalities are not affected by the drug. Its use as a sole agent in preparation for thyroidectomy is not recommended; propranolol does not render the patient euthyroid, and a surgically induced crisis may result. In doses of 40 to 120 mg daily, the drug may be useful while waiting for a response to conventional antithyroid agents and in the management of thyrotoxic crisis.

d. ***Radioactive iodine (^{131}I)*** is a simple, effective, and economical means of treating thyrotoxicosis. It limits the secretion of thyroid hormone by destroying thyroid tissue. The principal disadvantage of this therapy is its tendency to produce hypothyroidism in 40 to 70% of patients within 10 years of treatment. The insidious onset of this complication may obscure diagnosis, and therapy may not be instituted until serious complications have already developed. It may be helpful to give all patients treated with

^{131}I permanent physiologic replacement doses of thyroid hormone.

2. **Surgical therapy** usually includes a subtotal thyroidectomy and is an effective means of treating this condition. Surgical therapy is indicated when medical therapy fails or when one suspects the presence of a malignant tumor. One may thus avoid exposing younger individuals to radiation. Surgical treatment is sometimes indicated for cosmetic effect in patients with a large neck mass.
   a. ***Preparation*** It is important to attempt to operate on the euthyroid patient. SSKI and thiourea derivatives can be given concurrently for 1 to 2 weeks preoperatively. This regimen decreases the vascularity of the gland and the incidence of thyroid storm.
   b. ***Complications*** include vocal cord paralysis, hypoparathyroidism, recurrence of hyperthyroidism, the risks of anesthesia, postoperative thyroid storm, hemorrhage, and wound infection.

3. **Complications of Hyperthyroidism**
   a. ***Cardiac complications*** of hyperthyroidism include tachycardia, congestive heart failure, and arrhythmias. Standard digitalis or diuretic therapy for congestive heart failure or arrhythmias is usually adequate, but attention must be directed to the hyperthyroid state. Propranolol is usually helpful in this situation.
   b. ***Malignant exophthalmos*** must be distinguished from the stare, lid lag, and retraction that frequently accompany hyperthyroidism. Ocular proptosis due to an increase in the volume of retroglobal tissue usually accompanies Graves' disease. The course of the exophthalmos is unpredictable; however, malignant exophthalmos may develop rapidly over several weeks. This disease should be treated in consultation with an ophthalmologist and an endocrinologist, with particular attention directed toward visual acuity and extraocular muscle functioning. In general, artificial tears and ointments are helpful, and corticosteroids (60 to 80 mg prednisone per day) may be of value. Occasionally, tarsorrhaphy is necessary. Orbital decompression may be necessary in the presence of corneal ulceration, progressive loss of visual acuity, or progressive loss of extraocular muscle function. This decompression may be performed by a transantral, transethmoid, lateral, or supraorbital approach. Preoperatively, the patient should be in a euthyroid state.
   c. ***Thyrotoxic crisis (thyroid storm)*** is a medical emergency manifested by a fulminating increase in all the signs and symptoms of hyperthyroidism. It is characterized by marked irritability, severe hyperpyrexia, tachycardia and other arrhythmias, vomiting and diarrhea, and a delirium

that may progress to coma, shock, and death. Vigorous, prompt treatment is essential and should not be delayed for laboratory confirmation of thyrotoxicosis. Predisposing factors include infection in an untreated or inadequately treated patient with hyperthyroidism. These infections must be identified and treated appropriately. Other stresses, such as surgical, may also induce thyroid storm. Postsurgical thyroid storm is rare today because patients are properly prepared, as previously discussed. One must treat patients in shock with fluids and vasopressor agents as necessary. Hyperpyrexia and cardiac problems must be corrected, and oxygen therapy may be required. As previously discussed, propranolol may be helpful in the management of the peripheral effects of hyperthyroidism. The drug should be given intravenously, with careful monitoring of the patient's electrocardiographic and vital signs. Propranolol may also be given by nasogastric tube. Corticosteroids, in the form of dexamethasone (Decadron), 10 mg intravenously every 6 to 8 hours, are used to treat the relative adrenal insufficiency that may occur in this condition. The dose should be tapered as soon as hypothyroidism is under control. The synthesis and release of thyroid hormone can be inhibited by propylthiouracil, 300 to 400 mg, or methimazole, 30 to 40 mg, administered by nasogastric tube. The initial dose should be repeated every 8 hours and decreased as necessary. Sodium iodide should be given in the form of SSKI, 5 to 10 drops every 8 hours, if the patient is able to take fluids by mouth. Sodium iodide may also be given by slow intravenous infusion 1 to 2 g every 24 hours, starting 1 to 3 hours after thiourea administration. Broad-spectrum intravenous antibiotics should be given after appropriate cultures have been obtained.

D. Thyroiditis

This nonspecific term implies inflammation of the thyroid gland and embraces several disorders of differing origin. Treatment depends on the cause of the condition.

1. **Subacute or de Quervain's thyroiditis** is a distinct disease that appears to be viral in origin. It has been reported in association with mumps, measles, influenza, the common cold, adenovirus, Coxsackie virus, infectious mononucleosis, and cat-scratch fever. The disease is much more common in the female, by a ratio of about 5 to 1. Signs and symptoms include sore throat, malaise, odynophagia, dysphagia, and pain in the thyroid gland. Tenderness of the gland is the most important physical sign. Twenty percent of the cases are unilateral. Laboratory findings include an increased erythrocyte sedimentation rate, low RAIU on scan, absent or low levels of antithyroid anti-

bodies, and minimal leukocytosis. The disease usually has a well-defined self-limited course lasting about 1 to 3 months. Aspirin and corticosteroids, such as 20 to 40 mg prednisone per day, seem to control the symptoms. A return of the RAIU to normal indicates when therapy can be withdrawn without recurrence of symptoms.

2. **Chronic thyroiditis** This term denotes a disorder with a self-limited bout of thyrotoxicosis and has been referred to as painless thyroiditis, silent thyroiditis, chronic thyroiditis with spontaneously resolving hyperthyroidism, or chronic thyroiditis with transient thyrotoxicosis. The production of thyroid hormone is negligible, and the RAIU is decreased in this condition. The syndrome mainly occurs in women and is manifested by mild thyrotoxicosis. The thyroid gland is nontender, firm, symmetric, and frequently not enlarged. Elevations of T_4 and T_3 levels are noted, but the RAIU is depressed. The erythrocyte sedimentation rate is normal or only slightly elevated. The thyrotoxicosis results from leakage of hormone from the gland, as in subacute thyroiditis. Because the thyroid gland is not hyperfunctioning, measures used in the treatment of hyperthyroidism are useless. Symptomatic treatment with propranolol or sedatives is indicated until the thyrotoxicosis abates. In patients with frequently recurrent disease, thyroid ablation with ^{131}I may be necessary.

3. **Hashimoto's thyroiditis** is also known as autoimmune thyroiditis, struma lymphomatosa, or lymphadenoid goiter. This condition predominates in females and is often associated with Graves' disease. It appears to be mediated by both cellular and humoral immune factors. Signs and symptoms include insidious onset with gradual thyroid enlargement, pressure in the throat, dysphagia, and hoarseness. The nontender thyroid gland is usually enlarged bilaterally and feels firm and rubbery. The titer of antithyroid antibodies is high. T_4 levels are usually low, although the protein-bound iodine level is frequently elevated. The disorder coexists with other disease of a presumed autoimmune nature, such as pernicious anemia, Sjögren's syndrome, chronic active hepatitis, systemic lupus erythematosus, rheumatoid arthritis, nontuberculous Addison's disease, and diabetes. Goiter is the outstanding feature. Early in the disease, the patient is metabolically normal; as the disease persists, however, serum T_3 and T_4 concentrations decline, and the patient becomes hypothyroid. Therapy is usually by replacement with levothyroxine, .15 mg per day.

4. **Riedel's struma** This rare condition is also known as invasive fibrous thyroiditis. The signs and symptoms are caused by pressure secondary to gland enlargement, often unilateral. Shortness of breath and cough may be present. Laboratory tests are not helpful, and no effective medical therapy exists. Surgical intervention may be indicated for diagnosis and for

relief of symptoms caused by pressure. A wedge resection of the thyroid isthmus may be necessary, and tracheotomy is occasionally required.

5. **Acute infectious thyroiditis** is also rare and is seen in patients recovering from infections of the pharynx and upper respiratory tract. The infecting organism is usually Streptococcus haemolyticus, Staphylococcus aureus, or pneumococcus. This disorder has also been seen in patients recovering from chickenpox, measles, and cat-scratch fever. The signs and symptoms include sudden fever, chills, and pain with marked local tenderness and swelling. Computed tomographic (CT) scanning may demonstrate an abscess within the visceral space. Therapy should include intensive intravenous antibiotics, followed by incision and drainage of an abscess, if present. Tracheotomy may be necessary (see Chapter 28).

6. **Chronic infectious thyroiditis** Tuberculosis may involve the thyroid gland; however, such involvement is usually seen in patients with disseminated disease. Diffuse enlargement with nodular formation is common. Therapy must be directed against the tubercle bacillus, with antitubercular medications, incision and drainage of any abscesses that develop, and subtotal thyroidectomy if medical therapy fails. The patient may also have syphilitic involvement of the thyroid gland manifested as a unilateral nodular swelling with cervical lymph node involvement. Diagnosis is based on histologic and serologic testing, and therapy is with antisyphilitic medication. Actinomycosis and echinococcosis may also involve the thyroid gland.

E. Thyroid Carcinoma

A wide spectrum of malignant lesions may involve the thyroid gland. Possible etiologic factors include radiation exposure, heredity, and long-term TSH stimulation. Carcinomas are more frequent in females; the ratio is about 2 to 1.

1. **Papillary adenocarcinoma,** the most common and least aggressive type of thyroid carcinoma, represents at least 50% of all malignant tumors of the thyroid gland. In spite of the usually benign course of this lesion, the 20-year mortality rates range from 10 to 16%. The prognosis is worse in patients with primary lesions larger than 1.5 cm in diameter. The female-to-male ratio is 3 to 1, and the disease is frequently multicentric. Signs and symptoms usually include asymptomatic goiter; however, 10% of these patients have only a neck mass. The incidence of neck metastases is high. From 30 to 40% of these patients have clinically apparent lymph-node involvement, and 30 to 70% have ipsilateral occult nodal involvement. Distant metastasis is rare. The surgical therapy of this lesion is controversial. Some workers recommend complete lobectomy on the side of the lesion with a near-total lobectomy on the opposite side; others opt for total thyroidectomy, and still others

prefer unilateral lobectomy. Therapy of the neck is also controversial, although most workers agree that the anterosuperior mediastinum must be carefully evaluated for metastatic disease. Modified or standard radical neck dissections and "node picking" may yield similar results (Medicine, *56*:171, 1978). Medical therapy of this disease includes thyroid hormone suppression and radiotherapy with ^{131}I (RAI therapy). RAI therapy is indicated in patients whose lesions are inoperable, who have had incomplete excision, or who have distant metastases. Eighty-five percent of differentiated tumors demonstrate uptake with elevated TSH levels. Thyroid hormone must be withheld for approximately 2 weeks prior to therapy with ^{131}I. External radiation may be helpful in alleviating pain from distant metastases. The prognosis in general is favorable at 5-year follow-up, but the mortality rate increases to 10 to 20% at 20-year follow-up. Most deaths are due to local recurrence of the tumor, usually seen in patients treated by lobectomy rather than sub-total or total thyroidectomy. The prognosis is worse in prepubertal children, in patients over 40 years of age, in patients with tumors larger than 1.5 cm in diameter or with extracapsular invasion, and in patients receiving a limited thyroidectomy (lobectomy). Neck metastases do not appear to affect prognosis if therapy is directed toward cervical lymph nodes.

2. **Follicular adenocarcinoma,** the second most common malignant tumor of the thyroid gland, occurs in females at a ratio of 3 to 1 over males. It is usually seen in older patients and is more aggressive than the papillary lesion. Signs and symptoms include pressure symptoms in the neck, neck mass, or distant metastasis. The incidence of nodal metastasis is less than 20%; however, distant metastases to bone or lung have been reported in 15 to 65% of patients. Therapy of these lesions is controversial and is similar to that described for papillary lesions. The prognosis is much poorer than for papillary tumors; the mortality rate at 20 years is 40 to 60%.

3. **Hürthle cell carcinoma** Most classifications of thyroid carcinomas exclude Hürthle cell carcinomas, which are usually considered to be variants of follicular or papillary carcinomas. The presence of the Hürthle cell, however, makes the histologic evaluation of lesions difficult. Nodular lesions composed of Hürthle cells are found in the thyroid glands of patients with Graves' disease, Hashimoto's disease, and nodular goiters. The problem arises in a large, solitary, solid, and encapsulated mass composed entirely of Hürthle cells. It is difficult to histologically differentiate benign from malignant Hürthle cell lesions of this type. It has been suggested that any well-encapsulated Hürthle cell lesion that is solid and enlarged be treated as carcinoma. These lesions rarely take up ^{131}I; otherwise, however, they should be treated as a follicular carcinoma. These

tumors comprise about 6% of all malignant thyroid lesions and usually occur in the sixth decade of life. Survival rates have been estimated at 75% at 5 years and 40% at 25 years.

4. **Medullary carcinoma** represents about 10% of all malignant tumors of the thyroid and has a propensity for metastasizing early to cervical and mediastinal lymph nodes. Direct extension to the larynx and esophagus is common. Unfortunately, this tumor responds poorly to therapy with radioactive iodine, radiation, hormones, and chemotherapeutic agents. The incidence of neck metastasis is in the range of 75%, and mediastinal involvement is present in about 25% of patients. These tumors produce calcitonin and histaminase, which may be used as biochemical markers for the presence of the tumor. They appear to be associated with the development of parathyroid adenomas, pheochromocytomas, and mucosal neuromas. Both familial and sporadic types of medullary thyroid carcinoma are seen. The familial lesion usually involves both lobes and occurs in the second decade of life, but it may be diagnosed much earlier. The sporadic type, which generally only involves a single lobe, is not usually diagnosed until the fifth or sixth decade of life. The sporadic form accounts for 90% of all medullary thyroid carcinomas. The signs and symptoms center around a firm neck mass in the thyroid gland or cervical lymph nodes. About one-third of these patients have significant diarrhea. Characteristic radiographic features, if present, include a dense, irregular calcification of the tumor mass on lateral soft tissue roentgenograms of the neck and widening of the superior mediastinum on chest films. This sign is due to early metastasis to the mediastinal soft tissues. Urinary vanillylmandelic acid levels and levels of metanephrine, serum calcium, and phosphorus should be obtained preoperatively in all patients with familial disease, to rule out the presence of a pheochromocytoma or parathyroid disorder. Treatment is surgical, including total thyroidectomy and a standard neck dissection. Cervical metastasis present at the time of diagnosis worsens the prognosis. The prognosis for the familial type of medullary carcinoma is usually better than that for the sporadic type, probably because it is usually diagnosed earlier.

5. **Undifferentiated carcinoma** or poorly differentiated carcinoma of the thyroid is an aggressive lesion. It spreads rapidly and early beyond the thyroid capsule and the regional lymph nodes to involve the deep muscles and other soft tissues of the neck. These carcinomas may arise from pre-existing differentiated tumors and are often found in older persons. Such lesions comprise about 10 to 15% of thyroid carcinomas and are usually first seen as an obviously malignant thyroid mass. The patient notes pressure, cough, hoarseness, vocal cord paralysis, or dysphagia. Widespread cervical and distant metastases are often present at the time of diagnosis. Therapy is usually unsuccessful, and survival rates are 10% or less at the end of a year. The average duration of the patient's life after

diagnosis is 6 months. Death is caused by both local disease and distant metastasis.

F. Thyroid Nodules

The problem facing the physician in the treatment of thyroid nodules is one of diagnosis. One must be familiar enough with thyroid diseases to make an educated estimate of the likelihood that a particular nodule may be malignant. One must also determine whether a solitary thyroid nodule should undergo biopsy.

1. **Evaluation** must, of course, include the patient's medical history. One must carefully question the patient regarding symptoms, and the duration of such symptoms, related to the thyroid nodules. Prior radiation exposure and a family history of thyroid disease are important. On physical examination, one must search for lymph nodes in the neck and estimate the thyroid gland's size and consistency. A careful search for recurrent nerve dysfunction is necessary. Elevated calcitonin levels help in the diagnosis of medullary carcinoma of the thyroid. Laboratory tests in the evaluation of thyroid disease are described previously in this chapter.

2. **Risk factors associated with malignant disease** The patient's age is of extreme importance; 50% of isolated thyroid nodules in children are malignant. Because thyroid disease is more common in females than in males, an isolated thyroid nodule in a man, particularly a young man, is most likely to be cancer. Solitary, nontoxic thyroid nodules are malignant about 30% of the time, and the incidence of malignant lesions in patients under 40 years of age with nodules is about 35%. Any patient with a history of radiation to the head and neck or mediastinum who has a palpable abnormality of the thyroid gland should undergo excisional biopsy; such prior radiotherapy increases the chances that the lesion is malignant. A "cold" nodule is more likely to harbor cancer than a "hot" nodule. The incidence of malignancy in "cold" nodules is between 10 and 25%. Malignant nodules are likely to be firm or hard, and regional cervical lymphadenopathy may be the presenting sign. Thyroid cancer is unlikely to decrease in size as a result of T_4- or T_3-suppressant therapy for 6 months. Totally cystic lesions are rarely malignant. Mixed cystic and solid lesions have an incidence of malignancy similar to totally solid lesions, although it is possible for a cystic lesion to harbor malignant disease. Antithyroid antibodies in high titers suggest Hashimoto's thyroiditis; 3% of these patients have malignant disease, however. Rapid or recent growth of a lesion increases the chances of malignancy. Needle aspirations are sometimes helpful, and excisional biopsy is best performed by lobectomy.

3. **Therapy of "hot" nodules** Up to 25% of solitary nodules are hyperfunctioning and appear on a scan as "hot" nodules. One should attempt to determine whether the nodule is autonomous, that is, whether it functions independently of TSH control and is not suppressible by the administration of thyroid

hormone. If the nodule is nonautonomous and is functioning under TSH control, it will be suppressible by thyroid hormone. This effect can be achieved by administering triiodothyronine (Cytomel), .025 mg 3 times daily for 1 to 2 weeks; one should then repeat the scan. Autonomous lesions continue to function and appear as "hot" nodules on repeated scans, whereas nonautonomous lesions appear as "cold" nodules on repeated scans. In treating a nonautonomous nodule, full thyroid hormone replacement is indicated. If the lesion progressively enlarges or if hyperthyroidism develops, treatment may require lobectomy, antithyroid medication, or ^{131}I therapy. If the nodule is autonomous, antithyroid medication, ^{131}I therapy, or lobectomy will be indicated.

4. **Therapy of "cold" nodules** Seventy-five percent of isolated nodules are considered "cold" or isofunctioning nodules. Full thyroid replacement should be attempted for 3 to 6 months, and the patient's response should be monitored by changes in the size of the nodule. Occasionally, malignant lesions decrease in size, however. Nodules that are most likely to regress with this therapy include lesions smaller than 2.5 cm in diameter, those of recent origin, those occurring in females, and those seen in patients under 40 years of age. Controversy exists concerning the treatment of the "cold" nodule, but most workers agree that excisional biopsy is indicated at an earlier date in children and in males with solid, solitary lesions. If a malignant tumor is suspected on clinical grounds, excisional biopsy (lobectomy) or fine-needle aspiration should be performed immediately.
5. **Therapy of solitary cystic nodules** Such nodules should be suppressed with thyroid medication. Fine-needle aspiration and cytologic study should be attempted. Lobectomy is probably indicated if the nodule progressively enlarges, if the patient has compressive symptoms, or if the physician suspects a malignant lesion. Such nodules may increase to such a degree that the patient desires their removal for cosmetic reasons. Lesions under 3 cm in diameter, however, have a 2% incidence of malignancy.

G. Therapy of Patients with Prior Radiation Exposure

Patients with a documented history of prior radiation exposure should be examined every 2 years. Initially, they should have a thyroid scan, which should be repeated if any clinical changes are noted in the thyroid gland. Patients who have a normal physical examination and a "cold" nodule should undergo biopsy (lobectomy) of that lesion because 20 to 30% of such lesions are malignant. Careful re-examination and frequent follow-up or thyroid suppression may also be indicated in patients with a "cold" nodule and a normal physical examination. If the patient has a palpable nodule, regardless of the results of the scan, surgical exploration and excision should be performed to rule out the presence of a malignant lesion.

31

SKIN DISORDERS IN OTOLARYNGOLOGY

MAX E. REDDICK

It is important for the physician to observe skin lesions in the patient firsthand. Description, slides, and pictures are helpful, but they do not make one a reliable clinician.

I. TUMORS OF THE SKIN

Physicians who choose not to perform a biopsy on a skin tumor must instruct patients to return should the lesion change in size, color, character, or symptoms. That patients have been thus instructed should be noted in the chart along with the medical history, clinical description, size, and location of the lesion, and the physician's clinical impression of that lesion. Location can be better documented by using a tracing or stamp of the area and drawing in the lesion. Such a tracing is helpful when the patient is seen at a later date or by another physician.

A. Malignant Tumors

1. **Malignant melanoma** The most significant feature in the medical history of a pigmented lesion is recent change.
   a. ***Clinical features*** include a recent change in size; color; shape, often including an irregular border or halo pigment; surface, such as scaling, papular or irregular growth, ulceration, crusting, or bleeding; and symptoms of itching, pain, tenderness, or a vague sensation of its presence. Because the early changes are subtle, any positive history should direct one's attention to a careful clinical examination of the lesion. Excision or biopsy are indicated if any question exists. The important clinical

features of melanomas are variegated color, irregular and often notched border, and irregular surface (N. Engl. J. Med., *289*:989, 1973). Melanoma is a dangerous skin lesion, and its incidence is increasing. Except for nodular melanoma, this lesion has an early horizontal growth phase involving lateral spread along the skin plane. This phase is followed by a vertical or downward growth expressed as an anatomic level or as the measured thickness of the lesion (Cancer Res., *29*:705, 1969; Ann. Surg., *172*:902, 1970).

b. ***Types of melanoma*** The 3 major clinical types of primary malignant melanoma are lentigo maligna melanoma, superficial spreading melanoma, and nodular melanoma. **Lentigo maligna** melanoma, which occurs late in life, often in the eighth decade, has a prolonged preceding horizontal phase of growth of about 8 to 10 years' duration as a precancerous Hutchinson's melanotic freckle and is usually located on the sun-exposed areas of the face. It generally appears as an irregular, tan macule with minute, dark brown or black flecks and an overall size of several centimeters with an area of elevation and deeper pigmentation. The elevated papular or nodular portion is the clinical sign of dermal invasion and the beginning of true melanoma. This area should undergo biopsy if the lesion is not easily excised. **Superficial spreading** melanoma has a shorter horizontal growth period than lentigo maligna melanoma and, therefore, a worse prognosis. The tumor is noted for its variegation in pigments. A single lesion often exhibits shades from black to blue to red to pink to white. These lesions are generally greater than 0.5 cm in size and may reach 2 to 3 cm. It is important that most acquired, not congenital, benign nevi grow no larger than 7 to 10 mm. **Nodular** melanomas grow vertically from the start, have a more uniform coloring, and have the worst prognosis of the melanomas. They are often bluish black, bluish gray, or bluish red.

c. ***Diagnosis*** of melanoma is made from tissue examination. A biopsy should be performed on all lesions that are suspicious from either a clinical or a historical aspect. Excisional biopsy is preferred when it can be done simply. To avoid excessive surgical manipulation of a large benign lesion, a smaller biopsy of the clinically positive area can be performed. No convincing evidence in the literature suggests that a limited biopsy of a melanoma worsens its prognosis. A shave biopsy should not be done on a lesion thought to be a melanoma because the procedure complicates later determinations of the level of tumor invasion and of the appropriate treatment.

d. ***Treatment of melanoma*** is involved and undergoing evolution. Physicians should not treat melanoma unless they are abreast of the literature and experienced in this area.

2. **Squamous cell carcinoma** of the skin is common in actinic-damaged skin in which the incidence of metastasis is low (0 to 0.5%). When the tumor arises from normal skin, scar tissue, chronic sinus tracts, radiation-damaged skin, or the lip and mucous membranes, the rate of metastasis can be as high as 20 to 30%. A low degree of differentiation, a high degree of dermal invasiveness, and a large overall tumor size all seem to indicate a tendency to metastasis (Arch. Dermatol., *107*:395, 1973).
   a. ***Clinical features*** Clinically, the lesion usually has a firm, raised, smooth border with central hyperkeratosis, crusting, or ulceration. The size ranges from a few millimeters to 2 cm or larger.
   b. ***Treatment*** Squamous cell carcinoma on actinic-damaged skin is easily treated by curettage and electrodesiccation, when lesions are under 2 cm in diameter, or by surgical excision with 3- to 5-mm margins. Invasive lesions and those larger than 2 cm in diameter should be excised. All excised lesions should have clear margins checked by the pathologist. Smaller lesions of recent onset on actinic-damaged skin may metastasize, however (Arch. Dermatol., *108*:670, 1973).

3. **Basal cell epithelioma** occurs almost exclusively in sun-exposed areas of the skin and is a common skin cancer. It rarely metastasizes, according to reports in the literature of about 90 such cases.
   a. ***Types*** Three main clinical types are known. **Nodular** basal cell epitheliomas are the most common and start as a translucent-looking papule, often with small dilated vessels (ectasia) overlying it. As the lesion enlarges, the border takes on a rolled appearance and is composed of multiple confluent papules, whereas the center is flattened, atrophic, or ulcerated. This feature is often referred to as a rolled "pearly" border. At times, the lesion is pigmented and must be differentiated from melanoma. In a blue-eyed person with such a pigmented lesion, the diagnosis is more likely to be melanoma than basal cell epithelioma. **Morphea-like** or **fibrosing** basal cell epithelioma is an indurated, skin-colored, yellowish plaque with a diffuse border; the overlying skin is often intact. Because the lesions are usually subtle, they are not often diagnosed early. In the scalp, the lesion may cause scarring alopecia, and biopsy is almost always necessary for diagnosis. **Superficial** basal cell epithelioma consists of an erythematous or scaling patch of skin with little induration and a sharp border that is only slightly raised. Other lesions in the differential diagnosis are squamous cell carcinoma in situ (Bowen's

disease), actinic keratoses, or in certain anatomic areas, extramammary Paget's disease.

b. ***Treatment*** Most basal cells can be simply curetted and desiccated, provided they do not invade the dermis of the skin into deeper structures such as cutaneous fat, cartilage, or bone. This procedure should not be used on the morphea-like sclerosing basal cell epithelioma or on recurrent lesions in which prior scarring prevents proper curettage. Excision of tumors is easily done; one should take a 3- to 5-mm border and have a pathologist check the surgical margins. This is the treatment of choice for recurrent lesions with scars, sclerosing basal cell epithelioma, and large or invasive tumors. Freezing with liquid nitrogen, using a thermocouple needle monitor under the lesion, is recommended by some experts, especially over cartilage. Mohs' chemosurgery, more accurately described as microscopically controlled excision of malignant skin tumors, is useful in treating advanced and certain recurrent lesions. It is particularly effective against lesions that tend to invade deeply and large lesions with uncertain borders. Deep invasion of basal cell epithelioma often occurs at the junction of the ear and scalp, around the eyes, at the junction of the nose and face, and on the nose. Recurrent lesions in these areas should be considered for microscopically controlled surgical excision. The cure rate with this procedure approaches 100%.

4. Metastatic tumor to the skin generally appears as a nodule or group of nodules, most often skin-colored, firm, nontender lesions that grow rapidly to 1 to 2 cm and then remain stationary. The other forms of skin metastases may be seen as diffuse erythema or as sclerodermoid plaques (Arch. Dermatol., *107*:80, 1973). The erythematous lesions usually resemble an infection clinically, except for the absence of toxic symptoms, such as fever and leukocytosis, and the prolonged duration. When metastatic sclerodermoid plaques occur on the scalp, the primary tumor is often of the breast. The lesion resembles localized alopecia and must be differentiated from morphea-like basal cell epithelioma, discoid lupus erythematosus, and alopecia areata, which is nonscarring.

B. Benign Tumors

1. Actinic keratoses are rough, erythematous or brownish in color, and have variable amounts of keratin scale. They are generally small in size, ranging from about 1 to 5 mm on sun-exposed areas. If left untreated, these lesions may progress to squamous cell carcinoma. Actinic keratoses are best frozen with liquid nitrogen spray, probe, or swab. They may be lightly curetted or electrodesiccated, but this procedure is more likely to scar or depigment the skin. 5-Fluorouracil, 1 or 5% cream or solution, may be applied twice daily for 2 weeks and the patient checked in 3 to 6 weeks. Remaining lesions should then undergo either biopsy or treatment with liquid nitrogen or electrodesiccation. The face of a patient with early lesions that are not clinically perceptible will become red, but a risk also exists of allergic contact dermatitis from 5-fluorouracil. Patients with actinic keratosis should be checked at 6- to 12-month intervals for new or advancing disease. At this time, other types of skin cancer may also be sought.

2. **Seborrheic keratoses** are rough-to-smooth keratotic lesions ranging in color from light tan to black. They are common about the head, neck, and trunk, and it is necessary to be able to recognize them clinically. When such lesions cause itching or soreness or when they resemble melanoma in appearance or history, they should be removed or should undergo biopsy. Seborrheic keratoses need no therapy, except for cosmetic purposes, unless they are symptomatic or clinically suggestive of a malignant lesion. The simplest surgical approach is to shave the lesion flush with the surrounding skin using a no. 15 scalpel blade. It may help to rim the lesion with a marker such as gentian violet prior to injection of local anesthesia. The denuded base can be treated with 20% aluminum chloride (Drysol solution), or light electrodesiccation. Partial biopsy or surgical excision with primary closure is best for lesions suspected of being melanoma. These pigmented lesions respond to freezing with nitrogen, but a small biopsy specimen should be obtained if the diagnosis is not clinically certain.

3. **Cutaneous horns** are a localized outgrowth of hard keratin from the skin, with or without a papule at its base. The histologic picture is that of an actinic keratosis, a seborrheic keratosis, a wart, or rarely a squamous cell carcinoma. Therefore, cutaneous horns, including the base, should either be removed or should undergo biopsy. Cutaneous horns are best treated by punch biopsy or elliptic excision that includes the base of the lesion for diagnosis. A shave biopsy may be done if it includes the base of the lesion for the pathologist's inspection.

4. **Chondrodermatitis nodularis chronica helicis** is a painful, dome-shaped papule, often hyperkeratotic, that appears over the cartilage of the ear and is sometimes associated with pressure in this area. At times, the surface becomes ulcerated and resembles a skin cancer. Histologically, the lesion is composed of keratosis, necrotic debris, and inflammatory tissue, with a spicule of cartilage in the center that appears to play a role in pathogenesis. This lesion is best treated by excision of the lesion with inclusion of a small rim of underlying cartilage. Tissue should be sent for histologic examination.

5. **Warts** are caused by a group of similar DNA viruses.
   a. ***Types*** The three types are classified by their gross mor-

phologic features. Papular warts have an irregular surface and often dark dots, which are capillary thrombi. Filiform warts resemble skin tags, except for the warty irregular top. Flat warts are small, discrete lesions that are skin colored, approximately 1 to 2 mm in size, and may be numerous over the face.

b. ***Treatment*** Warts respond well to light freezing with nitrogen. A salicylic acid preparation, Duofilm, can be applied daily for a week at a time. It is best to soak the skin in water 5 minutes and then apply the Duofilm. Larger lesions should be covered with an adhesive bandage, to increase the penetration into the wart. Flat warts should be treated carefully with light liquid nitrogen spray or a mild irritant such as Duofilm, every other day. Warts can be treated with electrodesiccation or a snip with scissors and desiccation of the base. This procedure is adequate for filiform warts on the nasal mucosa, but it should be avoided on the face because of possible scar formation or loss of pigment. Small, flat warts about the face present a special therapeutic problem in that they are resistant to treatment and are often recurrent. It is important not to be too aggressive in therapy; hypopigmentation or scarring is an undesirable result. These warts should be carefully, lightly frozen with liquid nitrogen or treated with Duofilm without occlusion every other day for a week at a time.

II. BACTERIAL INFECTIONS

Most bacterial infections of the skin of the head and neck region are due to Staphylococcus aureus or group A beta-hemolytic streptococci. These infections are further classified on an anatomic basis. For most superficial pyodermas with no associated toxic symptoms or fever, a bacterial culture is not necessary. In cases of failure of therapy, unusual medical history or clinical presentation, or toxic symptoms, a culture should be obtained to rule out such organisms as gram-negative bacteria, sporothrix, actinomycetes, and atypical acid-fast bacteria.

A. Infectious Lesions

1. **Furuncles** are usually the result of Staphylococcus aureus infection involving individual hair follicles. These lesions appear as single or multiple small pustules, erosions, or crusts. They are prevalent over the bearded area, posterior neck, and scalp.
2. **Boils or carbuncles** are of the same origin as furuncles, but they represent deeper invasion into the surrounding dermis and, often, a coalescence of adjacent infected follicles to produce a central core of purulent material.
3. **Cellulitis** can start from a local furuncle or boil and represents deep dermal and subcutaneous involvement with bacteria. The

borders are indistinct; the lesion appears as a diffuse erythema of the skin, often with a central focal abscess. The lesions are hot and tender.

4. **Erysipelas** is usually due to group A streptococci, but it has been described with staphylococcal infection. It represents involvement of superficial lymphatic vessels with adjacent connective tissue. The borders are sharp, and the lesion is edematous and raised, at times vesicular or bullous. It may become hemorrhagic. The patient is generally seriously ill and febrile, with an elevated white blood cell count. It is difficult to culture organisms. A common location is on the malar area of the face. Often, no portal of entry of the infection is found. Repeated episodes may occur, resulting in chronic edema (elephantiasis nostras).
5. **Impetigo** is a superficial infection of the outermost skin, not necessarily related to hair follicles. Its clinical appearance ranges from a yellow, crusting, weeping lesion to a varnish-like lesion of the skin. It can be associated with, or progress to, any of the foregoing types of infection. Most of the time, impetigo represents a combination of Staphylococcus aureus and group A beta-hemolytic streptococcal infection.

B. Principles of Therapy

1. **Surgical incision and drainage** of abscesses are indicated, with saline irrigation and, sometimes, packing with iodoform gauze for larger wounds. It is best to incise a boil quickly, without prior injection of local anesthetic, using a no. 11 scalpel blade.
2. **Dressings** Aluminum chloride hexahydrate (Aluwets), aluminum sulfate and calcium acetate (Domeboro), or normal saline solution can be applied to open and crusted lesions as a "wet-to-dry dressing." It is best to use a gauze-type dressing without cotton padding in 4 to 6 layers. This dressing is saturated with a soaking solution to almost dripping wet and is applied to the affected area. The dressing should be open to the air and should be rewetted with solution to avoid concentration of the solute. Generally, such dressings are applied 30 to 60 minutes 2 to 4 times a day, stopping when the lesion becomes dry.
3. **Antibiotics** Bacterial culture and sensitivity studies, when indicated, should guide antibiotic administration. For streptococcal and staphylococcal infections, erythromycin is economical and almost always effective, in an adult dose of 250 mg 4 times daily for 7 to 10 days. Cephalosporins or dicloxacillin are suitable alternatives. Patients allergic to penicillin may also be allergic to the cephalosporins. For less common infections not due to gram-positive cocci, therapy should be based on culture, sensitivity studies, and knowledge of the specific disease. Penicillin and ampicillin are ineffective against a high

percent of staphylococcal organisms, and they do not penetrate the hair follicles as well as erythromycin.

C. Complications

Complications rarely occur from superficial bacterial infections of the skin. Possible complications of bacterial infections include septicemia from infection in the middle of the face, with extension of bacteria by the venous route into the central nervous system; necrotizing fasciitis; deep abscess formation with the development of sinus tracts, tetanus, and gangrene.

III. VIRAL INFECTIONS

A. Herpes Simplex

Infection with this virus is common about the face and produces umbilicated, clear vesicles on an inflamed base. Often, one sees only a group of small, crusted, superficial ulcers, the result of the vesicles rupturing. The infection is frequently recurrent, and no effective therapy is known. Such therapies as smallpox vaccination, bacille Calmette Guérin, dye and light, levamisole, and herpes vaccine are all ineffective. The disease is usually benign, except in newborns and in persons with generalized eczema; both groups may have a severe, generalized infection.

B. Herpes Zoster

1. **Clinical features** Infection with this virus produces a group of erythematous papules and umbilicated vesicles in the distribution of a peripheral sensory nerve. The area is usually painful. At times, however, the pain of herpes zoster appears with no rash or only a few papules without vesicles, and the diagnosis is thereby made difficult. **Ramsay Hunt syndrome** is the term applied to total seventh-nerve involvement (motor and sensory), resulting in ear pain and facial paralysis on the affected side. **Herpes zoster ophthalmicus** can be a serious form of localized disease involving the ophthalmic division of the fifth cranial nerve. Because vision can be lost, consultation with an ophthalmologist is indicated. In debilitated patients with altered cellular immunity, generalized herpes zoster infection can result.

2. **Treatment**
   a. ***Dressings*** All vesicles and ulcers respond to topical wet dressings, which help to promote their healing. One should soak lesions 30 min twice daily, stopping when they appear dry, usually in 2 to 5 days. Normal saline soaks (½ teaspoon of salt in 8 oz of water) are adequate for this purpose.
   b. ***Ointments*** Acyclovir (Zovirax) ointment for herpes simplex and Silvadene Cream for herpes zoster promote healing.

c. ***Antibiotics*** Acyclovir (Zovirax) capsules or I.V. is for initial herpes simplex attacks, for intermittent outbreaks, and can be used in long-term prevention. It is useful for some cases of generalized herpes zoster. Rapid or bolus injections must be avoided.

d. ***Analgesics*** Herpes zoster infection may be painful, and analgesics usually need to be prescribed. Aspirin, codeine and aspirin, or oxycodone hydrochloride (Percodan) can be given initially. If severe pain persists for more than 2 weeks, a neurologist may need to be consulted. Such pain is most likely to occur in the elderly patient.

e. ***Corticosteroids*** Systemic corticosteroids given early in the course of a herpes zoster infection have been reported to relieve postherpetic neuralgia in elderly patients. This type of therapy should be used with caution and by someone experienced with it.

IV. FUNGAL INFECTIONS

Fungal infections involve the skin and can invade the hair, with resulting alopecia. Deep fungal infections are discussed in Chapter 23.

A. Clinical Features and Diagnosis

Infections of the skin result in an erythematous, scaly patch that clears in the center as it enlarges, giving the characteristic "ringworm" appearance. The border is raised and scaly, with a clear center. When the infection comes from an animal, a more inflammatory lesion is often seen; such a lesion has a plaque of edema and small abscess formation that may or may not show central clearing. This lesion is difficult to differentiate from a bacterial infection. Often, the patient has a history of exposure to a cat or dog or, less often, to another infected person. To make the diagnosis, a scraping of scale from the active border or scaly abscess area is placed on a glass slide. A drop of 10% potassium hydroxide is added to the scraping, and a cover slip is placed on top. Fungi can be seen at a magnification of 100 times, but generally, a magnification of 400 times is needed. If much scale is present, the slide can be warmed to promote dissolution of the keratin, to render the hyphal elements clearly visible. Fungal culture can be done, preferably on mycosel agar to inhibit the growth of contaminant bacteria. Scrapings or infected hairs are placed on the medium and are incubated at room temperature with a loose top. The dermatophytes grow as molds that are fluffy in appearance, whereas the yeasts grow as a dull, white, pasty colony.

1. **Tinea capitis** Infection of the hair (tinea capitis) results in alopecia, either with no inflammation or with scaling, or in a boggy, erythematous, edematous lesion of the scalp, depending on the infecting organism. To diagnose tinea of the scalp, it is best to pluck broken hairs carefully for examination on glass slide using potassium hydroxide. Scale from the scalp can

be examined in a potassium hydroxide solution. A fungal culture may be helpful. Rarely, the hair fluoresces under Wood's light because of the presence of certain fungi that invade the outer hair shaft. A negative result with Wood's light does not rule out tinea capitis. The causative organism in all these infections is varied, but treatment is the same, once the diagnosis of fungal infection has been established.

2. **Yeast infection** is generally confined to the angle of the mouth, where it is known as perlèche. It is seen as an erythematous, cracking, exudative lesion, often with a white coating. The infection is secondary to dentures, tooth braces, excessive drooling, or an anatomic configuration that causes a fold of skin to develop in this area and to trap moisture. A potassium hydroxide slide of a scraping can be made, to enable one to look for spores and pseudohyphae. The yeast can also be grown on fungal culture. Other causes of cracking at the corners of the mouth are vitamin B deficiency and secondary syphilis, both rare.

B. Treatment

1. **Dermatophyte (ringworm) infections**
   a. ***Localized superficial fungal infections*** of the skin generally respond to topical therapy. Topical clotrimazole (Lotrimin) solution placed thinly on the lesion 2 to 3 times daily for 3 to 6 weeks clears most infections. The rule of thumb is to treat the area for a week after it appears healed. The cream form of this drug is helpful if the area is irritated.
   b. ***Recurrent, chronic, or widespread disease*** requires griseofulvin (microsize), 250 mg orally twice a day with meals for 30 to 45 days, to clear adult infections. Pediatric doses are based on weight.
   c. ***Hair infection*** is a special problem requiring griseofulvin (microsize), 500 mg twice daily with meals for 45 days for adults. Pediatric doses are based on weight. A large single dose of griseofulvin can be administered if patients or their parents are unreliable.
2. **Yeast infections** Plain nystatin (Mycostatin) cream or ointment is the best therapy. One should apply it thinly 2 to 4 times a day for 3 to 6 weeks. Clotrimazole (Lotrimin) cream is an alternative.

V. ECZEMATOUS ERUPTIONS

Eczema is an inflammatory condition of the skin that appears as a pruritic eruption with features ranging from redness and oozing to dry scaliness. It is caused by contact allergens, exposure to sunlight, and irritants, but is often of unknown origin.

A. Types of Eruption

1. **Atopic eczema** is a hereditary form associated with asthma and hayfever, but the eczema is independent of the other components and its cause is unknown. When eczematous lesions develop atrophy, papules or nodules, ulceration, or induration, they should undergo biopsy, to rule out other pathologic processes.
2. **Contact allergy** causes a rash in the area of exposure to the allergen. Often, sharp, straight "cutoff" lines are present. Eyelid dermatitis, an exception, can result from eye makeup, shampoos, nail polish, and other allergens. The sensitive eyelids react, whereas the main primary site of exposure does not. It is often difficult to distinguish among seborrheic dermatitis, eczema, and contact dermatitis of the eyelids. Seborrheic dermatitis often appears in its other usual areas, with less redness and more scaliness.
3. **Light eruptions** may be caused by allergy to certain phototoxic or photoallergenic topical or systemic medications. Such eruptions usually involve most of the face and neck, but spare behind the ear lobes, the upper eyelids, and under the chin, where the sun's rays are blocked. Eyeglasses or hats may add additional areas of protection. Among the other disease processes that can manifest as light eruptions are lupus erythematosus, polymorphic light eruption, and porphyrias.
4. **Irritant and idiopathic eczemas** are usually chronic, scaly, and mildly erythematous, with a diffuse border. All degrees of caustics can be encountered, however; one may see a mild irritation or a frank chemical burn with ulceration. The usual, mild, irritant eczemas are made worse by scratching, by cold, dry weather, and by excessive washing. Over-the-counter medications may be irritants or may cause a superimposed allergic contact dermatitis.

B. Treatment

1. **Dressings** For weeping lesions, applications of saline or aluminum chloride hexahydrate (Aluwets) dressings, wet to dry, for 30 min 2 to 4 times daily, are helpful. They can usually be discontinued in 2 to 4 days as the eruption drys.
2. **Topical corticosteroids** are the mainstay of therapy. For acute lesions, a mild-base potent cream, such as Wescort-Cream 0.2% (15 or 45 g) works well. One must instruct the patient to apply the cream thinly to the rash only 2 to 4 times daily and to keep the cream out of the eyes. Strong fluorinated corticosteroids should not be used on the face for a prolonged period. Therefore, they are not for chronic conditions. Atrophy with ectasia has been associated with the long-term use of fluorinated corticosteroids on the face (Br. J. Dermatol., *87*:548, 1972).

3. **Ointments** For milder conditions and for chronic conditions, 1% hydrocortisone cream (Hytone), 30 g, applied thinly once or twice a day, is best. If a stronger medication is needed, 2½% hydrocortisone (Hytone) cream can be used. The physician should instruct the patient to keep the cream out of the eyes, to avoid raising the intraocular pressure; in addition, the creams are not formulated for use in the eye.
4. **Antihistamines** are helpful to control itching. Hydroxyzine (Atarax), 10- or 25-mg tablets 1 to 2 times daily, or cyproheptadine (Periactin), 4-mg tablets, ½ to 1 tablet 3 times daily, can be given to adults.
5. **Systemic corticosteroids** are effective, but their use should be limited to acute, severe reactions for which long-term therapy is not needed. The physician should inquire whether the patient has diabetes, high blood pressure, ulcer disease, glaucoma, or tuberculosis or other infections, is taking medications, or is pregnant or breast feeding. The drug is given in a single morning dose for 6 to 12 days. No problems have been reported with sudden withdrawal from a short course of these agents, but some adrenal suppression occurs. Therefore, patients should be warned to advise a physician that they have taken corticosteroids if they become ill or if they are to undergo a surgical procedure. Prednisone (Deltasone), 5-mg tablets, or methylprednisolone (Medrol), 4-mg tablets, can be given in daily morning doses, as follows: 6 for 2 days, 4 for 2 days, and 2 for 2 days; 8 for 2 days, 6 for 2 days, 4 for 2 days, and 2 for 2 days; or 12 for 2 days, 10 for 2 days, 8 for 2 days, 4 for 2 days, and 2 for 2 days.

VI. SEBORRHEIC DERMATITIS

A. Clinical Features

Seborrheic dermatitis is a scaly, erythematous rash with little or no induration. It may itch, as does eczema, or it may not. The lesions come and go, with no known cause or permanent cure. Typically, the scalp is most commonly involved and the eyebrows, eyelids, nasolabial folds, and ears are often affected. Despite its chronicity, the disorder responds rapidly to treatment with topical corticosteroids and shampoos.

B. Treatment

1. **Shampoos** are the first line of therapy. Commercial preparations, such as Ionil T (with tar) or plain Ionil, Head and Shoulders, or Selsun, all work. Depending on severity, the shampoos should be sudsed into the scalp for 5 to 10 min and then rinsed well. This procedure can be repeated daily. Often, patients believe that the scaliness is due to dryness, and therefore, they fail to use the shampoo frequently enough. The shampoos may also be applied to the rash on the face; one

must take care to keep the shampoo out of the eyes and to rinse well.

2. **Ointments** Topical 1% hydrocortisone cream (Hytone), applied daily or twice daily, is effective. The label should instruct the patient to keep the cream out of the eyes. A stronger nonfluorinated corticosteroid is Westcort Cream.

3. **Lotions** Barseb 1% HC Scalp Lotion can be applied to the worst rash of the scalp once or twice a day for extra therapy for a stubborn or severe case. Valisone solution, applied similarly, is a stronger fluorinated corticosteroid that is safe on the scalp.

4. **Tar** Rarely, a topical tar as Estar can be applied to stubborn areas in addition to corticosteroid lotions. Such a regimen can be irritating and is not the usual therapy for seborrheic dermatitis.

VII. PSORIASIS

A. Clinical Features

Psoriasis occurs most commonly as chronic, scaly, erythematous plaques with a sharp border. On scraping the lesion with a tongue blade, one may see silvery scales and one may elicit bleeding points. When psoriasis involves the scalp, it may occur around the margins and adjacent neck, as well as the face. Lesions elsewhere are usually found on elbows, knees, and the trunk. The patient may have pitting of the nails, nail separation, arthritis, and nonspecific intertrigo that may not be scaly because of the moisture of the skin in this area. Psoriasis does not atrophy and does not usually itch. It is less responsive to therapy than seborrheic dermatitis and eczema and often requires specialized care. Partially treated or resolving lesions may resemble eczema, neurodermatitis, or seborrheic dermatitis.

B. Treatment

Only local therapy is considered here. The application of topical corticosteroids is the best single therapy. On the face, one should apply 1 to 2½% hydrocortisone (Hytone) cream or Westcort Cream 2 to 4 times daily. On the scalp, Valisone solution or fluocinonide (Topsyn Gel) may be applied twice a day. Estar can be added at bedtime, and Pentrax or Ionil T tar shampoos may be used daily. A shower cap can be worn over the scalp for 4 to 8 hours after applying Valisone solution, to increase penetration of the drug. A triple topical regimen for stubborn plaques of the scalp is as follows: 1 drop Keralyt Gel (6% salicylic acid gel), 1 drop Estar Gel, and 1 drop Topsyn Gel, rubbed in well at bedtime and shampooed out in the morning. Careful exposure to sunlight without burning helps most lesions that are exposed.

VIII. ACNE VULGARIS AND ACNEIFORM ERUPTIONS

A. Types of Eruption

1. **Acne vulgaris** is a comedonal papular and pustular condition that normally manifests itself at puberty on the face and trunk. The lesions result from a keratin plug, which blocks the normal pilosebaceous openings on the face. This process produces a small, white papule known as a whitehead or closed comedone filled with sebum. Treatment is aimed at opening the follicle and reducing the activity of the bacteria, which converts the sebum to irritating fatty acids.

2. **Acneiform eruptions** can result from the ingestion of corticosteroids, iodide and bromide, and exogenous androgens, including some birth control pills whose progestational agent is androgenic and dominant in effect, as well as the endogenous production of androgens and industrial exposure to oils and chlorinated hydrocarbons. Corticosteroids and halogens usually produce inflammatory pustules in the same stage of development that predominate over the trunk. This form of acne is atypical in appearance. The patient who has acne of sudden onset or worsening of existing acne that is accompanied by hirsutism, abnormal menstrual periods, or other constitutional signs and symptoms may have an androgen-producing adrenal, ovarian, or testicular tumor. This possibility also applies to older individuals who suddenly develop acne for the first time. Some judgment and experience are needed in such cases because acne is a common and variable disease. Industrial acne consists of papules, nodules, and deep cysts and can occur over wide areas of the body. It may persist when exposure to the causative agent has been discontinued.

B. Treatment

1. **Topical benzoyl peroxide** 5 or 10%, or Desquam-X Lotion can be applied to acne lesions once or twice a day, to open comedones and to reduce bacteria.

2. **Topical antibiotics** can be applied once or twice a day. An example is clindamycin (Cleocin), 150-mg no. 4 capsules. Mix the powder from the 4 capsules in Neutrogena vehicle in lotion qs 50 ml applied twice daily. This type of preparation is also available as Cleocin-T solution.

3. **Tetracycline,** 250 mg, can be given systemically and is an older form of therapy to control bacteria. This drug should not be given to pregnant women or nursing mothers, nor should it be given to people with renal or hepatic disease, depressed white blood cell counts, or a tendency to develop vaginal yeast infections while taking antibiotics.

4. **Comedone extraction** It is generally necessary and important to open larger, deeper pustules and to drain them with a

comedone extractor. Numerous comedones can also be emptied in this manner.

5. **Other therapeutic techniques** and special combinations of therapy are often necessary to control acne, but such techniques should only be used by people who specialize in this type of care. Accutane is such a medication.

IX. ACNE ROSACEA

A. Clinical Features

Acne rosacea, a condition occurring in middle-aged individuals, resembles acne vulgaris. Erythema, telangiectasia, and the presence of papules and pustules may be observed in patients with this illness. Patients may notice flushing when ingesting alcohol, caffeine, hot liquids, or spicy foods. At times, this flushing must be differentiated from the carcinoid syndrome, or from menopausal estrogen deficiency.

B. Treatment

For acne rosacea, tetracycline, 250 mg twice daily, controls the disease well. Because systemic antibiotics are less desirable than topical agents, however, topical tetracycline (Topicycline), applied once or twice a day, may help to control the pustules.

X. PERIORAL DERMATITIS

A. Clinical Features

This condition occurs around the mouth at the vestibule of the nose and perioral area in teenagers and adults. It manifests as erythema with tiny papule vesicles less than 1 mm in diameter. At some times, the condition is purely erythematous with some scaling, and at other times, the papule vesicles predominate. The pinpoint vesicles occur at the top of the papules. This condition is not caused by any known allergy. It may be difficult to treat.

B. Treatment

1. **Ointment** Vytone Cream, applied to the rash twice daily, is helpful in lessening the erythema.
2. **Lotion** Topical Sulfacet-R lotion, applied to the papules only at bedtime, is helpful to reduce the papular component. Apply this under the Vytone Cream.
3. **Tetracycline** It may be necessary to administer tetracycline, 250 mg twice daily or another antibiotic to diminish the papules.
4. **Contraindication** It is important to avoid fluorinated corticosteroids in treating this condition because such agents often exacerbate the rash.

VI.

GENERAL CONCEPTS

32

GERIATRIC OTOLARYNGOLOGY

CHARLES F. KOOPMANN, JR.

As the population of industrial societies grows, a larger percentage of the total populace is 65 years old or older. This figure is rapidly approaching 20% in the United States. Geriatric patients present special challenges to each individual medical specialty. This chapter attempts to deal with the various general tissue changes that occur in aging, the dermatologic, otologic, vestibular, nasal, oropharyngeal, and laryngeal manifestations of aging, and some pharmacologic and oncologic considerations.

I. GENERAL TISSUE CHANGES

A. Epidermis

Generally speaking, the epidermis does not thicken with age. An exception is that exposed skin may increase in depth.

B. Dermis

Various elements of the dermis undergo changes during aging. Collagen, a main component of the dermis, makes up 75% of this layer by weight. Each decade, the collagen content decreases by approximately 17%. Also decreasing is water content, elasticity, and cellularity of the dermis, especially the fibroblasts, elastin, and ground substance. Stiffness and the tensile properties of collagen increase. These various changes in the general condition of the skin produce a decrease in strength of the skin and loss of elasticity. The result of the connective tissue changes is seen throughout each system discussed. Certain skin changes result from the cumulative effects of ultraviolet radiation, which, combined with the general physiologic aging process, are the major causes of pathologic changes in aging skin. A combination of these two elements contributes to senile elastosis, keratoacanthoma, premalignant diseases such as leukoplakia, and basal and squamous cell carcinomas. Moreover, the increase in skin wrinkles originates in the dermis secondary to a decrease in ground substance, decreases in skin elasticity, and collagen changes. Thus, the aged patient begins to have facial wrinkles, accentuation of forehead lines and nasolabial folds, droopy eyelids, and circumoral wrinkles. These changes are the basis for facial cosmetic operations in this age group.

C. Sebaceous and Eccrine Glands

Sebaceous and eccrine glandular production is decreased. This change predisposes the elderly to xerosis or dry skin. Xerosis is exacerbated by constant bathing, which leads to severe pruritus in the nasolabial and circumoral areas, as well as the scalp, postauricular areas, and the external auditory canal. The patient should be counseled to avoid warm baths and to use bath oils such as Alpha-Keri and ointments such as Aquaphor.

II. SPECIFIC DERMATOLOGIC MANIFESTATIONS

A. Seborrheic Keratosis

This disorder is basically of unknown origin. Lesions occur predominantly in unexposed areas of the skin in Caucasian persons. Most commonly, these lesions do not enlarge and are of a papillomatous or warty consistency. They are benign and are easily removed with a curette to confirm the diagnosis.

B. Actinic Keratosis (Senile Keratosis)

As the name of this disorder implies, it usually occurs in exposed areas of the skin. The most common sites are the forehead, cheeks, ears, and, in men, the bald scalp. This entity is due to the effects of ultraviolet light on the dermis and collagen. These lesions must be considered premalignant because between 10 and 25% have malignant components or become frank, invasive tumors. One of the most common signs of malignant change is induration. The best treatment is prevention with topical sun-screen ointments such as Solar Cream or PreSun lotion. Premalignant actinic keratoses may be destroyed by curettage, cryosurgical treatment, topical 5-fluorouracil application, or more recently, chemical peeling with either a concentrated phenol solution or trichloracetic acid. Excisional biopsy is indicated when strong suspicion of malignant change exists.

C. Cutaneous Horns

These lesions are thick collections of keratin, usually occurring over the face or auricle. They should all be considered worthy of excisional biopsy because of reports of malignant changes in the base. Cutaneous horns should undergo local excision.

D. Senile Lentigines

Senile lentigo and senile purpura are common on the face and the forearms. These lesions are well demarcated, irregularly shaped, and variable in size. Senile lentigo is persistent and displays an even yellowish brown to black contour. Most commonly, it is darker than one would expect of freckles. Unlike freckles, senile lentigo does not fade when exposed to light. Curettage, cryosurgical treatment, local excision, and chemical peeling are the treatments of choice. A variant is lentigo maligna, which bears a strong resemblance to senile lentigo, with the exception of irregularities and the development of invasive melanoma in approximately 33% of cases. This malignant degeneration usually has a latency period of 10 years or longer. Pigmentation ranges from black and dark to pale brown. The treatment of choice is surgical excision. The differential diagnosis is between keratosis and senile lentigo.

E. Basal Cell Carcinoma or Basal Cell Epithelioma

This lesion is the most common skin cancer in the Caucasian race. Metastasis is rare, but local destruction and invasion can occur. The most common site of basal cell epithelioma is the face. Clinically, this lesion is seen initially as a small, smooth, pearly papule covered with a thin epidermis and containing slightly dilated blood vessels. As the lesion enlarges, it may form a mass of pearly nodules along the outer aspects with central ulceration and may resemble squamous cell carcinoma or keratoacanthoma. Keratoacanthoma usually grows more rapidly and has a center of keratin rather than a central area of dried serum and blood, however. Squamous cell carcinoma has a rougher edge. Morphea-like basal cell carcinoma appears as a plaque of tissue with a fine, nodular border often mistaken for scar tissue. The treatment of basal cell carcinoma is varied. Some dermatologic surgeons consider curettage or cautery satisfactory. Because of the propensity for local destruction and recurrence, however, excision with the creation of free tissue margins is desired. In patients with extensive lesions of the eyelid or certain areas along the nose, one may consider chemosurgical treatment or radiation therapy (see Chapter 31).

F. Squamous Cell Carcinoma or Squamous Cell Epithelioma

This malignant lesion of the epidermis has a tendency for lymphatic metastasis. It usually appears in sun-damaged skin, especially in skin involved by actinic keratosis or leukoplakia. The initial signs of squamous cell carcinoma are induration and erythema, the presence of a small, hard, reddened nodule that is enlarged in more than one direction, and possibly, an ulcerated lesion with a raised, yellow edge. Squamous cell carcinomas are most commonly seen in the head and neck, on the lower lip, and in the auricle. Again, some dermatologic surgeons recommend curettage and cautery even of large lesions; however, because of the tendency for lymphatic spread, this author prefers either radiation therapy or primary, total excision, with the creation of free margins of tissue. Unless the lesion is unusually large or unless clinical evidence exists of regional metastasis, the lymphatic drainage areas may be merely observed closely.

III. OTOLOGIC MANIFESTATIONS

A. Auricle and External Auditory Canal

1. **Carcinoma** The auricle is a common site for basal cell and squamous cell carcinomas. The treatment of these lesions is as outlined previously.
2. **Chondrodermatitis nodularis chronica helicis** is another lesion of the auricle that may occur in the elderly. The presenting symptom is pain of the involved auricle, especially when lying on that side of the head. Such pain may be due to a necrotic spicule of cartilage, which may be palpable. A trial of corticosteroid therapy for 1 to 2 weeks is warranted, but if this regimen fails, then surgical excision is recommended.
3. **Otitis externa** occurs in the elderly more frequently than in young and middle-aged adults. One reason for this incidence is the decrease in the glandular elements in the external auditory canal, along with the drying of the skin, the tendency toward seborrheic keratosis, and the generalized pruritus seen in the elderly.
   a. ***Acute otitis externa*** usually causes erythema of the external ear and external auditory canal, pain on moving the auricle, and otorrhea. Treatment is directed toward removal of inciting agents such as hair spray or the ear mold of a hearing aid, the recommendation that the patient cease traumatizing the external auditory canal with objects such as cotton swabs or bobby pins, and avoidance of water in the ear until the symptoms have subsided. The external auditory canal should be cleaned of all debris and purulent drainage. Topical drainage is then initiated with a variety of otic drops (Cortisporin solution, Vasocidin, Domeboro, or Vōsol-HC) placed either in the ear canal or on a cotton wick. Another method of treating otitis externa in patients with a swollen ear canal is the instillation of Mycolog ointment into the entire canal using a small syringe and plastic venipuncture tubing. This ointment is removed every 2 to 3 days, and new applications are made until signs and symptoms have resolved.
   b. ***Malignant otitis externa*** has been described in elderly individuals with diabetes, progressive otitis externa, and osteomyelitis of the external auditory canal and temporal bone. In the initial descriptions of this disease, high mortality rates were reported. Treatment should be based on vigorous systemic antibiotic therapy, along with surgical debridement. The initial mode of therapy was a combi-

nation of Gentamicin and carbenicillin; however, in treating elderly patients, one must be aware of the sodium load, and it is therefore well to consider an alternate combination of tobramycin and ticarcillin. One should avoid prescribing carbenicillin in combination with the cephalosporins or penicillins because these agents interact with one another.

B. Middle Ear

1. **Otitis media** The general principles of treatment of otitis media in any other age group apply to the geriatric patient, with few exceptions. In a patient who develops unilateral serous otitis media without evidence of an upper respiratory tract infection, barotrauma, or allergy, one must suspect a nasopharyngeal neoplasm. Treatment of acute suppurative otitis media with antibiotics is valid in this age group, as in others. In the elderly, one may be inclined to be less aggressive in the treatment of chronic suppurative otitis media if no evidence suggests an impending complication; however, strong reasons exist for aggressive closure of tympanic membrane perforations and for reconstruction of the middle ear in all age groups. Therefore, one should follow the general principles of pediatric and adult therapy for otitis media in treating geriatric patients. The same criteria for exploration of the mastoid cavity and for closure of tympanic membrane perforations should be maintained. The elderly patient deserves to lead a full life without the continued annoyance of recurrent suppurative otitis media due to contamination of the middle ear space with water through a pre-existing perforation.
2. **Degenerative joint disease** The incudomalleal and incudostapedial joints are synovial, diarthrodial articular joints. Just as degenerative arthritis can affect the cervical spine, hip, or other cartilaginous articulations, so can it affect the joints in the middle ear. Although rare, this disorder may cause a conductive hearing loss that is amenable to surgical correction, either by ossicular replacement or by rotation.

C. Inner Ear

Presbycusis is loosely defined as deterioration in auditory function associated with aging. More specifically, it is a sensorineural hearing loss that may be of many types. Various factors may be involved in presbycusis, such as the following:

1. **Causes of presbycusis**
   a. ***Atrophy of the organ of Corti*** usually involves the basilar turn of the cochlea and may also be termed sensory presbycusis. The audiometric findings in this type of hearing disorder are abrupt high-frequency losses. The speech-reception threshold is usually adequate.

b. ***Hair cell changes*** A second factor in presbycusis is the decrease with age of the hair cells of the inner ear.

c. ***Mechanical presbycusis*** A third factor is the basilar membrane, which various authorities say atrophies, ruptures, or becomes thin. In patients with this disorder, the audiogram shows a progressive loss in the high frequencies, with no abrupt drop.

d. ***Metabolic presbycusis*** refers to defects in the biochemical or biophysical processes in the cochlea and is directly linked to atrophy in the stria vascularis ductus cochlearis. In this instance, the audiogram is a flat configuration.

e. ***Neural presbycusis*** takes into consideration the auditory nerves and has been described as neural atrophy. One finds the loss of ganglion cells in the spiral ganglia, as well as degeneration of the neurons in higher auditory pathways. The audiogram reveals phonemic regression. This refers to the situation in which a patient has much poorer speech discrimination than one would expect from the pure-tone audiogram.

2. **Treatment of presbycusis** In general, treatment of sensorineural hearing loss of the aged involves counseling concerning the environment and the potential usefulness of amplification. A few general suggestions may be given to patients with presbycusis. One should suggest that patients initiate conversations, rather than wait for other persons to speak. Patients should position themselves with the better ear toward the speaker, and they should ask a spouse or friend to tell them when the topic of a conversation changes. They should also position themselves so that strong light shines on the face of the speaker. A telephone amplifier with volume control should be installed at home. In counseling, the spouse or friends of patients should be told to talk at a moderate rate in a normal tone of voice and to use long phrases, which are more easily understood. These persons should make every attempt to ensure that the hearing-impaired patient is able to follow changes in the conversation. As a general rule, if the patient's hearing loss is 25 db or less, amplification is not necessary. Between 25 and 40 db, the patient has a minimal need for amplification, perhaps only on special occasions. Between 40 and 55 db, a frequent need exists for amplification. A patient with a hearing loss between 55 and 80 db has the greatest need for a hearing aid. Above 80 db, the need for amplification is great, but a hearing aid may not be effective (see Chapter 11).

IV. VESTIBULAR MANIFESTATIONS

The elderly patient who complains of dizziness or vertigo requires a complete medical history and physical examination. Equilibrium is based on the interdependence of the vestibular, visual, and proprioceptive systems. Most patients can tolerate a disturbance in one of these three areas, but a disturbance in two or more is incapacitating. Fifty percent of elderly patients living at home complain of "dizziness." As with any other patient, the medical history is of the utmost importance. The spell should be described in an attempt to distinguish true vertigo, with nausea and vomiting from lightheaded sensations. Special attention should be paid to precipitating factors, such as hyperextension of the neck or sudden changes of position, that may point to a vascular origin. The pattern of the spell is important. One should determine whether the patient has any associated neurologic symptoms such as blind spots or sensory deficits. Finally, special attention should be placed on any medications the patient may be taking because elderly patients are more likely to take antiarrhythmic agents, sedatives, or antihypertensive drugs than patients in other age groups. The most common causes of vertigo in the elderly are postural hypotension, vertebrobasilar insufficiency, cardiac arrhythmias, cerebrovascular insufficiency, overuse of or reaction to medications such as quinidine, antihypertensives, salicylates, or barbiturates, and diabetes mellitus. During the workup of these patients, one must take note of electrocardiographic findings, auscultation of the carotid arteries, and cardiac irregularities. Moreover, one must be aware of dietary insufficiencies that can have neurologic sequelae, such as vitamin-B or iron-deficiency anemia. The radiographic and laboratory evaluations are similar to those for any other patient with vertigo, (see Chapter 10).

V. NASAL MANIFESTATIONS

A. General Changes

As one ages, several general changes occur in the nasal composition that affect physiology and appearance. A loss of internal moisture in the nose predisposes the patient to atrophic rhinitis. Other changes are loss of hydration in the subcutaneous tissue of the skin, a loss of elastic fibers, and atrophy of the collagen. The adipose tissue is absorbed. Increased fragility of the blood vessels and a tendency to sclerosis are noted. Finally, evidence of muscle atrophy is present.

B. Epistaxis

1. **Predisposing factors** The loss of internal moisture and the increased fragility and sclerosis of the blood vessels predispose the elderly patient to epistaxis. As in other age groups, the most common site of epistaxis is in Kiesselbach's plexus. Because of the foregoing factors, however, the elderly patient is also more susceptible to posterior nose bleeds.

2. **Treatment** of epistaxis in the elderly should follow the general principles of treatment of epistaxis in any other patient. Therapy is predicated on the identification of the bleeding site. Anterior epistaxis may be treated with cautery, either thermal or chemical, using silver nitrate, light packing using petrolatum

gauze or a hemostatic agent such as oxidized cellulose (Oxycel) cotton, digital compression, or the application of topical vasoconstrictors such as cocaine. Posterior epistaxis must be treated by anterior and posterior nasal packing. If posterior nasal packing is necessary, one must remember that any patient with a posterior nasal pack in place is prone to hypoxia. Therefore, blood-gas determinations and close observation of the elderly patient during the first 24 to 48 hours are important. For this reason, if patients show evidence of respiratory complications, one should consider arterial ligation of the involved vessels, such as the ethmoidal or internal maxillary arteries. In many cases, surgical intervention is not only less risky, but also allows earlier discharge from the hospital. Another method of treatment of epistaxis from the internal maxillary system is embolization of the involved artery with absorbable gelatin sponge (Gelfoam), muscle, or silicone pellets through the angiographic approach (see Chapter 14).

C. Cosmetic Changes

Cartilaginous changes in the nose affect both cosmetic appearance and functional capacity. The upper and lower lateral cartilages separate and eventually fragment as age advances. The upper lateral cartilage softens along its inferior margin, as does the superior aspect of the lower lateral cartilage. Partial, and occasionally total, fragmentation of the superior border of the lower lateral cartilage and of the inferior border of the upper lateral cartilage occurs. The columella becomes retracted, and the medial crura show a tendency to diverge. These changes alter the air flow current and may cause symptoms of airway obstruction as the years progress. The treatment for such symptoms is by septoplasty, with preservation of a cartilaginous septum, and by cartilaginous rhinoplasty. In the rhinoplasty, 2 to 4 mm of lower lateral cartilage (cephalic end) are resected, as is a strip of the anterior caudal portion of the septum. Autogenous cartilage is placed anterior to the nasal spine, and the skin overlying the nasal dorsum is undermined and elevated by retaping. Elevation of the nasal tip allows air flow to approach physiologic levels.

VI. ORAL MANIFESTATIONS

A. Loss of Dentition

As is easily noted, elderly patients have an increased incidence of loss of dentition. Various studies have shown that 50 to 75% of patients over 60 years of age are completely edentulous. This loss of dentition may be secondary to dental caries, periodontal disease, diminished salivary flow, food retention, or bruxism. A slowly progressive loss of alveolar bone also occurs and has been termed "senile atrophy." Other contributing factors to alveolar bone loss are poor oral hygiene, osteoporosis, and the physiologic aging of skeletal bone after age 40. Xerostomia is common in the elderly because of salivary gland atrophy or fibrosis. This dryness may cause severe dental problems, as well as complaints of burning in the mouth, oral or hypopharyngeal pain, or hoarseness. Xerostomia is treated by increased fluid intake, stimulation of remaining salivary flow with lozenges or sialagogues, or the use of artificial saliva (see Chapter 18).

B. Changes in the Oral Mucosa

The epithelial layer of the mucous membrane in the oral cavity becomes thinner with age. The connective tissue becomes less elastic, and the blood supply is diminished. These changes, combined with the loss of salivary gland function, contribute to atrophic glossitis, which is treated in the same manner as xerostomia.

C. Atrophic Tongue

The elderly patient with atrophic mucosa over the tongue may indeed have a geographic tongue, may exhibit lichen planus, or may have iron-deficiency anemia. The geographic tongue may be caused by local irritation from smoking. In such an instance, one should advise the patient to stop smoking. A complete blood count and a serum iron level determination assist in the diagnosis of iron-deficiency anemia. More generalized atrophy of the tongue and oral mucosa must cause the physician to suspect vitamin-B deficiency, lichen planus, iron-deficiency anemia, and if xerostomia and dysphagia are present, Plummer-Vinson syndrome, or finally, amyloidosis. Patients with vitamin-B deficiency usually also have angular stomatitis (see Chapter 16).

D. Temporomandibular Joint Syndrome

Elderly patients lose elasticity in the temporomandibular joint ligaments. They also have decreased excursion of the mandibular condyle as it moves in the articular surface of the glenoid fossa. Finally, a marked change in occlusion is usual because of the previously mentioned changes in the patient's dentition and oral cavity. These factors predispose the elderly patient to temporomandibular joint symptoms. Usually, the patient complains of pain, which is most intense in the early morning and slowly abates as the day progresses. The joint may become dislocated. If the disease is unilateral, the mandible may drift away from the involved side. Treatment is by equilibration of the dental occlusion, if possible. Patients whose symptoms are acute and severe should be treated as one would treat patients with arthritis in any other joint; that is, one should prescribe joint rest with a liquid diet and minimal talking, anti-inflammatory agents such as aspirin, muscle relaxants, and local applications of moist heat. Corticosteroid injections into the temporomandibular joint are not usually warranted. In patients with severe degenerative changes in the temporomandibular joint who have difficulty in opening the mouth, it may be advisable to perform a condylectomy, including replacement with a prosthesis such as Proplast.

E. Pemphigus

The oral manifestations of pemphigus include vesiculobullous lesions that often precede skin involvement. Any or all areas of the mouth may be involved. Development of these lesions may be stimulated by abrasion of the oral mucosa with food or other traumatic factors. Bullae form on what appears to be normal oral mucosa. If the bullae become poorly demarcated and if some loss of epithelium is noted near the periphery, then the oral counterpart of Nikolsky's sign is present. Hemorrhage may occur at any stage. The ulcerated lesions may have a pseudomembranous covering, which is easily removed to reveal a raw surface that bleeds easily. Patients with oral pemphigus are usually treated with corticosteroids.

F. Leukoplakia

This plaque-like lesion may appear in the oral cavity as a result of the body's response to local irritation, most commonly caused by smoking. This disorder may be either localized or widespread. Histologically, leukoplakia has varying degrees of hyperkeratosis and chronic inflammation. Up to 10% of these lesions also reveal dysplasia and may be considered precancerous. The differential diagnosis of leukoplakia includes lichen planus, early invasive carcinoma, and discoid lupus erythematosus. When the clinician is unsure whether invasion has occurred, an incisional biopsy is advisable. Localized leukoplakia may be excised, and the patient may be advised to remove the inciting factor. Widespread leukoplakia of the oral mucosa may be treated adequately with superficial cryosurgical procedures (see Chapter 16).

G. Candidiasis

Infestations with Candida albicans appear as a creamy, whitish exudate over the oral cavity with bright, reddened bases. When the exudate is removed, usually with moderate difficulty, the raw surface may or may not bleed. Frequently, patients complain of a hot, burning sensation in the oral cavity. Among the underlying conditions that may predispose a patient to candidiasis are carcinoma, diabetes, broad-spectrum antibiotic therapy, immunosuppression or chemotherapy, radiation therapy, and hormone deficiencies. Should one of these underlying conditions be present, the inciting cause should be eliminated, if possible, and the oral cavity should be treated with nystatin (Mycostatin) suspension. Oral candidal infections are not reported to be contraindications to continued radiation therapy unless the patient is too uncomfortable because of the burning sensation. The high incidence of candidiasis is one reason that broad-spectrum antibiotics should be prescribed with extreme caution in the elderly patient. If a patient with candidiasis has lost weight, with or without dysphagia, a barium swallow will be essential because the entire upper gastrointestinal tract may be involved by the disease (see Chapter 16).

VII. LARYNGEAL MANIFESTATIONS

A. Atrophic Laryngitis

This disorder produces hoarseness, a sensation of a lump in the throat that requires the patient to clear his throat constantly, and cough. Findings include a dry mucosa with an occasional foul-smelling crust in the supraglottic region. Treatment is directed at increasing humidification and intake of fluids (see Chapter 23).

B. Cricoarytenoid Joint Fixation

Up to 20% of all patients with rheumatoid arthritis may have laryngeal manifestations. In the acute stages of the disease, such laryngeal features include red, swollen arytenoid cartilages. Patients with chronic disease have thickened arytenoid cartilages with reduced vocal cord mobility. Patients frequently complain of dysphagia, odynophagia, and if the joints are fixed, severe respiratory distress with hoarseness. Initial treatment is directed toward reducing the inflammatory stage and includes tapered doses of oral corticosteroids. It may be necessary to treat the patient on a long-term basis with corticosteroids or other anti-inflammatory agents such as aspirin. Should medical management fail, tracheostomy and, eventually, arytenoidopexy will be required (see Chapter 23).

C. Morphologic Changes

1. **The epiglottis** undergoes degeneration of the cartilaginous ground substance.
2. **Laryngeal cartilages** Ossification progresses after the age of 20 years.
3. **False vocal cords** Aging is manifested by squamous metaplasia in the false vocal cords. Moreover, diminished mucous production causes atrophic changes in the mucosa and decreases protection to the underlying cellular tissue.
4. **Thyroarytenoid muscles** Aging decreases muscle fiber mass.
5. **Vocal cords** Aging decreases elasticity.
6. **General vocal changes**
   a. ***Clinical features*** The foregoing factors, when taken as a whole, manifest themselves in a reduced vibratory mass in the larynx secondary to muscle atrophy. Abductor strength is noticeably reduced. Factors such as vocal pitch, quality, and volume are changed as one grows older. Volume is reduced because of a decrease in thyroarytenoid muscle fibers and because of bowing of the true vocal cords secondary to loss of connective tissue support. Drying of the laryngeal mucosa contributes to hoarseness.
   b. ***Treatment*** of vocal problems in the aged depends on the

cause. Vocal abuse, as in any other age group, should be treated with voice rest and counseling by a speech pathologist. Neurologic manifestations of laryngeal involvement in patients who have had cerebrovascular accidents may be treated by a speech pathologist and, in the case of unilateral and bilateral vocal cord paralysis, by Teflon injection. Morphologic changes secondary to the aging process, such as senile bowing and atrophic laryngitis, must be treated by counseling and by the use of throat lozenges, saline sprays, or humidification, especially at bedtime.

7. **Functional dysphonia** may cause a patient to complain of chronic sore throat with an aching, tingling, or burning sensation. Not only may the foregoing morphologic changes be present, but older persons may also show signs of increased generalized body fatigue. Functional dysphonia may become worse during periods of emotional upset (see Chapter 23).

D. Spastic Dysphonia

1. **Diagnosis** Spastic dysphonia was initially described in 1871 by Traube, who believed that the disease was of psychogenic origin. The disease was originally described as "stuttering with the vocal cords." The age of onset is usually over 40 years. Diagnosis is made by listening to the quality of the patient's voice, which has a tight, hoarse, soft sound low in the throat. Grimacing is associated with speech, as is often seen in severe stutterers. Evaluation of the patient should include a tape recording of the voice before and after the injection of the recurrent laryngeal nerve with 1% lidocaine. Usually, the right recurrent nerve is selected. If the injection causes an improvement in the quality of the voice, then spastic dysphonia may be diagnosed. This diagnosis should also be made by indirect laryngoscopic study, in which the vocal cords frequently appear to be in spasm during phonation.

2. **Cause** No clear cause of spastic dysphonia is known. Some workers believe that the disease is psychogenic in origin because the spasticity usually increases with stress or fatigue, and patients may talk more normally when intoxicated. Other investigators believe that the disease is of neuromuscular origin. Investigators at the Mayo Clinic found that 20 of 27 patients had one or more of the following neurologic signs: tremor, hyperreflexia, reduced rapid alternating motion, and faciolingual asymmetry. Finally, one investigator has reported that a disturbance in the proprioceptive control of the vocal cords may be a factor.

3. **Treatment** is aimed at improvement of vocal quality. Psychotherapy has not been useful, and speech therapy is of limited value. Currently, the recommended treatment involves surgical section of one of the recurrent laryngeal nerves. This

procedure usually provides a noticeable improvement in the quality of the patient's voice (see Chapter 23).

E. Gastroesophageopharyngeal Reflux

1. **Diagnosis** The symptoms of this disorder include hoarseness, a globus (pharyngeal tightness) sensation, paroxysmal cough, dysphagia, pharyngeal clearing, laryngospasm, "heartburn," otalgia, and cervical pain in the thyrohyoid area. Usually, symptoms are worse in the morning and occur in middle-aged to elderly, obese patients. Physical findings include arytenoid erythema, granulomas, and occasionally, point tenderness over one superior laryngeal nerve. Diagnosis is made by medical history, the foregoing physical findings, and radiographic studies, which may include a reflux acid barium meal.
2. **Treatment** is strictly medical. The head of the patient's bed should be elevated on blocks. The patient should be instructed to take antacids after meals, especially before retiring at night. When symptoms become worse, voice rest should be prescribed. Finally, if the foregoing suggestions fail, propantheline bromide (Pro-Banthine) should be added to the regimen. Complications of this disease include esophageal webbing, contact granulomas of the larynx, and occasionally, hyperkeratosis of the vocal cords (see Chapter 22).

VIII. PHARYNGEAL AND ESOPHAGEAL MANIFESTATIONS

A. Incidence of Dysphagia

Dysphagia is a frequent complaint in the geriatric patient. Peristalsis is impaired in 90% of the elderly; 50% of these patients have diminished contractions.

B. Oropharyngeal Dysphagia

This disorder involves transfer of material from the pharynx and involuntary contraction of the pharyngeal constrictors past the cricopharyngeus muscle. In oropharyngeal dysphagia, liquids are poorly tolerated. Causes of acute oral pharyngeal dysphagia include pharyngitis, stomatitis secondary to viral infections, fungal infections, vitamin deficiency, iron-deficiency anemia, the presence of foreign bodies, trauma, and retropharyngeal abscesses. Chronic oropharyngeal dysphagia in the elderly is frequently caused by neuromuscular dysfunction, such as from cerebrovascular accident, amyotrophic lateral sclerosis, myasthenia gravis, or diabetic neuropathy. Other causes of chronic dysphagia of the upper gastrointestinal tract include oropharyngeal or laryngeal tumors, amyloidosis, xerostomia, hypertrophic cervical vertebrae, previous surgical procedures, and globus hystericus. If amyloidosis is found in the elderly, one should suspect multiple myeloma as an underlying cause (see Chapter 22).

C. Middle and Lower Esophageal Dysphagia

Benign and malignant esophageal tumors must be considered. Moreover, distal esophageal structures secondary to reflux esophagitis, a lower esophageal (Schatzki) ring, or achalasia may be encountered in the elderly patient. In the edentulous patient, an obstruction secondary to a meat impaction or foreign body may be present. Diverticuli in the upper esophagus (Zenker's) are most common in elderly patients. Another cause of dysphagia in this age group is obstruction secondary to a vascular disorder. Possible causes include cardiac hypertrophy secondary to congestive heart failure, a tortuous, calcific descending aorta, or a thoracic aortic aneurysm. Treatment is most frequently medical, including a soft diet and medical control of congestive heart failure or hypertension in patients with a calcific descending aorta. Surgical resection of a thoracic aortic aneurysm is indicated, however (see Chapter 22).

IX. ONCOLOGIC CONSIDERATIONS

A. Conservation Operations on the Larynx

Until 1977, it was frequently written that patients over 65 years of age were not to undergo conservation operations on the larynx, such as vertical hemilaryngectomy or supraglottic laryngectomy. At this time, however, it appears that age alone should not be considered an absolute contraindication for such a procedure.

B. Composite Resections

All too frequently, referring physicians and consultants in medical or radiation oncology report that elderly patients tolerate composite resections in the head and neck poorly. It appears that if medical problems, both cardiac and pulmonary, are treated vigorously pre- and postoperatively, however, the mortality rate in the elderly who undergo composite resections may be 7% or less. Associated medical complications may be kept under 20%, as compared with a rate of 5 to 10% in patients under 65 years of age. The incidence of surgical complications in patients 70 years of age and older who undergo radical neck dissection appears to be no greater than in patients under age 70. The incidence of medical complications is only 8% more in patients over 70 years (Laryngoscope, *87*:1378, 1977). Thus, failure to perform ablative surgical procedures in the elderly patient with head and neck cancer may, ultimately, be the most radical course of treatment. Advanced age should not be considered an absolute contraindication to major surgical procedures for head and neck cancer.

X. PHARMACOLOGIC CONSIDERATIONS

A. Pharyngeal Symptoms

Symptoms that may occur with the use of antimetabolite agents include oral ulceration and severe oral pain.

B. Esophageal Problems

Anticholinergic drugs delay gastric emptying and decrease the lower esophageal sphincter tone. These changes may increase symptoms of reflux esophagitis. In addition, antibiotics and immunosuppressive agents predispose patients to candidal infection.

C. Gastric Complications

Nausea, vomiting, and epigastric discomfort may occur with the commonly prescribed anti-inflammatory drugs. Antacids must be prescribed with great caution in patients with impaired renal function because of their calcium and magnesium levels. Moreover, the sodium content of the common antacids is high, and such agents should therefore be prescribed with caution in patients with cardiac failure. Finally, antacids raise the pH of the stomach and cause poor absorption of penicillin G, tetracycline, sulfa drugs, ferrous sulfate, and ferrous gluconate.

D. Disorders of the Small Intestine

Enteric-coated potassium, frequently prescribed in patients receiving diuretic therapy for hypertension or Ménière's disease, may cause stenotic ulcerations of the jejunum.

E. Congestive Heart Failure

Patients who have a history of congestive heart failure are susceptible to a sodium load. Thus, the physician should not prescribe such drugs as carbenicillin, sodium penicillin, and ticarcillin. Diuretics such as ethacrynic acid and furosemide may potentiate the ototoxic effects of antibiotics and, indeed, may be ototoxic themselves. Finally, patients taking digitalis are at risk for digitalis toxicity when receiving sodium penicillin, carbenicillin, or ticarcillin.

F. Diabetes Mellitus

Patients with diabetes mellitus are susceptible to certain side effects of antibiotics. Sulfonamides and chloramphenicol may potentiate the action of oral hypoglycemic agents. Glycosuria occurs with cephalosporins, chloramphenicol, penicillin, and tetracycline. Therefore, one should advise the patient to use Dextrostix or Labstix, but not Clinitest, for urine glucose determinations.

G. Clotting Factors

Antibiotics such as ampicillin, tetracyclines, and chloramphenicol may interfere with clotting or may potentiate the action of anticoagulant agents.

33

DIAGNOSTIC RADIOLOGY

BARBARA CARTER

I. GENERAL PRINCIPLES

A. Indications for Use

Radiographs are a vital supplement to the medical history and physical examination in the diagnosis and treatment of patients with otorhinolaryngologic disorders. The number of x-ray studies should be kept to a minimum because of radiation exposure, especially in children and in pregnant women, and because of cost. Once the physician decides on the area to be studied, the radiologist will determine the appropriate projections. If one is in doubt, or if one has reason for modifying the examination, the radiologist should be consulted prior to the study. Plain films are usually adequate in establishing a diagnosis in most patients. Tomography, laryngography, sialography, barium studies, fistulography, xeroradiography, radionuclide techniques, ultrasound, computed tomography (CT), and magnetic resonance imaging (MRI) all have specific indications that are evolving with improved technology (Table 33–1).

B. Hazards of Radiation Exposure

Epidemiologic studies have shown an increased incidence of thyroid cancer in young persons treated for "thymic enlargement" during infancy. Leukemia has occurred with greater-than-average frequency in patients exposed to large doses of radiation in utero and in a general population exposed to the atomic bomb or a high background of radiation. The radiation exposure received by the patient under these and similar circumstances is at a much higher

TABLE 33–1

Recommended Diagnostic Radiographic Studies

Anatomic Area	Study	Specific Purpose
Paranasal sinuses and nose	Plain roentgenograms	
	Pluridirectional tomograms	Trauma
	CT*	Tumors
Nasopharynx and infratemporal fossa	CT*	Tumors
Orbit	CT* MRI†	Trauma Tumors Abscesses
Skull base	Plain roentgenograms	Trauma
	CT*	Tumors
	Tomograms	
Petrous and temporal bones	Plain roentgenograms	Inflammatory disease
	Tomograms	Congenital anomalies; trauma
	CT*	Tumors, benign and malignant
	Posterior fossa air cisternography, angiograms, and MRI†	Tumors
Mandible and temporomandibular joints	Plain roentgenograms	Trauma
	Tomograms, CT,* MRI†	Abnormalities of joints
Oropharynx and hypopharynx	Plain roentgenograms	Foreign bodies
	Barium swallows	Diverticula
	CT,* MRI†	Tumors
Larynx	Plain roentgenograms	Foreign bodies
	Tomograms	Subglottic extension
	CT,* MRI†	Moderate-to-large tumors
	Laryngograms	Polyps; lesions of laryngeal ventricle
Salivary glands	Plain roentgenograms	Stones
	Sialograms	Inflammatory disease
	CT,* MRI†	Tumors
	Radionuclide scans	Tumors

*CT = Computed tomograms
†MRI = Magnetic resonance imaging

level than that received from diagnostic x-ray films by a factor of at least a thousandfold. Much publicity in lay journals and newspapers has caused an unwarranted public scare. Some patients have consequently refused x-ray examinations needed for proper medical management. Such studies should not be requested, however, unless a strong clinical indication exists. Magnetic resonance imaging (MRI) presents no radiation exposure.

II. PLAIN ROENTGENOGRAMS

A. Sinuses and Surrounding Facial Bones

Soft tissue changes within the sinus, as well as the integrity of the bony wall and adjacent structures, must be assessed on all plain film examinations. The sharp white line representing the cortical bone forming the wall of the sinus can usually be seen, unless it is demineralized, and indicates the actual size of the sinus. This feature is important in the recognition of a hypoplastic sinus, which when suspected, should be confirmed by the base projection. A hypoplastic sinus must not be confused with an opaque sinus caused by infection or tumor. Septa within the sinus should also be identified because they may be complete and may thereby separate the sinuses into two discrete compartments, one of which may become infected and may go unrecognized. The most common soft tissue change within a sinus, especially in the maxillary area, is the retention cyst, a sharply defined mound of little clinical significance. A mucocele cannot be identified unless it actually expands the sinus; the frontal area is the most common site, but this lesion may occur in any of the sinsues. Any slowly growing tumor may expand the sinus and may push bone before it as it advances. This phenomenon is in contrast to the behavior of a malignant tumor, which usually destroys bone. A single opaque sinus is unusual in patients with sinusitis and should alert one to the possibility of a tumor or an abnormality of an adjacent structure, such as a tooth in the case of the maxillary sinus. The following projections are obtained for the paranasal sinuses.

1. **Waters projection** is used to visualize the maxillary sinuses and the frontal and anterior ethmoid sinuses.

2. **Posteroanterior or Caldwell projection** enables one to see the frontal and ethmoid sinuses, the superior orbital fissure, the foramen rotundum, and the maxillary ethmoidal plate.

3. **Lateral projection** is used for the sphenoid and ethmoid sinuses, the nasopharynx and pterygopalatine fossa, and the maxillary and frontal sinuses.

4. **Base projection,** in which the patient's neck is hyperextended with the mandible projected anterior to the frontal sinuses, allows visualization of the frontal sinuses, especially the posterior wall, and of the maxillary and sphenoid sinuses.

5. **Additional views**
   a. ***Decubitus Waters and supine lateral (brow-up) views*** enable one to confirm a fluid level.
   b. ***Townes projection*** is used in the evaluation of facial and mandibular trauma.
   c. ***Bucket-handle view,*** which is a base view exposed for the zygomatic arch, is also used in evaluating trauma.

B. Nasal Bone

1. **Coned-down lateral view** allows visualization of nasal bone and of the spinous process of the maxilla.
2. **Occlusal view** may also be indicated to evaluate nasal fractures.

C. Nasopharynx

Large masses of the nasopharynx are visible on plain film studies because of the interface between air and soft tissue. Normal structures, such as the adenoids, the palatine tonsils, and the muscles of the posterior pharyngeal wall (constrictor pharyngis, longus capitis, and longus colli) must not be confused with tumors. Tumors that are flat may not be visible on a roentgenogram, even though they may be ulcerating and locally invasive. Thus, a tumor can be identified, if seen, but the diagnosis may not be excluded if a tumor is not apparent on multiple projections with plain films or tomograms (see Chapter 29).

1. **Lateral projection,** using a high-kilovolt technique (100 to 120 kv), is helpful in the evaluation of bone as well as soft tissue.
2. **Anteroposterior view** may also be useful to evaluate nasopharyngeal masses.
3. **Base projection** is indicated to visualize bone and soft tissue detail.

D. Orbit

1. **Posteroanterior projection** enables one to see the anterior orbital rim, the medial and lateral walls, including the frontozygomatic suture, the superior orbital fissure, and the innominate line (cortical bone, greater wing of the sphenoid bone; its absence usually means destruction by tumor or congenital anomaly). One also needs posteroanterior views for evaluation of the lacrimal gland groove and for other congenital anomalies such as hypertelorism.
2. **Lateral projection** is used to evaluate patients with trauma, tumor, foreign body, and calcification.
3. **Optic canal views**
   a. ***"Three-point landing" or oblique Waters view*** Optic canal should be projected at four o'clock and eight o'clock for optimum visualization. This projection is also indicated for evaluating posterior ethmoid cells.
   b. ***Base view*** is used to visualize the entire length of the optic canal. The patient's head is hyperextended, to place the orbitomeatal line 10° below the baseline.

E. Skull Base

Roentgenograms are needed to evaluate the foramen ovale, foramen spinosum, greater wing of the sphenoid bone, petrous apices, and foramen magnum, as well as to visualize congenital anomalies, fractures, and destruction or hyperostosis by tumor. A base projection is also useful for temporomandibular joint (TMJ) abnormalities. Asymmetry of the skull base, including the foramen ovale, may be a variant of normal. Correlation with the clinical findings and comparison with previous roentgenograms help to determine the significance of this difference. If tumor is suspected, a CT scan should be obtained.

F. Temporal Bone

Roentgenographic evaluation of this area includes the tympanic cavity, the inner ear, the mastoid antrum and air cells, the internal and external auditory canals, the jugular fossa, and the carotid canal.

1. **Posteroanterior view** through the orbit allows one to evaluate the following:
   a. ***Internal auditory canal*** may be visualized, to determine asymmetry in height (within 2 mm), in length (within 2 to 3 mm), integrity of the wall, trumpeting appearance with widening of the porus acousticus, and the level of the crista falciformis (medial to superior third of the canal).
   b. ***Scutum*** may be seen, to ascertain erosion by cholesteatoma.
   c. ***Mastoid antrum*** may be opaque with fluid or infection.
   d. ***Congenital anomalies*** of the inner and middle ear may thus be visualized.
2. **Townes projection** enables one to assess aeration of the mastoid antrum and the degree of development of mastoid air cells, to detect destruction by infection or tumor, and to evaluate postoperative change. An open cavity mastoidectomy is normally sharply defined as it becomes epithelialized. A closed cavity has softer, poorly defined borders with healing. A closed cavity with sharply defined edges often indicates a recurrent cholesteatoma.
3. **Base projection** is used to assess the degree of development of mastoid air cells and the presence of bone destruction by infection or tumor.
4. **Schuller (or Rönstrom) projection** is a lateral view of the mastoid air cells with the opposite side projected inferiorly or caudad to the side adjacent to the film. This view is used primarily for the identification of soft tissue within the mastoid air cells due to infection or fluid and the detection of destruction of cell walls, especially in mastoiditis.
5. **Owens (30° oblique) projection,** with the opposite side projected caudad or inferiorly out of the area, is used to assess the tympanic cavity and bone destruction due to cholesteatoma. This view may be used instead of the Meyers projection because it is easier to reproduce.

6. **Chausse III projection,** the third Chausse projection, is an oblique view, for evaluation of the scutum and lateral wall of the attic.
7. **Stenvers' projection** has the petrous bone parallel to the film. This tangential view is used for visualization of the mastoid tip, as well as for en face projection of the porus acousticus to detect acoustic neuromas and en face projection of the hypoglossal canal, which is inferior to the internal auditory canal.
8. **Jugular fossa projection** is a basal view halfway between a true base and a Waters projection. Three roentgenograms taken with the angulation varied by 10° and the patient's head unchanged in position can be viewed simultaneously or in stereo, to show the jugular fossa best.

G. Mandible

1. **Posteroanterior view** is often helpful in visualizing the mandible.
2. **Steep Townes projection** is used to assess the condyles and the condylar neck.
3. **Oblique lateral projection** allows one to evaluate the ramus and the body of the mandible. The x-ray tube is angled to project one side above the other.
4. **Base projection** is especially useful to view the condyle and the condylar fossa.
5. **Occlusal projection** provides a tangential view of the symphysis.

H. Temporomandibular Joint (TMJ)

One should use the coned-down lateral view, with the tube angled to project one joint below the side next to the film. This projection may be obtained with the patient's mouth closed or open, using a bite for equal motion on both sides.

I. Oropharynx, Hypopharynx, and Larynx

1. **Lateral projection** is helpful, using high kilovolt techniques (100 to 120 kv).
   a. ***Quiet breathing or rest*** is best to visualize the nasopharynx, the retropharyngeal airway, the laryngeal surface of the epiglottis and trachea, the laryngeal cartilage, soft tissue calcification, the hyoid bone, and the cervical spine.
   b. ***Phonation*** is indicated to distend the laryngeal ventricle and hypopharynx, including the vallecula. The tip of the epiglottis is best seen with this maneuver.
2. **Anteroposterior projection** If taken with phonation, this view shows soft tissue detail of the hypopharynx, larynx, trachea, and surrounding soft tissue.

J. Parotid and Submandibular Glands

Roentgenograms of these structures are indicated to visualize opaque calculi (80% of submandibular calculi are opaque) and calcification in or adjacent to the glands.

1. **Lateral projection** is useful in evaluating these glands.
2. **Oblique projection** is also frequently necessary.
3. **Posteroanterior projection** In this tangential projection, the patient's cheek should be distended, to visualize a stone in Stensen's duct.
4. **Occlusal projection** reveals the presence of a stone near the orifice of Wharton's duct.

III. TOMOGRAMS

Sections 1-mm thin are most desirable to identify structures clearly in compact areas. That the exposure time is predetermined for various units necessitates sedation for young or uncooperative children. The hypocycloidal motion with the polytome takes 6 sec, and the trispiral motion takes 4.5 or 3 sec, depending on the particular unit. A rapid exposure time is desirable for moving structures such as the larynx. Linear motion with an exposure time of 0.5 to 1.0 sec is usually employed in laryngeal studies. Unfortunately, the linear motion has less blurring effect and thus more "carry over" artifacts from adjacent structures anterior and posterior to the area of interest. Most tomographic examinations should be made with 2 different projections, at 90° to each other, for better evaluation. Anteroposterior and lateral views are usually obtained and are supplemented by other projections, depending on the specific problem. Conventional pluridirectional tomography is most commonly used in the following areas, after a review of the plain radiographic findings.

A. Paranasal Sinuses and Facial Bones

Tomograms may reveal unusual congenital anomalies, complicated fractures, severe infections, mucoceles, and benign and malignant tumors. Benign tumors grow slowly and expand the sinus. Malignant tumors are invasive and destroy bone or cause reactive sclerosis.

B. Nasopharynx

Tomograms of this area are indicated to evaluate encephaloceles and tumors.

1. **Encephaloceles** which represent herniation of the dura and subarachnoid space with some neural elements, are associated with a defect in the skull base appearing either in the nasopharynx through the sphenoid bone or in or anterior to the nasal cavity through a defect in the cribriform plate or the ethmoid or frontal bone.
2. **Mucous retention cysts** along the wall of the nasopharynx or

midline cell rests (Thornwaldt's cyst) do not have an accompanying bone defect.

3. **Malignant tumors** usually invade and thus destroy bone or cause reactive sclerosis.

C. Orbit

Tomograms are helpful in the assessment of trauma and tumors. The base projection is used for the medial wall of the orbit and for the optic nerve canal.

D. Skull Base

Tomograms are indicated to evaluate trauma and tumors, of the floor of the anterior and middle cranial fossa. Anteroposterior and lateral projections are needed to assess the clivus, when CT is not available or to supplement CT scanning.

E. Petrous Bone, Tympanic Cavity, Internal Auditory Canal, and Jugular Fossa

1. **Internal auditory canal** Tomography is a primary screening procedure for this area.
2. **Congenital anomalies** Tomograms confirm the diagnosis and determine the feasibility of surgical correction. Anteroposterior and lateral projections are needed for evaluation of the external canal, the middle and inner ear, and the internal auditory canal. An axial pyramidal view (45° oblique toward side under study) or a base projection is useful in the assessment of the cochlea. It may be helpful to obtain clear tympanic images prior to any surgical procedures, to identify various landmarks such as the facial nerve canal.
3. **Trauma** Anteroposterior and lateral views are indicated.
   a. ***Stenvers' view*** should be obtained for questionable transverse fractures in the presence of cerebrospinal fluid leak.
   b. ***Axial pyramidal view*** ascertains possible longitudinal fracture or ossicular chain disruption.
   c. ***Base projection*** should be obtained when additional information is needed.
4. **Cholesteatoma** Anteroposterior and lateral views are indicated to assess the scutum, wall of the attic, aditus, and antrum, and to detect fistulas of the semicircular canal. The normal lateral wall of the horizontal canal is convex laterally, whereas a flat or concave wall is indicative of a fistula. These studies are also useful to identify erosion of the tegmen or the sigmoid sinus plate, to visualize ossicles, and to evaluate recurrent disease postoperatively.
5. **Chronic infection** Anteroposterior and lateral views are helpful in determining the degree of bone destruction and in identifying cells not adequately removed by previous surgical

procedures, such as cells arising from the hypotympanum or cells in the petrous apex.

6. **Tumor** Anteroposterior, lateral, and base projections should be obtained. Pluridirectional tomography is indicated if CT is not available; it may also supplement the CT scan. The degree of bone involvement and soft tissue mass within the tympanic cavity and mastoid air cells can be ascertained by conventional tomography. The intracranial extent of tumor invasion and soft tissue involvement outside the skull cannot be adequately assessed by this technique alone. CT and plain radiographic studies are needed to determine whether the entire tumor-bearing area is included in the examination and to facilitate follow-up of the course of the disease.

F. Mandible

Tomograms of the mandible are helpful in the evaluation of unusual tumors, particularly those in locations such as the coronoid process, the condyle, and the condylar neck. Orthopantomograms (Panorex) are commonly used to survey patients with extensive dental caries, congenital and developmental anomalies of the teeth or mandible, and tumors, and to obtain preliminary findings prior to a plastic surgical procedure.

G. Temporomandibular Joint

Anteroposterior and lateral views are indicated to evaluate arthritis or post-traumatic changes.

H. Larynx and Hypopharynx

1. **Anteroposterior projection** Linear (short time exposure) views are indicated to evaluate tumors, polyps, and inflammatory diseases. Serial cuts are obtained from the anterior to posterior portions of the larynx, with the vocal cords in abduction and adduction.

2. **Lateral projection** Plain films, rather than tomograms, taken during quiet breathing and phonation, are valuable for assessing the nasopharynx, soft palate, epiglottis (to the anterior commissure), valleculae, laryngeal ventricles, trachea, and retropharyngeal space.

IV. COMPUTED TOMOGRAPHY

Computed tomography (CT) is the study of choice for evaluating head injuries and tumors of the skull base, orbit, petrous and sphenoid bones, and face and neck. CT is also useful in selected cases when abscess or hematoma is suspected. Although plain CT images are often adequate, intravenous infusion may be needed to enhance visualization of vascular tumors and to identify vessels in the area of interest.

A. General Indications

The major indications for CT scans in the head and neck area are as follows:

1. **Detection of the presence and extent of tumor, abscess, or hematoma** is a valuable indication.
2. **Identification of direct extension of tumor or infection** into the orbit, intracranial cavity, and spinal canal is possible with CT, as well as determination of the extent of destruction of adjacent bone and the presence of metastatic nodes.
3. **Determination of the mode of therapy,** whether surgical, radiotherapeutic, or chemotherapeutic, may be based on CT findings.
4. **Assistance in planning radiotherapy** and, occasionally, in determining the best surgical approach is another use of CT.
5. **Follow-up scanning** determines the patient's response to radiotherapy or chemotherapy.
6. **Detection of the presence of recurrent disease** is possible months or years after initial treatment has been completed.

B. Sinuses

CT is the preferred supplement to plain roentgenograms for the evaluation of certain disorders.

1. **Intranasal encephalocele** is demonstrated by CT.
2. **Complications of sinusitis,** including proptosis due to ethmoiditis, meningitis, epidural or intracranial abscess, and osteomyelitis, are visible with CT.
3. **Head trauma** involving the facial bones, the orbit, and the neck may be evaluated by CT.
4. **Benign growths** CT reveals the presence of mucocele, inverted papilloma, angiofibroma, schwannoma, and giant-cell reparative granuloma.
5. **Malignant tumors** Primary and secondary tumors can be detected with CT.

C. Nasopharynx and Infratemporal Fossa

Transverse and coronal projections without, or with, contrast infusion may detect vascular tumors, especially angiofibromas, carcinomas, metastatic disease, granulomas, and cysts.

D. Orbit

Transverse scanning is indicated, coronal when feasible. Contrast infusion should be used as needed.

1. **Congenital anomalies** Maldevelopment of the globe and bony wall and agenesis of the optic nerve may be ascertained.
2. **Trauma** CT scanning detects fracture deformity, such as chip

fractures within the orbit, foreign bodies within or adjacent to the globe, and hematoma.

3. **Infection** Celullitis or abscess arising from the orbit or extending into orbit from adjacent sinuses may be diagnosed.
4. **Tumor** CT enables one to identify primary and metastatic tumors, whether intraconal, extraconal, or of the bony wall, as well as tumors of the orbital septum and lacrimal gland.
5. **Miscellaneous** Pseudotumor or Wegener's granulomatosis, either of which may result in sharply localized or diffuse mass effect, may be diagnosed by CT. One may also detect hypertrophy of the rectus muscles secondary to Graves' disease.

E. Skull Base

Hyperostosis and destruction of bone due to tumor are clearly discernible, as well as any adjacent soft tissue mass superior or inferior to the skull base. CT is therefore the study of choice for this area. Lateral tomography of the clivus may be needed as a supplementary study in isolated cases. Congenital anomalies, such as a small foramen magnum in an achondroplastic dwarf, fractures, and osteomyelitis are all visible on CT images.

F. Petrous and Temporal Bones

CT is the procedure of choice for all tumors arising within or adjacent to the petrous bone, such as acoustic neuroma, glomus jugulare, glomus tympanicum, carcinoma of the tympanic cavity or external auditory canal, or metastatic carcinoma. These tumors usually require studies in the transverse and coronal planes, with and without contrast infusion. Increasing use of CT as a screening procedure for suspected acoustic neuroma will result from the increased availability of high resolution, thin-slice (1 to 2 mm) scans and improved reconstruction in the sagittal and coronal planes. It may also replace pluridirectional tomography for the assessment of cholesteatoma, trauma, and congenital anomalies.

G. Mandible and Temporomandibular Joints

CT is indicated to evaluate malignant tumor extending into adjacent soft tissue.

H. Oropharynx, Hypopharynx, and Parapharyngeal Space

Transverse and occasional coronal scans are indicated with intravenous enhancement, for vascular tumors. This procedure is the best means available for determining the total extent of malignant neoplasms of the palatine fossa and retromolar trigone. It is not needed for more clearly visible, palpable, localized lesions. Occasionally, CT is useful to identify abscesses or hematomas.

I. Larynx

Transverse scans, without intravenous enhancement, are indicated primarily for large tumors extending into the pre-epiglottic space and other areas around the larynx. It has also been recommended for trauma to the larynx, to identify fracture of the thyroid cartilage and dislocation of the arytenoid cartilage.

J. Salivary Glands

Transverse and, occasionally, coronal scans combined with sialography are useful in the assessment of tumors within or adjacent to the parotid and submandibular glands. These images are not diagnostic for the specific type of tumor, except for lipomas and cysts. Increased vascularity is recognized by intravenous infusion, such as in the diagnosis of hemangiomas and carotid body tumors.

V. SIALOGRAPHY

Sialography is used to confirm the presence of stones, strictures, sialectasia, sialadenitis, and tumor (see Chapter 20).

A. Preparation for Study

Plain films are important as a preliminary examination, to identify an opaque stone, calcification, and bone destruction. Parotid examinations should include a tangential view of Stensen's duct, with the patient's cheek blown out, in addition to anteroposterior, lateral and oblique projections. An occlusal view is essential for the detection of stones at or near the orifice of Wharton's duct.

B. Procedure for Contrast Examination

After the injection of ethiodized oil (Ethiodol) or aqueous contrast material (Sinografin), spot films are taken with anteroposterior, lateral, and various degrees of oblique projections. Early roentgenograms are obtained during the filling phase, and subsequent films are taken after opacification of the primary, secondary, and tertiary branches. Complete filling is usually essential for an adequate diagnosis, but care must be taken not to extravasate contrast material within the gland or around the ducts. Extravasation causes pain and misdiagnosis and may result in foreign-body granulomas or fibrosis.

C. Supplemental Scanning

CT scanning is useful as a supplement to, and may be replacing, sialography for the diagnosis and assessment of the total extent of tumor involvement. A vascular tumor, such as hemangioma, may be diagnosed by CT alone, when the procedure is performed before and after rapid intravenous contrast infusion.

VI. RADIONUCLIDE SCANNING

A. Technetium Pertechnetate (^{99m}Tc)

This isotope is occasionally used in the assessment of salivary gland function. The isotope is taken up by the gland and is monitored over a period of 15 to 30 min after injection. The isotope is secreted into the mouth with the saliva. Secretion is hastened by a stimulant such as lemon juice. Poor uptake with a high background occurs in patients with sialadenitis or Sjögren's syndrome. Most tumors, such as mixed tumor or pleomorphic adenoma, are "cold" or take up little isotope. In contrast, Warthin's tumor (papillary cystadenoma lymphomatosum), oxyphilic adenoma, and acute inflammatory reactions are "hot" and have an increased uptake of isotope. Thus, technetium is used in the evaluation of function and detection of tumors.

B. Gallium-67 (Gallium Citrate)

This isotope is taken up preferentially by some tumors, such as melanomas and lymphomas, and by acute and chronic inflammatory processes.

C. Bleomycin-57 (CO-Bleomycin)

This isotope is specific for tumors, particularly of the head and neck, and is occasionally used to supplement other diagnostic examinations. A radionuclide taken up by a primary tumor of the face and neck is usually taken up by distant metastatic lesions as well.

VII. BARIUM SWALLOW

This technique is used for patients with dysphagia and suspected foreign bodies, and tumors. Preliminary anteroposterior and lateral roentgenograms are obtained to detect calcification, opaque foreign bodies, and soft tissue masses. Anteroposterior and lateral films are taken at the height of swallowing barium, to demonstrate maximum distension, reflux into the larynx or nasopharynx, and functional abnormalities. Anteroposterior and lateral films are then taken with the patient "at rest," to detect any abnormality of the mucosa, such as the presence of a tumor, inflammatory mass, or fistulous tract. Acid barium, barium mixed with dilute hydrochloric acid, has been used to reproduce symptoms in patients with diagnostic problems. Tertiary waves or esophageal spasms are evidence of abnormal motility.

VIII. LARYNGOGRAPHY

This procedure detects mucosal and subglottic lesions and should thus precede a biopsy if both tests are to be performed. Although mucosal abnormalities of the larynx are more clearly demonstrated with this technique than with conventional tomography, laryngography requires the use of an atropine-like drug, local anesthesia, and contrast material. Some institutions now use CT rather than laryngograms and conventional tomography.

IX. MISCELLANEOUS TECHNIQUES

A. Dacryocystography

Aqueous contrast material or ethiodized oil (Ethiodol) is injected into the lacrimal duct through a cannula or plastic tube under fluoroscopic guidance. Spot films are taken for assessment of stricture, malfunction, or tumor.

B. Fistulography

Aqueous contrast material or ethiodized oil (Ethiodol) is injected through plastic tubing or a cannula under fluoroscopic control for assessment of the size and extent of a fistulous tract.

C. Localization of a Cerebrospinal Fluid Leak, Otorrhea, or Rhinorrhea

The medical history must be obtained, and the clinical examination must be done first to localize the site and cause of the leak as closely as possible. Factors such as trauma to the skull base or to the frontal area must be taken into consideration. Plain roentgenograms and pluridirectional tomograms are performed next. Isotope cisternography is occasionally used for the gross localization of the defect. The isotope is injected into the lumbar subarachnoid space, and the patient's head is monitored directly by a gamma camera and indirectly with cotton batting in the nasopharynx or ear canal to collect cerebrospinal fluid. Isophendylate (Pantopaque) and metrizamide are also used occasionally with fluoroscopy or with CT scanning over the area of concern, to demonstrate the actual site of the leak.

X. MAGNETIC RESONANCE IMAGING (MRI)

This new imaging technique using surface coils now makes it possible to visualize the seventh and eighth cranial nerves within the internal auditory canal and in the cerebellopontine angle, which previously could only be accomplished with contrast cisternography. There is little doubt that MRI will have many applications in the evaluation of diseases of the head and neck.

34

CHEMOTHERAPY FOR HEAD AND NECK CANCER

WAUN KI HONG

I. GENERAL PRINCIPLES

A. Indications

The otolaryngologist evaluates and actively treats patients with head and neck cancer. The primary treatment of head and neck cancer traditionally has been surgical and radiotherapeutic. If the patient fails initial treatment, then chemotherapy is considered. Even though chemotherapy can cure many hematopoietic and testicular cancers, patients with other solid tumors have responded inconsistently to single-method treatment.

B. Prognosis

The prognosis for patients with recurrent tumors of the head and neck is dismal. Survival times usually range from 4 to 6 months, despite the tumor-shrinking ability of several drugs. The site of recurrence is usually local and impairs adequate nutrition, handling of secretions, and maintenance of an airway because of defects created surgically and by radiation-induced fibrosis. Therefore, the role of chemotherapy in palliation has been limited.

C. Response to Treatment

Several factors modify response rates to chemotherapeutic agents in patients with head and neck cancer (Table 34–1). The primary site of disease is important because head and neck cancer comprises a heterogenous group of diseases. Bertino has shown variations in response to methotrexate as a function of the site of the tumor's

TABLE 34–1

Factors Affecting Response Rates in Head and Neck Cancer Patients	
Performance status	Patients with a low Karnofsky performance status are often unable to tolerate aggressive chemotherapy
Site of cancer origin	Lesions of the oral cavity and oropharynx respond to drug therapy most frequently, followed by laryngeal lesions; hypopharyngeal lesions respond less frequently
Prior treatment	Patients previously treated surgically or with radiotherapy respond less well to chemotherapy than those who have received no prior treatment
Nutritional status	Patients with a compromised nutritional status tolerate chemotherapy poorly

origin (Cancer, *46*:752, 1975). The highest response rate occurs in the oropharynx and oral cavity, followed by the larynx, and the lowest response rate is seen in the hypopharynx. The patient's performance status and nutritional status, as well as prior treatment, are important factors in predicting the response to chemotherapy.

D. Goals of Therapy

The majority of patients with persistent or recurrent head and neck cancer after surgical or radiation therapy have far-advanced disease, either locally or systemically. Only palliative measures can be considered for these patients. Traditionally, such patients have been given chemotherapeutic agents to slow tumor growth and to relieve pain and obstructive symptoms. In these situations, both patient and physician must understand the goals of therapy.

E. Adjuvant Chemotherapy

Chemotherapeutic agents used in conjunction with other methods of treatment, either simultaneously or sequentially, often increase the antitumor effect; this technique is known as adjuvant chemotherapy. The reduction of gross tumor mass by surgical intervention decreases the total number of tumor cells to a level at which chemotherapy is more effective. Adjuvant chemotherapy is the subject of many current experiments.

F. Monitoring of Patients

Once the implications of chemotherapy administration have been reviewed and the decision has been made to start treatment, the patient should receive a nutritious diet and should be monitored frequently for weight loss, possible infection, and biochemical and hematologic problems. Most chemotherapeutic agents are immunosuppressive and render the patient susceptible to infection.

G. Route of Administration

Most drugs used in the treatment of head and neck cancer are given systemically, most often by the intravenous route.

II. CHEMOTHERAPY FOR PATIENTS WITH RECURRENT TUMOR

A. Single Agent Chemotherapy

Cancer chemotherapy is barely 3 decades old. In the 30-year period since this discipline was initiated by giving methotrexate to patients with acute leukemia, many chemotherapeutic agents have been developed. Several of these, including methotrexate, bleomycin, hydroxyurea, *cis*-platinum, cyclophosphamide, 5-fluorouracil, vinblastine, and doxorubicin (Adriamycin), induce regression of head and neck squamous cell cancers (Table 34–2).

1. **Methotrexate (MTX)** This agent interferes with the biosynthetic steps that involve the folate coenzymes. It acts either by competition with or by inhibition of these coenzymes. This agent binds to or inhibits the enzyme dihydrofolate reductase, which catalyzes the reduction of folates to dihydro- and tetrahydro- forms, and thus inhibits DNA synthesis. Methotrexate reduces DNA synthesis in both normal and neoplastic cells. The number of cells affected is directly proportional to the number of cells that are replicating. Methotrexate is commercially available for both parenteral and oral administration. The organ systems most affected are the bone marrow and the gastrointestinal tract. A single dose of this agent induces leukopenia and thrombocytopenia, which reach a maximum in 9 to 10 days. The effect on the bone marrow lasts for a short time and reverses in several days. Mucositis occurs between 2 and 7 days following administration of the drug. Less common toxic effects are gastrointestinal ulceration and bleeding, dermatitis, and liver damage. Excretion of methotrexate occurs through the kidney in amounts from 50 to 95% within 24

TABLE 34–2

Single-Agent Activity in Head and Neck Cancer

Drug	*Evaluable Cases*	*Response Rate (%)*
Methotrexate (weekly)	100	50
Bleomycin	298	18
Cis-platinum	65	35
Hydroxyurea	18	39
Cyclophosphamide	77	36
Vinblastine	35	29
Doxorubicin (Adriamycin)	34	23
5-Fluorouracil	118	15

(Adapted from Wittes, R.E.: Chemotherapy of head and neck cancer. Otolaryngol. Clin. North Am., *13*:515, 1980.)

hours. The drug is retained in the presence of impaired renal function and may reach high concentrations rapidly in the serum. During treatment, frequent blood counts must be performed. Methotrexate is the most effective single drug against squamous cell cancer of the head and neck. Intermittent weekly schedules of 40 to 60 mg/m^2 have better response rates and fewer toxic effects than either daily or low-dose regimens. No conclusive evidence suggests that high doses of methotrexate with citrovorum rescue are more effective than conventional doses in patients with recurrent tumor.

2. **Bleomycin** Bleomycin is an antibiotic produced by Streptomyces verticillis. The exact mechanism of action is not clearly established, but bleomycin inhibits DNA synthesis in vitro by binding to DNA and causing splitting or scission of DNA strands. The drug is usually given intravenously, but it may be administered subcutaneously or intramuscularly. The use of bleomycin by continuous infusion may improve its efficacy because bleomycin has an inhibiting effect in the G-S_1 phase of the cell cycle, as well as a short serum half-life. Bleomycin concentrates in the epithelial tissues, particularly in skin, lung, and lymphatic tissue. The usual dose is 15 to 30 U once or twice per week. A total cumulative dose of more than 300 U is likely to result in a severe, irreversible pulmonary fibrosis that is often fatal. Hyperpigmentation and scaling of the skin occur frequently. Fever and chills can usually be controlled by an antipyretic agent. Pulmonary toxicity is the most serious consequence. Bleomycin has occasionally induced dramatic regressions in squamous cell cancer of the head and neck, although these remissions are short in duration.

3. ***Cis*-platinum (*cis*-diammine dichloroplatinum)** *Cis*-platinum is the most recently introduced chemotherapeutic drug with significant activity against head and neck cancer. The mechanism of action of this agent is thought to be similar to that of bifunctional alkylating agents. Dose-limiting renal toxicity has been minimized by vigorous hydration, with or without diuretic administration. Other toxic effects include marked nausea and vomiting, anemia, and neurosensory hearing loss. The nature of the dose-response curve for *cis*-platinum in head and neck cancer has not been well defined, but intravenous doses of 50 mg/m^2 on days 1 to 8 every month, or 80 to 120 mg/m^2 every month, are probably most appropriate. Overall response rates in previously treated patients range from 25 to 35%, with a short duration.

4. **New drugs** New drugs such as vindesine, dibromodulcitol, 4′-E piadriamycin, trimetrexate, and gallium nitrate are currently under evaluation for use in treating head and neck squamous cell cancer.

B. Combination Chemotherapy

Medical oncologists have been using drug combinations to increase response rates and duration of response in patients with various types of tumors, particularly in hematologic and some solid tumors. It is logical to select agents without overlapping toxicities, to allow simultaneous use of two or more drugs. Drug interactions within combinations can have synergistic effects. Given the many single agents that are at least active against head and neck tumors, combination regimens have been developed. Despite their theoretic benefits, combination regimens other than those incorporating *cis*-platinum have not yet improved the outlook for patients with recurrent head and neck cancer. The morbidity associated with intensive combination regimens must be carefully weighed against any improvement in the patient's quality of life.

III. ALTERNATIVE FORMS OF CHEMOTHERAPY

A. Intra-arterial Chemotherapy

Intra-arterial chemotherapy in the management of advanced head and neck cancer has been used for some time. The method consists of the continuous arterial infusion of chemotherapeutic agents into the accessible blood supply of the tumor site by means of a small, portable, ambulatory infusion pump. The procedure allows a high concentration of antitumor agents to perfuse the tumor bed without necessitating excessive systemic dosage. It was hoped that the effect of the local concentrations achieved with intra-arterial infusions would enhance local tumor regression with minimal toxicity. Some controversy exists regarding intra-arterial treatment because of inconsistencies in treatment techniques, drug and dosage schedule differences, and variations in the duration of treatment. Intra-arterial chemotherapy requires careful case selection, expertise, and close follow-up of patients. A review of the literature shows that the overall cumulative response rate is not much different from the cumulative response rate reported with systemic methotrexate. Infused drugs include methotrexate, *cis*-platinum, and 5-fluorouracil used as single agents, as well as combinations of 5-fluorouracil, methotrexate, cyclophosphamide, and actinomycin D. Treatment-related toxic effects of the infusions include alopecia, local erythema, mucositis, local pain, and hemorrhage and major embolization.

B. Chemotherapy Combined with Radiotherapy

The effects of single-agent chemotherapy combined with radiation therapy in the treatment of patients with head and neck carcinoma have been extensively investigated. The rationale for these studies is based on the potential radiosensitizing effects of certain chemotherapeutic agents. In addition, the cytotoxicity of these drugs may be enhanced when the vascular system of the tumor is not interfered with surgically, but is left intact. Chemotherapy may also induce a therapeutic or prophylactic effect on subclinical distant metastases. Many oncologists have therefore administered combinations of drugs simultaneously with radiation therapy. The results of randomized trials of single agents such as methotrexate, bleomycin, and hydroxyurea in multidrug chemotherapy with simultaneous radiotherapy have not reported consistent benefits from this approach, however.

C. Initial Chemotherapy

Intensive chemotherapy in patients with previously untreated head and neck cancer can induce dramatic tumor regression with acceptable toxicity. Drug delivery to primary tumors with an adequate blood supply is better than to tumors in previously operated or irradiated areas, which are replete with scar tissue. It is also likely that previously untreated patients with a high performance status and a satisfactory nutritional status can tolerate intensive chemotherapy and have fewer toxic effects. Tumor response rates are generally higher in these patients than in previously treated patients if one uses the same chemotherapeutic regimen. *Cis*-platinum, methotrexate, bleomycin, and 5-fluorouracil, either alone or in combination, are being used for induction chemotherapy. A response rate of 60 to 90% has been documented with an induction regimen in previously untreated patients. Recent combinations of *cis*-platinum and 5-fluorouracil have achieved clinically complete responses in 30 to 50% of patients after 2 or more cycles of treatment. Most studies have demonstrated tolerable levels of toxicity and a lack of surgical complications attributable to the chemotherapeutic regimens (Cancer, *51*:1353, 1983).

Several studies have demonstrated that T and N tumor staging characteristics are directly related to complete response rates from preoperative chemotherapy, with smaller tumors responding more frequently. In a recent trial sponsored by the National Cancer Institute, patients were prospectively randomized to standard local treatment with or without induction chemotherapy, consisting of only one cycle of *cis*-platinum and bleomycin. Survival was not improved in patients receiving the adjuvant chemotherapy; however, several pilot studies have reported significant improvement in survival for patients who obtain complete response to chemotherapy, and further trials are being directed toward improving chemotherapeutic regimens, either by adding other drugs or by alternating noncross-resistant drug combinations. The therapeutic value of these drugs has not been established at this writing.

35

CARBON DIOXIDE LASER IN OTOLARYNGOLOGY

STANLEY M. SHAPSHAY

The carbon dioxide (CO_2) laser is currently an accepted therapeutic technique in otolaryngology and other surgical fields. It was first clinically applied to treat lesions in the larynx in 1971, coupled to the operating microscope for greater accuracy (Ann. Otol. Rhinol. Laryngol., *81*:781, 1972). Further successful applications of this technique have been in the oral cavity, the trachea and bronchi, the pediatric airway, and the soft tissues of the head and neck (Int. Adv. Surg. Oncol., *1*:265, 1978). Basic laser physics, current instrumentation, guidelines for safe application, and indications for use are presented in this chapter.

I. BASIC PHYSICAL PROPERTIES

The word "laser" is an acronym for light amplification by stimulated emission of radiation. Several types of medical lasers are in current use, but the unique properties of the CO_2 laser make it ideal for soft tissue surgery.

A. Definition

When electrical energy is applied to molecular particles, such as CO_2, excitation results in photon emissions. Mirrors are used to reflect and further excite photon emissions, which are directed as a coherent beam of light (electromagnetic) energy. The CO_2 laser generates a beam of invisible light energy in the infrared wave length (10.6 μm). It can be reflected by mirrors and brought to a sharp focus by special lenses, and it has no ionizing effect on tissue.

B. Interaction with Soft Tissue

Absorption of the CO_2 laser energy by biologic tissue is practically complete; therefore, in contrast to many other lasers, the amount of tissue destruction is independent of its pigmentation. Tissue destruction is accomplished by water evaporization (steam production) secondary to energy absorption in the cells. Solid particles are also burned by the beam, leaving flecks of carbon as products of incomplete combustion. The most important variables are the power setting and the duration of exposure. For example, a low power setting, such as 10 w, for a short exposure time, such as 0.10 sec, produces a shallow tissue vaporization of 500 μ or less in depth (Ann. N.Y. Acad. Sci., *267*:263, 1976). The most important variable is exposure time, and therefore, short bursts of energy are used when one is close to an important structure such as the vocal cord muscle.

C. Advantages

1. **Minimal bleeding** Vessels less than 0.5 mm in diameter can be divided with the laser without any bleeding because of the coagulating heat effect. Vessels larger than 0.5 mm need to be ligated or electrocoagulated. Special instruments have been designed to facilitate endoscopic control of hemorrhage.
2. **Minimal postoperative edema** The CO_2 laser itself does not produce tissue edema as a result of vaporization. Edema may appear in response to blunt trauma from probes, retraction instruments, and suction tips. Intravenous, rapidly acting corticosteroids such as dexamethasone (Decadron) are routinely administered during laryngeal laser procedures.
3. **Excellent wound healing** Wound healing is similar to that occurring in scalpel-produced wounds. Because soft tissue destruction outside the 1- to 2-mm laser "spot" size is minimal, scarring of laser wounds is diminished, and healing progresses rapidly. Epithelial migration from the edges of the wound occurs early in the postoperative period.

II. LASER INSTRUMENTATION

A. Delivery Systems

A continuous-wave CO_2 laser apparatus can be used through a variety of different delivery systems. When coupled to the operating microscope, a 400-mm lens is usually used to allow for adequate working distance. A micromanipulator is used to direct the laser beam made "visible" by a superimposed visible aiming light. The laser spot size is 1 to 2 mm at the usual operating distance of 400 mm. An endoscopic attachment joins the laser manipulating arm to a specially prepared ventilating bronchoscope (Ann. Otol. Rhinol. Laryngol., *83*:769, 1974). A special handpiece containing a focusing lens can also be used. A hand-held stainless steel mirror may redirect the beam into confined or hard-to-reach areas such as the nasopharynx and subglottic space.

B. Special Instruments

Several specially made instruments for laser surgery are currently available. Standard microsurgical instruments used in suspension microlaryngoscopy are also used. Vocal cord retractors and protectors with built-in suction to remove the smoke of vaporization are helpful, especially in protecting the anterior commissure. Stainless steel laser mirrors, hand held with suction connection, allow the surgeon access to the undersurface of the vocal cords and nasopharynx.

III. ANESTHETIC CONSIDERATIONS

General anesthesia with noninflammable gases is routinely used for removal of laryngeal and oral cavity lesions with the CO_2 laser. Local anesthesia has been used when treating nasal or soft tissue lesions in adults.

A. Larynx

Microlaryngoscopy, in general, requires undersized endotracheal tubes for a better view of the larynx. A risk of fire exists during CO_2 laser procedures in the larynx and trachea if the laser beam repeatedly hits the endotracheal tube (Ann. Otol. Rhinol. Laryngol., *85*:656, 1976). Wrapping of red rubber endotracheal tubes with aluminum foil tape is necessary to prevent inadvertent endotracheal tube combustion. Flexible metal endotracheal tubes with rubber inflatable balloon cuffs are also available and are essential for safety. It is important to protect the endotracheal balloon cuff from the laser beam with moistened neurosurgical sponge "patties," with attached strings for control. The endotracheal tube can be removed when all visible lesions have been vaporized and replaced by a Venturi system clamp mounted within the lumen of the laryngoscopes. This maneuver provides access to the posterior third of the vocal cords and the interarytenoid space. Adequate ventilation with the Venturi system has been documented by arterial blood-gas measurement during anesthesia.

B. Trachea and Bronchial Airway

A specially prepared, ventilating, rigid bronchoscope is used to intubate the patient and is the delivery system for anesthesia. A noninflammable balloon cuff is currently being designed to fit over the distal part of the bronchoscope.

IV. PRECAUTIONS IN LASER SURGERY

A. General Precautions

The patient's eyes should be taped shut and covered with moist sponges to prevent injury in the unlikely event of an inadvertent reflection of the beam from a metal surface toward the eyes. Operating room personnel in the immediate area of the operative field should wear glasses.

B. Specific Measures against Fires

1. **Anesthetic gas mixtures** must be noncombustible.
2. **Avoidance of combustible materials in the operative field** Gauze wrapping or sponges must be kept moist with saline solution at all times.
3. **Selection of endotracheal tube** The endotracheal tube must be noninflammable. Flexible metal tubes are best, but red rubber wrapped with reflective self-adhering aluminum tape can be used (Ann. Otol. Rhinol. Laryngol., *87*:554, 1978). Polyvinyl chloride tubes should not be used because of their known heat lability.

V. INDICATIONS FOR USE

The indications for use of the CO_2 laser in otolaryngology have expanded since the first clinical application in the larynx in 1971. Table 35–1 is a summary of current indications, which are selectively described in greater detail.

A. Larynx

The most useful application of the CO_2 laser is in the larynx. Originally used to keep the pediatric airway free of obstructing recurrent respiratory papillomatosis, this application is still the most frequent. Although it does not cure respiratory papillomatosis, the CO_2 laser technique is the most accurate method for maintaining airway patency. The CO_2 laser's unique hemostatic abilities, along with minimal postoperative edema, make this an ideal instrument, especially in the pediatric larynx (Pediatrics, *61*:380, 1978). Excellent results have been obtained by careful excision of selected T_1 carcinomas of the membranous portions of the vocal cord. Tissue specimens can be examined by the pathologist to determine adequacy of the tissue margins. If these margins are free of tumor, further surgical treatment or radiotherapy will constitute overtreatment. Inadequate exposure and extension of the carcinoma to the arytenoid or subglottic areas are contraindications to laser cordectomy (Laryngoscope, *88*:1399, 1978).

B. Oral Cavity

The CO_2 laser is an excellent surgical tool for the transoral management of T_1 carcinomas, multiple superficial carcinomas, extensive leukoplakia, and verrucous carcinomas. The laser allows precise excision of the lesion and involved mucosa and provides a good specimen for histologic examination of the tissue margins. Edema is minimal, so tracheotomy is not usually needed, and the patient can often be discharged the next day. Usually, little pain is asso-

TABLE 35–1

Indications for Use

- Larynx
  - Benign tumors and lesions
    - Recurrent respiratory papillomatosis
    - Vocal cord nodules and polyps
    - Granuloma of the vocal process
    - Lymphangiomas and hemangiomas, including subglottic hemangiomas
    - Benign tumors such as neurofibromas and granular cell myoblastomas
  - Bilateral vocal cord paralysis
    - Transoral arytenoidectomy (subsequent scarring lateralizes the paralyzed vocal cord)
  - Malignant tumors (for curative treatment of early neoplasms or debulking prior to definitive therapy)
    - Endoscopic treatment of carcinoma in situ or mobile membranous vocal cord T_1 cancer
    - Epiglottectomy (transoral) for T_1 carcinoma of epiglottis and to facilitate indirect laryngoscopic visualization of the vocal cords
    - Removal of obstructing cancer of the larynx, to achieve airway endoscopically to prevent tracheotomy
    - Debulking of tumor, to reduce "tumor burden" prior to radiotherapy
- Oral cavity and oropharynx (exposure obtained with retractors and mouth gags)
  - Benign lesions
    - Leukoplakia and hyperkeratosis
  - Malignant tumors
    - Early cancers such as carcinoma in situ, T_1 carcinoma, verrucous carcinoma
      - Floor of mouth
      - Tongue
      - Buccal mucosa
      - Soft palate
      - Tonsil pillars
- Nasopharynx (exposure through palatal split or mirror deflection of beam into nasopharynx)
  - Benign tumors
    - Papillomas
    - Removal of adenoid tissue
  - Malignant tumors (palliation of fungating masses or debulking prior to definitive radiation or chemotherapy)
- Choanal atresia (Ann. Otol. Rhinol. Laryngol., *87*:658, 1978) (successful management possible by removal of stenosis with the laser and stenting)
- Nose (lesions of anterior nasal cavity, nasal vestibule, and nasal septum)
  - Benign lesions
    - Hereditary telangiectasis
    - Recurrent papillomas
- Facial soft tissue
  - Rhinophyma
  - Telangiectasis
  - Nevi
  - Tattoos (use reported for both CO_2 and argon lasers)
  - Keratoses
- Trachea and bronchi
  - Benign recurrent respiratory papillomas
  - Malignant tumors (palliation of endotracheal or bronchial obstruction from slower-growing tumors)
    - Adenoid cystic carcinoma
    - Low-grade mucoepidermoid carcinoma
    - Adenocarcinoma
    - Metastatic carcinoma such as hypernephroma
- Subglottic and tracheal stenosis (laser excision of stenosis and stent placement endoscopically; stent fixation by percutaneous wires over buttons)
- Tonsillectomy and adenoidectomy

ciated with the laser wound (the reason for this phenomenon is unknown) unless infection ensues. Strong and colleagues presented a series of 57 patients with early, localized, oral cavity carcinomas treated by laser excision (Laryngoscope, *89*:897, 1979). A 76% "cure rate" was noted in 21 patients at risk for 2.5 years.

C. Pediatric Airway

Lesions narrowing the pediatric airway present a challenging problem for the clinician. Avoidance of a tracheotomy in a young child is desirable because of the potential morbidity. Subglottic stenosis from prolonged or traumatic endotracheal intubation has been successfully managed in selected cases by laser excision and endoscopic stenting (Pediatrics, *61*:380, 1978). Subglottic hemangioma may be removed endoscopically by laser with minimal bleeding, obviating the need for tracheotomy, prolonged corticosteroid therapy, or irradiation (Laryngoscope, *90*:809, 1980).

D. Obstructing Neoplasms of Trachea and Bronchus

The CO_2 laser, attached to specially prepared, rigid, ventilating bronchoscopes, has mainly been used to remove potentially obstructing recurrent respiratory papillomas (Ann. Otol. Rhinol. Laryngol., *83*:769, 1974). Palliative management of obstructing, slower-growing malignant tumors of the trachea and major bronchi is also possible with the laser bronchoscope. Three previously treated patients with adenoid cystic and low-grade mucoepidermoid carcinoma have undergone palliative treatment for up to 36 months with repeated laser bronchoscopies.

VI. COMPLICATIONS

The major complication of CO_2 laser surgery is fire hazard. Several cases of endotracheal tube ignition and fire have been reported. This complication should be rare if proper precautions, as outlined previously, are taken. The transoral approach to laryngeal surgical procedures, especially when performed through the confines of a laryngoscope, demands considerable experience. Excessive tissue destruction can result from inexperience. With practice, mucosa, cartilage, bone, and tumor tissue can be differentiated when using the laser apparatus. One should obtain preliminary experience by operating on animals prior to clinical application of this technique.

36

PSYCHIATRIC PROBLEMS IN OTOLARYNGOLOGY

RUSSELL NOYES

A brief chapter cannot deal with all the psychiatric problems encountered in the practice of otolaryngology. Only the most common and serious conditions, including alcoholism, depression, delirium and hysteria, are presented. Because proper management of these disorders is based on accurate diagnosis, specific diagnostic criteria are emphasized (*Diagnostic and Statistical Manual,* 3rd ed. Washington, D.C., American Psychiatric Association, 1980). For the most part, these disorders are managed by nonpsychiatric physicians, who should be alert to possible serious complications that may require psychiatric consultation. Many otolaryngologic disorders are associated with psychiatric disturbances or complications at some time or other. In patients with cancer of the head and neck and in those seeking cosmetic operations, such is often the case. Therefore, management of the dying patient and prevention of an unfavorable outcome following cosmetic surgical procedures are discussed.

I. DEPRESSION

This psychiatric disorder affects about 5% of the adult population in a form severe enough to warrant professional attention. It is encountered in up to 30% of general medical patients and complicates serious physical illness in many such patients. Because of the risk of suicide, depression must be considered a life-threatening illness.

A. Diagnostic Criteria

The criteria for the diagnosis of depression are as follows:

1. **Dysphoric mood** is characterized by feelings of sadness, hopelessness, worry, and irritability.
2. **Associated symptoms** At least four of the following symptoms must be present:
   a. ***Poor appetite or weight loss*** (or weight gain).
   b. ***Sleep disturbance*** (hypersomnia).
   c. ***Fatigue or loss of energy.***
   d. ***Agitation or retardation.***
   e. ***Loss of interest*** in usual activities.
   f. ***Feelings of self-reproach*** or guilt.
   g. ***Decreased ability to think*** or to concentrate.
   h. ***Recurrent thoughts of death*** or suicide.
3. **Persistence of symptoms** The diagnosis depends on the presence of a dysphoric mood lasting at least a month, although this dysphoria is not always prominent. Many patients attempt to justify their disturbance in mood on the basis of physical symptoms, such as fatigue or insomnia, and in so doing, they distract the physician from a correct diagnosis. When five or more symptoms are present, the patient is definitely depressed. When four are present, the diagnosis is probable. In patients with serious physical illness, it may be difficult to distinguish between the vegetative signs of depression such as weight loss or insomnia and the symptoms of the illness. The diagnosis should still be considered when the criteria are met, however, especially if the physical disorder has been treated.

B. Differential Diagnosis

1. **Physical disorders** The differential diagnosis of depression includes a variety of physical disorders. Among them are endocrine conditions involving the thyroid, adrenal, and parathyroid glands, viral illnesses, neurologic disorders such as multiple sclerosis, hematologic disorders such as vitamin B_{12} deficiency and anemia, pancreatic carcinoma, subdural hematoma, and cardiovascular disorders such as thrombosis and stenosis.
2. **Drug reactions** A variety of medications may be associated with depressive symptoms. These include antihypertensive agents such as reserpine, methyldopa, and propranolol. antiparkinsonian drugs such as levodopa, corticosteroids, oral contraceptives, stimulants such as amphetamine, diuretics such as spironolactone, and antianxiety agents such as diazepam and chlordiazepoxide. With the exception of reserpine, methyldopa, and possibly, the oral contraceptives, these drugs produce disturbances in mood without the vegetative signs of depression.
3. **Depressed mood** is ubiquitous, especially among the medically

ill, who commonly experience losses of morale and self-esteem. Such disturbances in mood usually follow the course of the patient's illness and are rarely persistent. Vegetative signs of depression are unusual.

C. Classification

The classification of depressions is uncertain, but the reactive-endogenous dichotomy remains clinically useful. Reactive depressions, which comprise about two-thirds of such illnesses, develop in response to stressful events in unstable personalities, such as immature or excitable persons. Endogenous depressions usually develop without obvious precipitants in more normal, premorbid personalities. Patients with endogenous depression are more responsive to drugs, whereas those with reactive depression respond to psychotherapy as well as drugs.

D. Management

1. **Awareness of the disorder** Social impairment associated with moderate-to-severe depression is commonly misinterpreted. Deterioration of performance and of social relationships is often attributed to personal shortcomings rather than to an illness over which the patient has little control. It is consequently important that the illness, including its biochemical substrate, be explained to the patient and the family. The resulting shift in interpretation of symptoms provides valuable reassurance and may prevent unfortunate consequences such as job loss and marital separation.
2. **Hospitalization** should be considered in severely depressed patients, as well as in patients who are suicidal, unresponsive to medications, or expressive of ideas of hopelessness. Patients who are a burden to their families or who have little social support should also be considered for hospital treatment. A psychiatric consultant may assist in arranging such treatment.
3. **Prevention of suicide** The risk of suicide among depressed patients is high and must be directly assessed; 15% of manic depressives eventually kill themselves, as compared to 1% of the general population. When a patient has frequent and persistent suicidal ideas or when plans for suicide have been formulated and seem difficult to resist, psychiatric referral or hospitalization should be considered. For outpatients, it is wise to alert a family member to the suicidal tendency of the depressed person and to ask that firearms, sharp objects, and unnecessary drugs be removed from the home and that suspicious behavior be reported to the physician. The physician should be aware of the low therapeutic index of the tricyclic antidepressants. Fatalities have been reported with overdoses of as little as 500 mg, and for this reason, prescriptions should be for small amounts only. Depressed patients are often pessimistic about their prospects of recovery. Their loss of hope

contributes to poor compliance as well as suicidal tendencies. Physicians and family should regard expressions of hopelessness as a danger signal and as cause for considering psychiatric referral or hospitalization.

4. **Tricyclic antidepressant drugs** are the most effective and widely used agents for the treatment of depression. The improvement rate for patients taking these drugs is approximately 75%, as compared to 40% for patients taking a placebo. Thus, although tricyclic antidepressants are 70% effective, a proportion of patients fail to respond.
   a. ***Imipramine versus amitriptyline*** None of the tricyclic antidepressants are more effective than others, but they differ with respect to sedation. Of the two most commonly prescribed, imipramine is less sedating. When initial insomnia and agitation are prominent features of the illness, amitriptyline is preferred; when retardation is prominent, imipramine may be better tolerated.
   b. ***Dosage*** Imipramine and amitriptyline are conveniently administered in a single, bedtime dose. This method increases compliance and allows side effects to dissipate during the night. An initial dose of 75 mg should be increased by 25 mg every other day until a dose of 150 mg is reached. If definite clinical improvement of symptoms is not observed in a week and if no toxic manifestations appear, the dose may be increased by 25 mg daily to a maximum of 300 mg, until improvement is observed or until intolerable side effects occur.
   c. ***Delayed action*** The improvement resulting from the administration of tricyclic antidepressants is delayed and may not be evident to the patient for 10 to 20 days. This delay must be explained to both patient and family, to ensure compliance. Moreover, the maximum tolerable dose should be maintained for 4 weeks before concluding that the drug is of no benefit.
   d. ***Duration of therapy*** Patients should continue to receive a tricyclic antidepressant for 6 months. At the end of this period, the dose should be reduced by 50 mg per week. If the drug is abruptly discontinued, withdrawal symptoms, including nausea, vomiting, sweating, restlessness, insomnia, diarrhea and abdominal cramps, may occur.
   e. ***Side effects*** usually result from the anticholinergic effects of these drugs. Effects on the peripheral autonomic nervous system are, in descending order of frequency, xerostomia, thirst, constipation, urinary retention, especially in the presence of prostatic hypertrophy, and blurred vision. Effects on the central nervous system include drowsiness, tremor, dysarthria, agitation, and at high doses, visual hallucinations and disorientation. Because tricyclic antidepressants are capable of precipitating manic epi-

sodes in individuals with a personal or family history of bipolar illness, these agents should be used with caution in such patients. Cardiovascular side effects of tricyclic antidepressants include tachycardia, palpitations, orthostatic hypotension, and electrocardiographic changes such as T wave depression, prolonged QT interval, and ST segment depression. Life-threatening arrhythmias may occur in patients with cardiac disease; however, depression is also a life-threatening illness and must be treated. In patients with significant cardiac disease, the physician may wish to obtain a psychiatric consultation, to assist in considering an alternate course of action.

f. ***Poor compliance*** is a major problem with antidepressant medications. Compliance can be improved by close supervision during the dose-adjustment period and by issuing strict instructions to a patient not to deviate from the prescribed regimen without contacting the physician first. Patients take added comfort from being urged to phone the physician should any question regarding medication arise.

g. ***Failure to respond*** If patients fail to respond to an adequate trial of a tricyclic antidepressant, usually 200 mg for 4 weeks, they should either be given another drug or considered as candidates for electrotherapy. At this point, a psychiatric consultation may be desirable. Nonresponding patients are commonly given a monoamine oxidase inhibitor. These drugs may be more effective in those with reactive depressions. Electrotherapy, however, remains the most effective treatment for depression; 90% of such patients respond.

5. **Psychotherapy or counseling** should be considered in patients with mild or reactive depression. Supportive counseling may involve once-weekly, 20-minute sessions designed to provide the patient with emotional support and an opportunity for ventilation and discussion of problems that have contributed to symptoms. Environmental manipulation may also be an important aspect of counseling. For example, one may elicit the support of a patient's spouse or employer. The physician may provide such counseling or may arrange for a skilled paraprofessional to undertake it. Alternately, a psychiatric consultation may be arranged.

II. ALCOHOLISM

Alcoholism is a common disorder with serious social and health complications. It is estimated that 15 to 30% of general medical inpatients suffer from alcoholism, a disorder that is often unrecognized by attending physicians. Although patients with alcohol dependence represent frustrating treatment prospects, appropriate medical care can scarcely be provided without recognition of this illness and its complications. It is very common in patients with head and neck cancer.

A. Definition

Alcohol dependence is characterized by continuous or episodic abuse of alcohol together with social complications of that use and psychologic dependence. In addition, prolonged exposure to alcohol results in tolerance and physical dependence manifested by a withdrawal syndrome consisting, in its mildest form, of tremulousness and, in its severest form, of delirium.

B. Diagnosis

Diagnostic criteria for alcohol dependence are as follows:

1. **Continuous or episodic abuse of alcohol.**
2. **Social or occupational impairment** includes arguments with family or friends over alcohol use, violence while intoxicated, absence from work, job loss, and legal difficulties such as arrests for intoxication or for driving while intoxicated.
3. **Psychologic dependence** is characterized by a compelling desire for alcohol, by an inability to cut down or to stop drinking, and by repeated efforts to control or reduce excessive drinking by "going on the wagon" or restriction of drinking to certain times of day; or the patient may have a pathologic pattern of use, which involves the drinking of nonbeverage alcohol, binges during which the patient remains intoxicated throughout the day for at least 2 days, occasionally the drinking of a fifth of spirits or its equivalent in wine or beer, and the occurrence of two or more blackouts (amnesia for events that take place while intoxicated).
4. **Tolerance** is characterized by an increase in the amount of alcohol required to achieve a desired effect or by a diminished effect with the regular use of the same amount; or the patient may experience alcohol withdrawal, which involves morning "shakes" and malaise relieved by drinking, after cessation or reduction of drinking.

C. Course and Complications

A number of persons discontinue drinking after many years with or without treatment. Such is the exception, however, and most experience progressive social impairment and deterioration of health. Complications of alcohol dependence are numerous. Medical complications include alcoholic gastritis, pancreatitis, carcinoma of the head and neck, and cirrhosis of the liver; neuropsychiatric complications include peripheral neuropathy, delirium tremens, alcoholic hallucinosis, and dementia. Accidents and suicide contribute to the increased mortality rates in these patients.

D. Treatment

Treatment of alcohol dependence involves the management of acute intoxication and withdrawal, followed by long-term management to achieve control or moderation of drinking.

1. **Management of withdrawal** should be undertaken in the hospital whenever a patient has a serious medical illness, severe withdrawal symptoms, whether past or present, or a desire to stop drinking without the necessary social support for such an effort. Regardless of the setting, the following principles should guide management of alcohol withdrawal.
   a. ***Discontinuance of alcohol*** Alcohol intake should be stopped abruptly.
   b. ***Improvement of nutritional status*** Nutritional problems associated with heavy alcohol intake must be treated. Dehydration and electrolyte imbalance may require parenteral fluids in the presence of vomiting. Otherwise, orally administered fluids monitored by intake-and-output records should produce adequate hydration within a few days. Nutritional deficits should be corrected by vitamin supplements. Thiamine, 50 to 100 mg daily, intramuscularly if indicated, and pyridoxine, 50 mg daily, should be given especially in patients with evidence of nervous system dysfunction. Other vitamins may be given in oral multivitamin preparations.
   c. ***Treatment of withdrawal syndrome*** When a withdrawal syndrome develops, it usually does so within 24 to 48 hours of the last alcohol intake. Management of delirium tremens is like that of postoperative delirium, described later in this chapter. Chlordiazepoxide and diazepam are safe and effective in preventing or ameliorating the withdrawal syndrome (Ann. Intern. Med., *90*:361, 1979). At the first sign of the syndrome, such as tremulousness, 50 to 100 mg chlordiazepoxide may be given and repeated every 2 to 6 hours intravenously or orally until the patient's condition has stabilized. The dose should not exceed 500 mg in the first 24 hours, and the dose required during the first 24 to 48 hours should be halved the following day, to prevent accumulation of the drug. Detoxification may proceed at a rate of 25 to 50 mg per day. No evidence suggests that prophylactic phenytoin prevents seizures; therefore, the drug should not be given. Complete recovery from withdrawal may not occur for 6 weeks. Tremulousness, irritability, and restlessness may persist and may contribute to a resumption of drinking.
2. **Long-term treatment** begins once withdrawal is complete. Such treatment aims at control of alcohol intake, with abstinence as its goal.
   a. ***Identification and treatment of underlying psychiatric disorders,*** such as depression, should have priority.

b. ***Counseling*** may identify personality or interpersonal difficulties related to drinking. Correction or modification of these factors may reduce the patient's desire to drink. In many areas, specially trained alcoholism counselors are available.

c. ***Social support*** for the alcoholic patient may be arranged, and living circumstances that support drinking may be modified. Halfway houses, if available, may provide social support for alcoholics seeking to re-establish themselves. Environmental manipulations designed to reduce access to alcohol and the social pressure to drink should be considered.

d. ***Alcoholics Anonymous*** is a national organization dedicated to helping alcoholics achieve sobriety. The influence of group support coupled with religious faith has proved successful for many and should be encouraged.

e. ***Disulfiram (Antabuse)*** may be administered in an outpatient setting and, for some patients, is a useful deterrent to impulsive drinking. The usual dose is 0.5 g daily for 10 days, followed by 0.25 g daily as a maintenance dose. The patient must not have been drinking for 24 hours and should not drink for a week after discontinuing the drug.

f. ***Suicide prevention*** The risk of suicide becomes high when the alcoholic develops a secondary depression or during times of important personal loss such as divorce or loss of job. This risk should be recognized.

III. HYSTERIA

This confusing term has, at one time or another, been used to refer to a symptom (conversion), a personality type (hysterical) and a syndrome (hysteria). Here, it applies to a disorder characterized by recurrent and multiple somatic complaints unrelated to any physical disorder but for which medical attention is sought. This common disorder, also known as somatization disorder or Briquet's syndrome, occurs predominantly in women, has an onset prior to age 25, and follows a chronic, fluctuating course. Recognition is critical for the prevention of a variety of iatrogenic complications that result from unnecessary medical or surgical treatment.

A. Clinical Features

Patients with hysteria present complaints in a dramatic, vague, or exaggerated manner. These complaints involve many organ systems and have been the object of medical attention from a number of physicians. Common complaints include headaches, fatigue, palpitations, fainting, nausea, vomiting, abdominal pain, bowel and bladder difficulties, allergies, menstrual and sexual difficulties, and conversion symptoms. Such symptoms are part of a complicated medical history. Individuals with hysteria often show histrionic personality traits and are dramatic, attention-seeking, excitable, demanding, manipulative, and self-centered. Marital difficulties are common, as are suicide attempts in times of crisis. Anxiety and depressive symptoms are also frequently reported.

B. Diagnostic Criteria

These patients have a dramatic, vague, and complicated medical history beginning prior to age 25. Such persons complain of at least 1 symptom in 5 or more of the following 6 groups (4 for men) of symptoms. The severity of these symptoms must have required medication, alteration of the patient's life pattern, or care by a physician. Symptoms explained by physical illness should not be counted.

1. **Belief in ill health** These individuals believe that they have been sickly for most of their lives.
2. **Loss of sensation,** aphonia, trouble in walking, any other pseudoneurologic conversion symptoms such as paralysis, blindness, seizures, deafness, or anesthesia, or dissociative symptoms such as amnesia and loss of consciousness may be present.
3. **Abdominal pain** and vomiting spells may be a feature in the patient's medical history.
4. **Dysmenorrhea and menstrual irregularities,** including amenorrhea or excessive bleeding, are judged by the patient to be more severe than experienced by most women.
5. **Sexual indifference** and lack of pleasure or pain during sexual intercourse for the major part of the patient's sexually active life are possible symptoms.
6. **Back pain,** joint pain, pain in the extremities, and headaches are more common than in most people.

C. Conversion Symptoms

Such symptoms may occur in hysteria or as a separate disorder. They represent a loss or alteration in physical function resembling a physical disorder. The most common conversion symptoms suggestive of neurologic disease are paralysis, aphonia, seizures, blindness, akinesia, and anesthesia. Usually, these symptoms develop in a setting of psychologic stress and are associated with secondary gain. Caution should be observed in labeling symptoms as conversion in the absence of such psychologic factors because many patients subsequently prove to have organic disease.

D. Course and Complications

Hysteria is a chronic disorder that follows a fluctuating course. Because medical attention is frequently sought, unnecessary evaluations and surgical procedures are often undertaken. For the same reason, many patients become dependent on prescribed medications, such as tranquilizers, hypnotic agents, and analgesics. Suicide attempts are frequent, as are marital conflict and divorce.

E. Management

Several principles should guide the physician in managing patients with hysteria.

1. **Prevention of iatrogenic complications** Such complications may be prevented once the diagnosis of hysteria is made: Drugs on which dependence may develop should be avoided whenever possible, and surgical treatment should be approached with extreme caution.
2. **Treatment of new complaints** When a patient with hysteria presents new complaints, the physician should be guided by objective signs rather than symptoms, repeated and extensive workups should be avoided if possible, and detailed reassurance should be offered in a way that conveys the physician's interest and non-judgmental attitude.
3. **Communication** is important in managing patients with hysteria. Communication of findings to family members reduces secondary gain and misrepresentations that serve manipulative ends, and communication with other physicians ensures a unified approach to treatment.
4. **Relationship with patients** Physicians should place a premium on maintaining a favorable doctor-patient relationship. They should express continuing interest in the patient, regardless of negative findings, perhaps by means of regular, if infrequent, follow-up visits. Limits must often be set on the patient's demanding or manipulative behavior. Gentle firmness helps to keep the relationship within tolerable bounds. "Doctor shopping" should be discouraged.
5. **Psychiatric consultation** may be useful. Patients should be encouraged to see their problems as emotional rather than physical and to solve them through discussion with a counselor or psychotherapist. Indeed, many patients are willing to consult a counselor or therapist during times of emotional crisis.
6. **Encouragement of independence** Dependence on medical care should be discouraged. Patients should understand that they suffer from a chronic disorder that they must learn to live with, and they should be urged to work and to remain active despite persisting symptoms.

IV. DISTURBANCES FOLLOWING COSMETIC SURGERY

Although psychiatric disturbances following cosmetic surgical procedures are rare, they are often severe and persistent (Br. J. Psychiatry, *132*:568, 1978; Br. Med. J., *1*:1099, 1981). Patients with these disturbances are characterized by a preoccupation with an unfavorable modification in appearance, by a belief in the surgeon's responsibility for this presumed injury, and most disturbingly, by an insatiable demand for revisions that prove no more satisfying than the original operation. Patients such as these return to haunt the plastic surgeon and are the more troublesome because of their lack of response to psychiatric treatment. Such results are, unfortunately, difficult to predict, but clinical experience and outcome studies are in agreement on a series of warning signs. In contrast to patients seeking reconstructive operations, those desiring cosmetic procedures have a high incidence of pre-existing psychopathologic manifestations. Many are attempting to solve long-standing personality problems accompanied by feelings of inferiority and social inadequacy. Such pathologic features are not, however, predictive of an unfavorable result because, even in patients with severe psychologic disturbances, cosmetic operations usually result in improved appearance and emotional satisfaction. Postsurgical psychoses, including delusional preoccupation with deformity, probably occur in no more than 2% of patients.

A. Criteria for Predicting Unfavorable Results

1. **Minimal physical defect or discrepancy between the defect and the patient's concern** Often, a minor defect is viewed unrealistically as a source of interpersonal difficulties and becomes a focus of morbid preoccupation.
2. **Patient's inability to define desired anatomic results** Such vagueness may be part of the communicative style of patients who are otherwise guarded, remote, and difficult to interview.
3. **Difficulty in communicating or establishing emotional contact with the patient** This difficulty may be evidence, directly observed, of a severe psychopathologic disturbance.
4. **Male sex** Although men seek cosmetic surgical procedures less commonly than women, they more often react adversely to such operations, especially when they blame their defect for long-standing inadequacies.
5. **A history of disappointment with previous physicians** Such a history is predictive of future dissatisfaction.
6. **Physician's discomfort** Surgeons who feel forced to act against their best judgment, or who believe that the patient is not prepared for a less-than-optimal result, should stop and reconsider the operation.
7. **Previous unsuccessful cosmetic operations** Such patients are often chronically dissatisfied, but demanding of further surgical procedures, and should be approached with caution.
8. **Paranoid tendencies** are reflected in the foregoing criteria. Individuals with such personality traits harbor long-standing and pervasive suspicion and mistrust of others. They are hypersensitive and are easily slighted. When interviewed, such persons are guarded, aloof, and vague, but often reveal a belief in having been victimized and treated unjustly. Frequently, these patients have initiated legal action. Under stress, such persons may develop paranoid psychoses.

B. Management

In case of doubt, the surgeon should obtain a psychiatric consultation and should keep in mind that patients most willing to accept such consultations are most apt to respond favorably to cosmetic surgical procedures. The presence of psychopathologic disturbances or a history of psychiatric treatment in a patient need not cause one to deny a request for a cosmetic operation, but the foregoing criteria should alert the surgeon to potential problems.

V. POSTOPERATIVE DELIRIUM

Also known as postoperative confusional state or psychosis, this disorder is a common and serious surgical complication. Delirious patients often injure themselves when falling from bed or when attempting to escape frightening hallucinations. Suicidal or homicidal incidents sometimes occur. Agitation may interfere with medical management, and if untreated, delirium may lead to permanent neurologic impairment or death. The incidence of postoperative delirium varies according to the type of operation and the type of patient. It increases with age, and approximately 25% of patients over 65 experience this complication. Delirium is also more frequent in patients with organic brain disease or alcohol dependence. The incidence of delirium following cardiac operation is particularly high and is probably related to cerebral ischemia.

A. Clinical Features

Disordered attention is manifested by an inability to attend to environmental stimuli and to engage in goal-directed thinking or behavior. Other cognitive disturbances associated with this impairment in attention are disordered memory and orientation. Short-term memory is usually impaired; for example, individuals may not be able to recall the names of three objects presented to them after 3 minutes. Inattention to surroundings leads to disorientation or inability to identify the date, day of the week, or time of day correctly. Frequently, unfamiliar places and persons are mistaken for familiar ones; for example, the hospital room may be mistaken for home. Commonly, diminished alertness is noted, ranging from drowsiness and stupor in some patients to excessive arousal and difficulty sleeping in others. Misinterpretations of environmental stimuli, together with illusions and hallucinations, are common. Many patients are restless and overactive, whereas others are sluggish and inert.

B. Diagnostic Criteria

1. **Disturbances in attention** are manifested by impairments in attention to the environment, goal-directed thinking, and goal-directed behavior.
2. **Disturbances of memory and orientation** may also be present.
3. **At least two of the following** are present: reduced wakefulness

or insomnia; misinterpretations, illusions, or hallucinations; or increased or decreased psychomotor activity.

4. **Rapid development and fluctuation** of clinical features may be noted.
5. **Evidence of a specific organic factor** may be judged to be etiologically related to the disorder.

C. Course

Postoperative delirium has a rapid onset and generally persists for several days to a week. Symptoms often first appear and are most severe at night. Prodromal symptoms include restlessness alternating with somnolence during the day and insomnia with vivid dreams at night. Impairment in attention fluctuates widely and may be interrupted by lucid intervals during the day.

D. Differential Diagnosis

Delirium should be distinguished from the much less common functional psychoses, chiefly schizophrenia and depression. Disturbances in memory and orientation that are characteristic of delirium are rarely present in patients with the functional psychoses. Hallucinations are typically visual among delirious patients, but are more commonly auditory among schizophrenics. In delirium, one notes generalized slowing of the electroencephalogram and an obvious organic cause of the syndrome, both of which are absent in functional disorders. Careful assessment of mental status is essential to the diagnosis of postoperative delirium. A recently developed technique for this purpose is the Mini-Mental Status Examination (Fig. 36–1). This brief assessment provides for testing and scoring of several areas of functioning. It includes 11 questions and may be administered in 5 to 10 minutes. The examination may be repeated at frequent intervals to show improvement or decline in function.

E. Management

1. **Search for cause** Management of postoperative delirium begins with a search for the cause, which may be infectious, metabolic (electrolyte imbalance), neoplastic (metastasis), vascular (thrombosis), hypoxic, hematologic (hemorrhage), or toxic (alcohol intoxication). Delirium represents an important clue to such complications because it does not occur in their absence.
2. **Safety measures** Because the patient's safety is a fundamental concern, steps must be taken to ensure it. Regardless of other measures, adequate supervision must be provided. Family members may help, and their presence often quiets the patient. Such patients should be placed close to the nurses' station, and the nursing staff should be mindful of the risk of self-injury, particularly at night. An occasional patient requires more supervision than the nursing staff is capable of providing.

Maximum score	Score	
		Orientation
		Ask the patient:
5	( )	What is the (year) (season) (date) (day) (month)?
5	( )	Where are we: (state) (county) (town) (hospital) (floor)?
		Registration
3	( )	Ask the patient to name 3 objects: 1 second to say each; then ask the patient all 3 after you have said them; give 1 point for each correct answer; then repeat them until he learns all 3; count trials and record. Trials ________
		Attention and calculation
5	( )	Ask the patient to count serial 7's; 1 point for each correct; stop after 5 answers; alternately, spell "world" backwards
		Recall
3	( )	Ask for the objects repeated above; give 1 point for each correct answer
		Language
9	( )	Ask the patient to: Name a pencil and a watch (2 points) Repeat the following "No ifs, ands or buts" (1 point) Follow a 3-stage command: "Take a paper in your right hand, fold it in half, and put it on the floor" (3 points) Read and obey the following: Close your eyes (1 point) Write a sentence (1 point) Copy a design (1 point)
		Total score
		ASSESS level of consciousness along a continuum ________ Alert Drowsy Stupor Coma

Fig. 36–1. Mini-Mental Status Examination. (Adapted from J. Psychiatr. Res., *12*:189, 1975.)

In such an instance, the physician must personally arrange for special assistance.

3. **Medication** Sedative and hypnotic medications should be avoided in delirious patients, when possible, because they may mask or aggravate mental abnormalities. If the patient's behavior becomes a problem, however, medication may be used to assist in management. For a mildly uncooperative or agitated patient, benzodiazepine may be tried. An initial oral or intramuscular dose of 5 mg diazepam may be administered and titrated according to its effects and the patient's level of arousal. For an agitated or unmanageable patient, phenothiazine derivative or butyrophenone may be preferable. Haloperidol, in an initial oral or intramuscular dose of 5 to 10 mg, may be

ordered 3 or 4 times daily, with additional doses as necessary. Do not sedate the hypoxic patient.

4. **Environment** The more familiar and simple the environment of delirious patients, the less disturbed they will be. For this reason, the following measures are important.
   a. ***Visits*** Family members should be encouraged to visit and to bring familiar items from home to place in the patient's room.
   b. ***Orienting devices,*** such as a calendar and a clock, should be placed in the patient's room.
   c. ***A light*** should remain on at night.
   d. ***Removal of excessive stimulation,*** whether from roommates, moving apparatus, or loud television, is indicated.
   e. ***The nursing staff*** should inquire repeatedly about the patient's orientation and should offer reminders to fill in the gaps.
   f. ***Communication*** Procedures should be explained simply, slowly, and repeatedly.

VI. PREPARATION FOR DEATH

When we attempt to define the "dying patient," we recognize immediately the tremendous ambiguity and uncertainty that patients, together with their families, face as they approach a terminal illness. If we say, arbitrarily, that a dying patient is one who is expected to die within a few months, we may help ourselves to think about the problems such a patient faces, but we shall still find it difficult to classify many patients according to this definition.

A. General Principles

1. **Adaptation** Most dying patients cope with the final months of life successfully. Despite the vicissitudes of serious illness, they maintain their morale and sense of meaningful participation in family life. Many give, as well as receive, emotional support during this difficult period. Most dying patients come to recognize that their illness is fatal and act in accordance with this realization in an individual manner. No correct way exists for a person to die.

2. **Physicians' initial discomfort** Physicians usually find their initial contacts with dying patients a source of considerable discomfort. They are bearers of bad news that is difficult to soften. Although physicians may be perplexed about what they should say or do, their presence and concern are generally more meaningful than their words.

3. **Physicians' participation** Physicians have been criticized, sometimes unjustly, for neglecting dying patients. They should, however, recognize the importance of their continued participation in the care of such patients and not delegate it

wholly to others. The physician's skillful involvement is a source of great comfort.

4. **Role of patients' families** Despite their vulnerability, families play a central role in the care of the dying patient. Relatives of dying patients must be guided and supported in their vital and meaningful participation.

B. Psychophysiologic Reaction

The psychologic reaction that accompanies the dying process is complex and subject to much individual variation, but a typical pattern has been described (Kübler-Ross, E.: *On Death and Dying.* New York, Macmillan, 1969).

1. **Pattern of reaction** The realization that a patient has a fatal disease is not accepted all at once. Denial serves as a buffer that allows this painful awareness to enter gradually. Initially, most patients react to physiologic clues or worried facial expressions with shock and denial. Over a matter of weeks, however, denial gives way to grief, not unlike that experienced by surviving family members. This emotion includes sadness, anger, guilt, preoccupation with anticipated losses, and physical distress including anxiety, insomnia, weakness, and loss of appetite.

2. **Fearful anticipation** of the dying process is usually greater than fear of death itself. Unrelieved pain is expected by many. Some fear becoming a burden to loved ones, whereas others dread a helpless and vulnerable state that may accompany loss of mental or bodily functions. Ultimately, patients fear abandonment by loved ones. Many of these fears may be relieved by specific reassurance; others are allayed by competent medical care and harmonious family relationships. Under favorable circumstances, a partial resolution of anticipatory grief occurs in a matter of weeks. In the process, the patient may experience a flood of memories that place his life in the perspective of its approaching end. A new self-image, modified by illness, impairment, and a limited future, takes shape as the patient prepares for activities that will bring his life to completion. Priorities are reassessed, and a process of social disengagement begins.

3. **Physiologic decline** is associated with regression in psychologic function. Loss of energy, interest, and attention is accompanied by increasing egocentricity and preoccupation with bodily functions. A further decline in vital energy may be accompanied by memory and orientation difficulties, together with fluctuations in level of consciousness. As strength and energy diminish, attachment to life is withdrawn, and the patient develops an attitude of resignation toward, even expectation of, death.

C. Communication

Communication with dying patients needs to be open and honest. Mistrust develops when information is withheld. Informed consent, active cooperation in treatment, and meaningful participation in the final affairs of life depend on such communication. Similarly, harmonious family relationships are based on shared information. Studies show that at least 80% of patients would prefer to know an unfavorable prognosis.

1. **Breaking bad news** may be undertaken as follows. Patients should be given advance warning of a discussion of findings and treatment, so they may express their wishes with respect to it. The physician should sit down with such a patient where privacy is ensured. An opening statement should be brief and designed to encourage further dialogue. Reassurance of continued care and attention should be offered. Silence and quiet observation of the patient's emotional reaction indicate the direction of further discussion.
2. **Ongoing participation** Communication with dying patients and their families should be viewed as an ongoing affair. It should be guided by respect for and interest in the patient, who often has much to teach about coping with fatal illness. The physician should, perhaps, be less concerned with what to say than with how to listen. Physicians who listen well convey their concern and learn what their patients would have them do to bring ease or comfort.

D. Medical Goals

Medical goals in the management of dying patients include the relief of symptoms and the maintenance of function.

1. **Psychologic objectives** have been proposed, including Kübler-Ross's adaptational goal of "acceptance" and Weisman's ideal of an "appropriate death;" the ethical concept of dying with dignity has been critically reviewed (JAMA, *239*:850, 1978).
2. **Relief of pain** and other physical discomforts should have the highest priority. Complete relief of pain can be achieved without sedation in over 90% of patients under favorable circumstances. This requires careful diagnosis, a range of therapeutic approaches, such as radiation, chemotherapy, and hormonal therapy for bone metastases, and continuing dedication to the task (Semin. Oncol., *2*:379, 1975). The following approach to narcotic administration is recommended.
   a. ***The goal*** should be complete pain relief without sedation.
   b. ***Reassurance*** The patient should be assured of the physician's intention to control pain, and his aid should be enlisted. This reassurance also contributes to relief of pain.
   c. ***Morphine*** should be administered every 4 hours in a dose sufficient to relieve pain completely. In this manner, pain

is continuously controlled and is not allowed to emerge. Psychologic dependence does not develop with this method, and according to the St. Christopher's Hospice experience, physical dependence does not interfere with dose reductions, nor does tolerance limit effectiveness over long periods of time.

d. ***Monitoring*** Pain should be carefully monitored, and the doses of narcotics and phenothiazine derivatives should be carefully titrated. Prochlorperazine, 10 mg, serves as an antiemetic and sedative that potentiates the analgesic effect of morphine.

e. ***Addiction*** The physician should have an attitude of "no concern" for addiction.

E. Relief of Emotional Distress

Emotional distress among dying patients is associated with family difficulties, depression, anxiety, and delirium, in that order.

1. **Awareness of the problem** The physician must remain alert to the development of disturbed family relationships. Often, a failure of communication temporarily disrupts family harmony. On the other hand, simmering discontent may develop into open conflict under the stress of serious illness. Occasionally, family members themselves are overwhelmed or unaccepting of a patient's illness. Most family problems may be resolved by timely conferences to improve communication and to provide mutual support.

2. **Treatment of depression** Depression may be difficult to distinguish from the symptoms of physical disease or from the patient's reaction to it. A number of chemotherapeutic agents may also be associated with depression in cancer patients. These include corticosteroids, vinca alkaloids, alkylating agents, and enzymes. Antidepressant medication should be reserved for patients whose symptoms are persistent and difficult to explain on the basis of response to illness. A cautiously administered trial of a tricyclic antidepressant should not be withheld from a patient who may benefit from it, however. These drugs may cause organic mental syndromes in seriously ill patients, but they may also contribute to relief of pain.

F. Hospice Concept

The hospice concept embodies a number of principles that should guide physicians and other professionals who care for dying patients. These principles are as follows:

1. **Relief of pain** and of associated physical discomforts is of primary importance. This goal requires persistence and devotion to detail.

2. **Family support** The unit of care is the family, and family members should be helped to support one another. When staff

members become personally acquainted with family members, they place themselves in a position to influence them favorably.

3. **Social interaction** and a sense of belonging should be maintained. Regular visits from physicians and others provide tangible proof of continued support and concern.
4. **Personal attention** The uniqueness of the person who is dying should be preserved. For the physician, this goal is often facilitated by listening to the story of the patient's life and by sharing certain features of it with the staff participating in the person's care.
5. **Independence of thought and action** should be maintained to the extent possible. The staff should encourage self-care and active participation in decisions regarding treatment.
6. **The spiritual aspect** of the dying person's experience should not be neglected. When staff members recognize religious conviction, they should encourage the visits of a minister or chaplain.

37

PSYCHIATRIC PROBLEMS IN CHILDREN

HOWARD B. ASHBY

Children make up a large part of otolaryngologic practice. This chapter discusses psychiatric syndromes such as mental retardation, conduct disorder, and hyperactivity, which are commonly encountered in children and may represent special management problems. Autistic and speech-disordered children are referred specifically to otolaryngologists for speech and hearing evaluations. The specialist should know how to recognize these problems and should be prepared to refer such patients for appropriate evaluation and treatment. In addition, the adolescent patient presents special management considerations, which are briefly discussed. A more complete, yet concise, medically oriented description of psychiatric problems of children can be found in Stewart and Gath's *Psychological Disorders of Children* (Baltimore, Williams & Wilkins, 1978) and in the third edition of *Diagnostic and Statistical Manual of Mental Disorders* (Washington, D.C., American Psychiatric Association, 1980).

I. INFANTILE AUTISM

Infantile autism, a syndrome beginning before 30 months of age, is characterized by a lack of social responsiveness, delayed and abnormal language, unusual response to environmental stimuli, and stereotypic behavior.

A. Clinical Features

1. **Abnormal social responsiveness**
   a. ***Lack of responsiveness to others.***
   b. ***Indifference to affection.***
   c. ***Lack of eye contact.***

d. ***Playing parallel to other children,*** rather than with them.

2. **Abnormal language development**
   a. ***Absence of speech,*** or use of single words or phrases.
   b. ***Echolalia*** or repetition of phrases.
   c. ***Pronominal reversal*** or use of third-person pronouns when referring to self.
   d. ***Perseverative speech.***
   e. ***Absence of gestures*** or facial expression.
3. **Unusual Response to Environment**
   a. ***Resistance to change.***
   b. ***Attachment to inanimate objects.***
4. **Stereotypic behaviors** may include rituals and posturing.
5. **Associated features** may be present, but they are not diagnostic.
   a. ***Self-stimulation.***
   b. ***Temper tantrums.***
   c. ***Enuresis.***
   d. ***Encopresis.***
   e. ***Feeding problems.***
   f. ***Mental retardation.***

B. Description

Many of these behaviors are noted from early infancy, and parents may suspect their child of being deaf because of the child's failure to respond to their comings and goings. Parents describe their autistic child as independent, seeking little social contact with themselves or other children. Eye contact is fleeting at best, and speech, when present, seems preprogrammed or obviously echolalic. During parallel play, an autistic child may exhibit no interest in the play of children about him. Although indifferent to others, autistic children may become attached to inanimate objects and may prefer to occupy their time in repetitive play. They may, for example, pour sand back and forth or watch spinning objects for extended periods. All symptoms may vary in intensity. For example, resistance to physical closeness may range from an indifference to cuddling to a complete rejection of closeness. As autistic children grow older, symptoms may diminish. Some children may begin to have eye contact or to respond to their parents.

C. Epidemiologic Features

Autism occurs in boys more commonly than in girls, with a sex ratio of 2.6 to 1 and with a prevalence of about 2 to 4 cases per 10,000 births. The disorder is identified by the second year in 75% of cases. An onset of autistic symptoms or a deterioration of development after the age of 4 years suggests an organic problem and calls for a thorough medical workup. It was believed earlier that autism resulted from parental rejection in infancy. More recent, controlled studies have disproved this view. Autism may be related to disorders such as encephalitis, meningitis, rubella, and phenylketonuria. About 25% of patients have evidence of definite brain damage. That autism occurs 50 times more often in the siblings of autistic children than in the general population suggests the probability of genetic influence.

D. Differential Diagnosis

Autistic children are often referred to an otolaryngologist because parents wonder whether their child may be deaf. Evaluating this possibility may be difficult because lack of language and social responsiveness may interfere with the usual audiologic examination. Evoked potential audiometry is often used to obtain definitive information. Children with **elective mutism** have one person, usually their mothers, with whom they interact and converse normally, and they show no other features of autism. Children with **developmental language disorders** (dysphasia) are usually of normal intelligence, relate normally to others, and lack resistance to change. Morever, they make full use of whatever ability to communicate they have. Their disorder of language may be either receptive or expressive; expressive disorders are most common. Whereas severely or **profoundly retarded** children may develop little language and may be difficult to evaluate, mildly or moderately retarded children develop speech and social awareness and make a lack of social responsiveness, abnormal use of language, or abnormal response to the environment easier to detect.

E. Treatment and Prognosis

Treatment usually centers around efforts to stimulate language, socialization, and self-care. Autistic children who develop speech by the age of 5 years or those with an intelligence quotient (I.Q.) above 50 (70% of autistic children have an I.Q. of 70 or below) have a better outlook, but even autistic children with a normal I.Q. have residual symptoms as adults. Seizures develop in about 20% of autistic children during adolescence, especially in those with an I.Q. below 50. In the office setting, autistic children are often active. They tolerate prolonged sitting or structure, such as an examination, poorly. If it is necessary to wait for an examination, these children will often be calmer in a quiet room. Breaking up the examination into small parts, with oral reinforcers of the child's cooperation, may be useful. Use of the papoose or restraining board in difficult cases helps to expedite the examination and decreases the prolonged frustration of the child.

II. HYPERACTIVITY

This complex of symptoms is currently referred to as attention-deficit syndrome. Increased activity or "hyperactivity" is not necessary for the diagnosis. Other terms used in the past include minimal brain dysfunction and hyperkinetic reaction of childhood.

A. Clinical Features

1. **Poor concentration.**
2. **Impulsivity.**
3. **Distractibility.**
4. **Other common features,** not essential for the diagnosis, include behavioral problems such as disobedience, aggressiveness, and antisocial behavior, soft neurologic signs such as uncoordinated rapid alternating movements or tandem walk, and specific learning disabilities.

B. Description

The symptoms of this disorder are not always constant, and diagnosis is usually based on the patient's medical history, as obtained from parents and teachers, rather than by observation in the office. For example, children with this disorder may be able to sustain attention in one-to-one situations such as a medical examination, but in less-structured situations, they may become distracted. Parents often describe their children as impulsive and unable to stay with an activity for more than a few minutes. If a child also has increased motor activity, parents may complain, for example, that the child runs instead of walking or that he is unable to sit still. Teachers describe poor concentration, constant talking, and distractibility. Behavioral problems associated with poor school performance commonly prompt evaluation of these children.

C. Prevalence and Prognosis

The prevalence of attention-deficit syndrome may be as high as 3%. Boys are affected much more often than girls. Symptoms appear as early as 3 years of age, but professional attention is not usually sought until school age. Steady improvement usually occurs, although mild cognitive impairment may persist into adolescence or adulthood. Most such patients eventually obtain employment and do well.

D. Treatment

Treatment consists of the administration of cerebral stimulants, such as dextroamphetamine or methylphenidate, although long-term follow-up study indicates no beneficial effect on learning. Sprague demonstrated that doses of methylphenidate (Ritalin) of 0.3 mg/kg body weight/day have the most effect on cognitive functioning, whereas higher doses, about 1 mg/kg/day, are most effective for decreasing undesirable social behavior and restlessness (Science, *198*:1274, 1977). Use of less than 0.8 mg/kg/day methylphenidate has not been associated with growth retardation. If cerebral stimulants are used, medication holidays on weekends and summer vacations should be routine. In addition, the discontinuance of cerebral stimulants well before epiphyseal closure helps to circumvent iatrogenic growth retardation. Other interventions include training in verbal self-cuing, impulse control, and social skills. These techniques are important adjuncts to pharmacotherapy and can be initiated by school psychologists or other mental-health workers. In the office setting, hyperactive children may do well because of the individual attention they receive. They may also be distractible and incapable of following instructions or attending to tasks for more than a few moments at a time, however. Handling equipment, getting up and down from the examination chair, and asking irrelevant questions may distract and frustrate the examiner. It is helpful to explain procedures in advance to all children, but particularly to inquisitive and restless children. During the examination, firm directions, avoidance of prolonged waiting, and verbal praise increase cooperation in most cases.

III. CONDUCT DISORDER

Persistent disobedience, fighting, quarrelsomeness, destructiveness, and meanness are the hallmarks of aggressive conduct disorder. Children with this disorder may be seen in otolaryngologic practice following accidents or voice changes due to shouting.

A. Clinical Features

1. **Aggressiveness.**
2. **Noncompliance.**
3. **Destructiveness.**
4. **Meanness.**

B. Description

Aggressiveness may be both physical and verbal. In addition to fighting with peers, children with conduct disorder may be physically and verbally abusive toward adults. Noncompliance is most frustrating to parents and teachers, who complain that such children are impossible to discipline. Destructiveness is common and may take the form of vandalism or fire setting. Meanness may be evidenced by cruelty to younger children or to animals. The families of these children are often chaotic. Low socioeconomic status, divorce, alcoholism, and a history of conduct disorder in the father are common. The parents of children with aggressive conduct disorder are often reluctant to describe antisocial behavior, but express frustration with and lack of control over their child. Once the parents have described this problem, additional questions usually elicit a history of the foregoing behavioral traits.

C. Epidemiologic Features

Conduct disorder is more common in boys than in girls. Aggressive behavior is usually noted by school age, but it may appear earlier. Robins found that 25% of children with aggressive and antisocial behavior received the diagnosis of antisocial personality disorder as adults (*Deviant Children Grown Up*. Baltimore, Williams & Wilkins,

1966). Children with conduct disorder may also be hyperactive, and when these problems are combined, the outcome is worse.

D. Differential Diagnosis

Aggressive behavior may be seen in children with encephalitis or other serious disorders of the brain. In such a case, however, rebellious or aggressive behavior is acute in onset and represents a definite change from the child's previous character. Moreover, signs of impaired intellectual functioning can be elicited in organically impaired children, to make the distinction possible. Epilepsy, particularly of the psychomotor type, may be associated with aggressive behavior. Aggressiveness may also be exacerbated by the use of anticonvulsant agents such as phenobarbital, and a change in medication often results in improved behavior.

E. Treatment

Behavior modification, training in social skills, assertiveness training, and instruction in self-control all have some positive effect. The use of drugs, including cerebral stimulants and major tranquilizers, is common despite little objective evidence of benefit and a considerable risk of side effects. In the office or hospital, firmness and clear explanation of procedures, both before and during examinations, reduce anxiety and lessen the tendency for rebellious behavior. Children with conduct disorder are used to manipulating and dominating adults to get their way. Hospital or office protocol and expectations of the child are best discussed with both nurse and parent present, to minimize the opportunity for one to be pitted against the other. As with most children, feeling involved and, in some measure, having a sense of control may help to alleviate undesirable power struggles.

IV. MENTAL RETARDATION

Because visual and auditory problems are often associated with mental retardation, these children are frequently seen by the otolaryngologist. In addition, autism, attention-deficit syndrome, and conduct disorder occur three to four times as often in mentally retarded children as in the normal population. Retarded children are often cooperative in office or hospital settings, but frequently present special problems.

A. Clinical Features

1. **Below-average intellectual function.**
2. **Deficits in adaptive behavior;** that is, independent living and social responsibility.
3. **Onset before age 18.**

B. Subtypes and Description

1. **Mild mental retardation** Children with an I.Q. between 50 and 70 are mildly retarded and constitute about 80% of the

total. They are educable and may develop skills to a sixth-grade level by their late teens.

2. **Moderate mental retardation** Those with an I.Q. between 35 and 49 are moderately retarded and represent about 12% of the total. They are considered trainable and may develop second-grade-level skills by their second decade. As adults, they may function well in structured settings such as sheltered workshops.

3. **Severe mental retardation** These children, who have an I.Q. of 20 to 34, represent 7% of the total. By school age, these children may have learned speech and self-care skills. As adults, they may perform simple vocational tasks under supervision.

4. **Profound mental retardation** represents 1% of the total. These children have an I.Q. of less than 20. As adults, they may develop some speech, but only minimal self-care skills. They require a structured and supervised setting.

C. Management

Retarded children are easily upset by changes in routine or new surroundings, and extra time may be required in the office and hospital for simple explanations, reassurance and "warm-up." A simplified setting and procedure should be considered, including covering of instruments until they are needed or until the patient is asleep. If repeated procedures, such as venipuncture, are needed during the course of extended treatment, simple explanations and walking through the procedure using dolls often reduce resistance and fear. Such an approach may help children of normal intelligence as well.

V. DISORDERS OF SPEECH AND LANGUAGE

Such disorders are often associated with mental retardation and behavior problems.

A. Stuttering

Stuttering is an exception and is not usually associated with behavior problems, reading difficulties, or psychiatric problems in parents. This finding suggests that it is not a psychogenic or neurotic disorder. Positive family histories indicate that stuttering may have genetic determinants. Transient stuttering that remits spontaneously is more common than persistent stuttering, which affects only about 1% of children. If stuttering persists beyond the age of 5 years, referral for speech therapy is indicated. This therapy is usually oriented toward increasing fluency and handling the psychosocial problems that result from the disorder.

B. Delayed Speech

Children who are without speech by the age of 2 years or who have no phrase speech by the age of 4 years have a significant developmental language delay. Mental retardation accounts for most delayed language, but some children with developmental dysphasia are of normal intelligence. Evaluation of all these children by educational and speech therapists is essential, to determine the proper intervention and school setting. Hearing must be evaluated.

VI. SPECIAL CONSIDERATIONS IN ADOLESCENT PATIENTS

Otolaryngologic problems may have a special impact on the adolescent because adolescents are particularly sensitive about their physical appearance. Their growing independence and increasing responsibility may also cause them to be more emotional, but on the whole, adolescence is a healthy period psychiatrically as well as medically.

A. Clinical Considerations

Psychiatric disorders in adolescents are similar to those seen in adults, especially patients in their middle and late teens. During early adolescence, for example, a fall in school performance and seclusiveness may be the only indications of significant depression, whereas later, a full depressive syndrome may be observed.

B. Common Disorders

Personality disorders such as antisocial behavior become more evident during this period as the adolescent begins employment and broadens social contacts. Conversion symptoms, such as loss of function, usually neurologically related without organic explanation, and other psychogenic disorders occur in adolescents. When confronted with vague symptoms, care should be taken to rule out somatization disorder (recurrent multiple somatic complaints of several years' duration for which medical care has been sought but for which no physical basis has been determined) or histrionic personality disorder.

C. Management

Care of adolescents can be facilitated by recognizing the need for careful explanation of their medical problems and by allowing time for questions. These patients should be helped to take responsibility for decisions about treatment and for their own care.

38

COUNSELING FOR COMMON OTOLARYNGOLOGIC DISORDERS

BARBARA A. MacLEAN AND ELLEN M. HOWARD

The following is a summary of information that should be included in the counseling of patients.

I. EAR

A. Water Precautions

An active ear infection may occur if patients with mastoid cavities, perforated tympanic membranes, ventilating tubes in place, or a recent ear operation allow water to enter the ear canal. When washing one's hair, the ear may be occluded with lambswool or cotton coated with petrolatum. This method is the safest, although even it may fail. Molded ear plugs, made by taking an impression of the ear canal, give a tight seal and can sometimes be used while the patient is swimming. No diving is allowed.

B. Myringotomy and Tube Placement

Counseling is necessary to enable the parents and child, if appropriate, to understand the cause, effects, and treatment of middle ear effusion. The physician should do the following:

1. **Describe the anatomic features** of the ear in simple terms: ear canal, ear drum, ossicles, middle ear, eustachian tube, cochlea, and inner ear.
2. **Explain eustachian tube function** in equalizing middle ear pressure and lack of function producing fluid accumulation.
3. **Describe the effects of middle ear fluid,** including the increased incidence of ear infections and conductive hearing loss.

4. **Show the parents and child an actual tube,** to dispel misconceptions about its size.
5. **Explain the procedure** for myringotomy and tube insertion.
6. **Instruct the patient and parents in water precautions** after the procedure.
7. **Review the symptoms of ear infection** Such symptoms include pain and fever without tubes and drainage once tubes are in place.
8. **Explain that possible speech delay may be prevented** if hearing is restored by removal of fluid.

C. Ear Protection

1. **Airplane flight** Inability to equalize middle ear pressure may cause bleeding into the middle ear during descent of an airplane. Children with functioning ventilating tubes in place are not at risk. Airplane travel should be discouraged if the eustachian tube is not functioning. Patients with an upper respiratory infection or poor eustachian tube function who must fly should take a decongestant an hour before descent. The physician should caution patient about driving and drinking alcohol with antihistamines. The patient should also use a nose spray twice just before descent of the aircraft.
2. **Scuba diving** Inability to equalize pressure in the air spaces of the head may cause pressure, pain, and bleeding while diving. A patient with eustachian tube dysfunction or upper respiratory infection should not dive. If a diver has occasional pressure problems due to nasal congestion, nose spray or drops should be used 1 to 2 hours before diving. Antihistamines are not recommended because of possible drowsiness.
3. **Unilateral hearing loss**
   a. ***Counseling session*** Once the diagnosis of severe unilateral hearing loss has been established, the patient and family should be counseled on special considerations because of the hearing loss, including the need to protect the hearing in the normal ear.
   b. ***Classroom modifications*** If the patient is a child, the school should be made aware of the hearing loss. The patient should sit in the front row of the classroom with the good ear facing the teacher.
   c. ***Protection from noise*** The hearing ear should not be subjected to noises of loud intensity, such as fireworks, loud music, or gunfire.
   d. ***Discouragement of contact sports*** is indicated.
   e. ***Examinations*** Hearing should be checked periodically.

D. Ménière's Disease

Patients with Ménière's disease may benefit from a low-sodium diet. The patient should know that all foods contain sodium. Meat, eggs, fish, and milk have greater amounts than fruit, vegetables, and cereal. On a low-sodium diet, no salt should be added to foods in cooking or at the table. Foods high in sodium that should *not* be used are: ham, bacon, and processed meat such as bologna and frankfurters; fat from meat; duck and goose; canned, salted, or smoked meat or fish; shellfish; cheese, except unsalted cottage cheese; canned baked beans or soup; pickles, olives, and prepared sauces; soft drinks and prepared beverage mixes; candy; baking powder and soda; and salted potato chips, popcorn, corn chips, pretzels, and peanuts. The physician should recommend the use of vegetable oil or margarine in place of butter. Meat and fish should be restricted to two servings daily of meat, fish, or poultry. Eggs should be limited to three per week. Foods may be flavored with herbs, spices, fresh lemon juice, onions, pepper, vinegar, dry mustard, or garlic. The patient must be sure to read the label of any canned or prepared foods (see Chapter 10).

II. NOSE

A. Epistaxis

The patient should be instructed not to pick his nose, insert anything into it, or blow his nose forcefully. One should sneeze with an open mouth. Strenuous exertion, hot beverages, and alcoholic drinks should be avoided. If the patient is constipated, a laxative should be taken to avoid straining. Humidification of room air is important. If the bleeding point is in the anterior portion of the nose the patient can be taught to apply pressure by pinching the nose below the nasal bone (see Chapter 14).

B. Nasal Surgical Procedures

Trauma to the nose for a few weeks after a nasal fracture or rhinoplasty may displace the nasal bones. The patient should be informed of this possibility and should avoid sports such as basketball, soccer, football, and hockey. The patient should also be advised not to sleep in a prone position. If an external splint or cast is used, the patient should know how long it should remain in place and how to reapply it if necessary. Postoperatively, the patient should apply pressure to the nose while looking in a mirror. Both index fingers should be held gently to the nose for one minute three times a day. If the nose appears to drift to one side, then more pressure should be applied to that side.

III. THROAT

A. Tonsillectomy or Adenoidectomy

1. **Instructions prior to hospital admission** Avoid aspirin (acetylsalicylic acid) or aspirin-containing drugs for 14 days prior to the operation. Aspirin retards blood coagulation and increases the risk of postoperative bleeding. Many drugs, such as Dristan, Coricidin, and Anacin, contain aspirin, so be sure to check the label before using. Contact the physician if a cold, cough, or elevated temperature develops just prior to hospital admission.
2. **General instructions after hospital discharge** Drink fluids. Rest in bed during the first day at home. Activity may be increased gradually thereafter, but do not run for 7 days. Avoid clearing the throat. The mouth may be rinsed with water. Ear pain is common after tonsillectomy and originates from the throat rather than from the ears. Low-grade fever (99 to 101° F) is usually due to insufficient oral intake of fluids.
3. **Dietary instructions** Avoid citrus fruit juices and hot or highly seasoned foods. Otherwise, the diet can be broadened as tolerated.
   a. ***First day*** Water, milk, ice cream, or sherbet are indicated.
   b. ***Second day*** Milk, cereal, ice cream, jello, pudding, and broth are recommended.
   c. ***Third and fourth days*** Soft foods may be added gradually, such as mashed potatoes, soft cereals, and eggs.
   d. ***Fifth day*** Regular diet is gradually resumed.
4. **Complications** Contact the physician if bleeding occurs, if persistent cough develops within 10 days, or if you have any questions. If you cannot contact the doctor, come to the hospital emergency ward.

B. Throat Irrigations

Throat irrigations, whether on an inpatient or an outpatient basis, can relieve throat pain associated with peritonsillar abscess. An irrigating container, such as a 1000- to 1500-ml disposable enema bag, should be filled with warm water to which is added a teaspoon of salt. The patient should be instructed to stand over a sink or basin and allow the water to irrigate the painful area of the throat while running out his mouth. This procedure should be repeated every 2 hours while awake until throat pain has decreased. This regimen should be advised along with appropriate treatment for the specific cause of the throat pain.

C. Esophageal Reflux

The following instructions are designed to help to neutralize the stomach contents, to reduce the production of acid, and to prevent acid from entering the esophagus.

1. **Take an antacid in liquid form,** such as Gelusil, Maalox, or

another of your choice, 20 to 30 minutes after meals and at bedtime.

2. **Dietary restrictions** help to control symptoms. A light, bland diet divided into multiple small feedings is recommended. Avoid highly seasoned food that is either extremely hot or very cold. Chew food properly.
3. **Avoidance of irritants** Alcohol, tobacco, and coffee are irritants to the esophagus and should be avoided. Alcohol and coffee also stimulate stomach secretions.
4. **Avoidance of food before bedtime** Do not eat for 3 or 4 hours before retiring.
5. **Sleeping with the head of the bed elevated** may provide night-time relief. Blocks or several pillows may be used.
6. **Lose weight** if you are overweight.
7. **Avoid tight clothing** around the waist.
8. **A relaxed attitude** during activities helps to reduce symptoms.

IV. HEAD AND NECK

A. Dietary Supplements for Cancer Patients

Patients with tumors of the head and neck have frequently lost considerable amounts of weight when they first undergo treatment. Because treatment often affects the oral cavity, nutritional maintenance becomes difficult. When dietary supplements such as Isocal or Ensure are too costly or unavailable, the patient should be advised to mix Instant Breakfast as directed, then add ice cream and an egg and blend together well. Two of these drinks a day are suggested in addition to regular meals, to help promote weight gain and healing. Soft, moist foods are swallowed most easily.

B. Dental Care for Cancer Patients

All patients with cancer of the head and neck should have a full dental evaluation prior to treatment. Vigorous dental care is important, to prevent radiation caries when xerostomia is present. The patient should be taught dental care and should be reminded periodically. This special care includes brushing three to four times a day with fluoride toothpaste, flossing daily, daily fluoride treatment with trays of fluoride gel, and regular dental visits. Radionecrosis of the mandible is painful and is difficult to treat. It usually follows poor dental care in the irradiated patient (see Chapter 19).

C. Postoperative Humidification

Extra humidity is necessary after tracheotomy or laryngectomy. The amount of extra humidity needed depends on the season and the climate. The heating season always increases the problem. Large home humidifiers are effective, but they may be costly. Small bedside humidifiers work well as long as they are kept nearby and the patient is consistent with their use. Hand-held atomizers with saline solution may be used as a supplement for extra thick secretions or when the patient is away from home. Home humidification is often helpful for nose and throat dryness as well.

D. Tube Feedings

1. **Care of feeding tubes** The patient with a feeding tube in place should know how to change the tape without dislodging the tube, how to check the tube for placement, and how to cope with a plugged tube.
2. **Procedure for tube feeding** Feeding oneself by tube may be frightening to both patient and family. Patients should be taught not only how to feed themselves, but also how to watch for potential problems. Before leaving the clinic or the hospital, the patient should be able to demonstrate the complete feeding procedure to the physician.
   a. ***Placement of the tube*** should be checked.
   b. ***Flow of gravity*** Feedings should be allowed to drain through the tube by gravity and should not be forced.
   c. ***Temperature*** Tube feeding should be given at room temperature or body temperature.
   d. ***Rinsing*** Feeding should be followed by free water to clear the tube. This procedure also aids in hydration.
   e. ***Clamping*** The tube should be clamped until the next feeding.
   f. ***Position*** The patient should not lie down immediately after feeding.
   g. ***Other liquids*** can be taken through the feeding tube, but they should not be given in place of prescribed feedings.

E. Tracheotomy Care

The patient and family members should be taught all aspects of caring for the tracheotomy and maintaining the airway, and they should be able to perform these procedures for a few days prior to the patient's hospital discharge.

1. **Anatomic features of the respiratory system** and parts of the tracheotomy tube must be taught.
2. **Cleaning** The patient must know how to clean and replace the inner tube using proper technique involving hand washing, tap water, and a small brush.
3. **Extra humidity** is needed.
4. **Suction technique** The physician should provide the patient with a suction machine. Such a machine may be rented from a medical supply house.
5. **Communication** The patient must be taught how to communicate whether by writing, with an electronic larynx, or by plugging the tracheotomy tube with the finger.

6. **Difficult Breathing** One should check the patency of the inner tube, use cough and suction techniques, increase humidity, go to the hospital emergency room, or call the physician if the problem is severe or if these measures do not help.
7. **Changing the entire tube** should be taught, if appropriate. A duplicate tube should be provided for home and always kept at the patient's bedside. This tube is to be used in an emergency.

F. Wound Care

Although care of wounds is individualized, basic instructions should be taught to each patient. Wounds should be cared for daily, with clean technique. They should be washed with half-strength hydrogen peroxide and then covered with bacitracin ointment. Closed wounds can be left without a dressing, but open wounds should be covered.

1. **Wash hands first.**
2. **Wash wound** with gauze pad and half-strength hydrogen peroxide.
3. **Dry wound.**
4. **Apply bacitracin ointment** with an applicator stick.
5. **Complicated dressing changes** may require the aid of a visiting nurses' association.

G. Exercises following Radical Neck Dissection

After radical neck dissection, many patients complain of shoulder stiffness or limitations in range of motion of the arm. The following are exercises that may help the patient to regain a full range of motion. All exercises should be done with a broomstick or cane in both hands, to let the stronger arm help the weaker arm.

1. **Lifting** Hold the cane in both hands in front of your body. Keeping your elbows straight, lift the cane up and over your head.
2. **Pushing out** Let the stronger arm push the weaker arm out to the side, with the cane held in both hands. Keep your arm in line with your body.
3. **Bending** With the cane up and over your head, bend your elbows and bring the cane down behind your head.
4. **Pushing back** Hold the cane in both hands behind your back. Keep your elbows straight, and push the cane back away from your body.
5. **Sliding** With the cane held in both hands behind your back, slide the cane up your back.
6. **Pulling** Hold the cane in the strong arm over your shoulder and down behind your back. Bring the weak arm behind your back and grab the other end of the cane. Pull the cane up with the strong arm.

H. Esophageal Bougienage

Esophageal bougienage is sometimes necessary after laryngectomy or caustic ingestion because of stricture formation. The initial bougienage should be done in the office, and the patient should be taught to use the bougie at home to maintain the patency of the esophagus. The procedure is as follows:

1. **Swallow lidocaine** (Xylocaine Viscous).
2. **Lubricate the bougie** with a lubricating agent (Lubafax).
3. **Pass the bougie** orally beyond the point of stricture.
4. **Allow to remain in place** one minute if tight.
5. **Repeat at home** twice daily.
6. **Use the wrist loop** at all times so that the entire bougie is not swallowed.
7. **Wash the bougie** in mild soap and water and store flat in a clean towel.
8. **Do not use the bougie if it is cracked** because it contains mercury.

V. FACIAL PARALYSIS

A. Cornea Protection

If the eyelid does not cover the cornea while sleeping and the patient is unable to blink, the cornea will have to be protected from drying. If a tarsorrhaphy is not done, the patient should be instructed to use artificial tears at least four times a day and to tape the eye shut at night. The tape should be applied vertically to the upper lid and then to the lower lid. A horizontal band of tape on the upper and lower lids can be applied first, to give a firm base if the vertical tape is not enough. An eye pad should not be used; if the eye opens with a pad in place, the pad may scratch the cornea.

B. Facial Massage

Passive exercise can be used to maintain muscle tone when the facial muscles are temporarily paralyzed. If function is expected to return in 5 to 6 weeks, no special exercises will be necessary. If the paralysis is expected to persist for a longer period, facial muscle tone may be preserved by massaging the muscles in a direction opposite to that of the deformity. For example, the angle of the mouth or forehead should be massaged in an upward direction. This massage should be gentle, to avoid stretching the muscles. If facial nerve recovery is delayed, a galvanic stimulator, which produces mild twitching of the muscle, can be used 5 to 6 times a day. The patient should be taught to use the stimulator by a physical therapist.

Index

Page numbers in italics refer to illustrations; page numbers followed by a t refer to tables.